HANDBOOK OF
NUCLEAR MEDICINE AND
MOLECULAR IMAGING
Principles and Clinical Applications

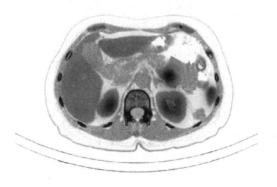

HANDBOOK OF NUCLEAR MEDICINE AND MOLECULAR IMAGING

Principles and Clinical Applications

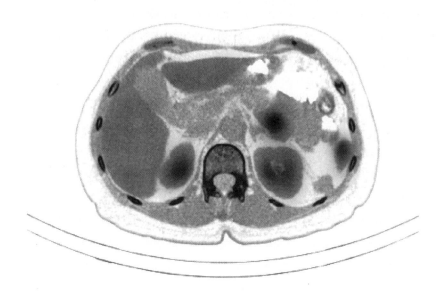

E. Edmund Kim (University of Texas, USA)

Dong-Soo Lee (Seoul National University, Korea)

Ukihide Tateishi (Zentralklinik Bad Berka GmbH, Germany)

Richard P. Baum (Yokohama City University, Japan)

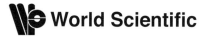 **World Scientific**

NEW JERSEY · LONDON · SINGAPORE · BEIJING · SHANGHAI · HONG KONG · TAIPEI · CHENNAI

Published by

World Scientific Publishing Co. Pte. Ltd.

5 Toh Tuck Link, Singapore 596224

USA office: 27 Warren Street, Suite 401-402, Hackensack, NJ 07601

UK office: 57 Shelton Street, Covent Garden, London WC2H 9HE

British Library Cataloguing-in-Publication Data
A catalogue record for this book is available from the British Library.

HANDBOOK OF NUCLEAR MEDICINE AND MOLECULAR IMAGING
Principles and Clinical Applications

ISBN-13 978-981-4366-23-6
ISBN-10 981-4366-23-4

Typeset by Stallion Press
Email: enquiries@stallionpress.com

Printed in Singapore by Mainland Press Pte Ltd.

Preface

Over the last decade, the field of nuclear medicine and molecular imaging has evolved considerably with advances in molecular biology, chemistry and engineering as well as hybrid PET/CT and SPECT/CT. Molecular imaging aims to explore the dynamics of molecules indicative of physiology and disease in a qualitative as well as quantitative manner. New agents and imaging techniques are steadily strengthening as well as refining of their clinical applications.

Many textbooks have been published in an attempt to educate not only the practitioners of our speciality, but also referring physicians and our trainees. Such a daunting array of continuous changes with the magnitude of complexities present a challenge to nuclear medicine practitioners. That is why this handbook offers an easily accessible approach to the clinical applications and also basic science ground work in a very pragmatic way.

We are very fortunate to invite many international collaborators in our field who are experienced experts in our field. We hope to achieve our goal to make this book a convenient ready reference of nuclear medicine and molecular imaging.

E. Edmund Kim
Houston, Texas

Contributor List

Bruce J. Barron, M.D.
Department of Radiology/Nuclear Medicine
Emory University School of Medicine
Atlanta, Georgia

Richard P. Baum, M.D.
Prof. and Chairman, Dept. of Nuclear Medicine
Center for PET/CT, Zentralklinic, Bad Berka
GmbH, Germany

David Brandon, M.D.
Department of Diagnostic and Interventional Radiology
University of Texas Health Science Center
Houston, Texas 77030

Gi-Jeong Cheon, M.D.
Department of Nuclear Medicine
Korea Cancer Center Hospital
Seoul, Korea

June-Key Chung, MD, PhD <jkchung@plaza.snu.ac.kr>
Professor
Department of Nuclear Medicine
Seoul National University College of Medicine
Seoul 110-744, Korea

Isis W. Gayed, M.D.
Chief, Div. of Nuclear Medicine
Univ. of Texas Medical School
Houston, Texas 77030

Tomio Inoue, MD, PhD
Professor and Chairman
Department of Radiology
Yokohama City University Graduate School of Medicine
Yokohama 236-0004, Japan

Usha A. Joseph, M.D.
Assist. Professor of Nuclear Medicine
Univ. of Texas Medical School
Houston, Texas 77030

Keon- Wook Kang, MD, PhD <kangkw@snu.ac.kr>
Associate Professor
Department of Nuclear Medicine
Seoul National University College of Medicine
Seoul 110-744, Korea

E. Edmund Kim, MD, MS <ekim@mdanderson.org>
Professor
Departments of Nuclear Medicine and Diagnostic Radiology
The University of Texas MD Anderson Cancer Center
    and Medical School
Houston, Texas 77030, USA
WCU Professor
Graduate School of Convergence Science and Technology
Seoul National University, Seoul, Korea

Seok-Ki Kim, MD <skim@ncc.re.kr>
Chairman
Department of Nuclear Medicine
National Cancer Center
323 Ilsan-ro, Ilsandong-gu, Goyang-si
Gyeonggi-do, 410-769, Korea

Yu- Kyeong Kim, MD, PhD <yk3181@snu.ac.kr>
Assistant Professor
Department of Nuclear Medicine
Seoul National University, Bundang Hospital

166 Gumi-ro, Bundang-gu, Seongnam-si,
Gyeonggi-Do 463-707, Korea

Dong Soo Lee, MD, PhD <dsl@snu.ac.kr>
Professor and Chairman
Department of Nuclear Medicine
Seoul National University College of Medicine
WCU Department of Molecular Medicine
    and Biopharmaceutical Sciences
Seoul National University
101 Daehang-ro, Jongno-gu
Seoul 110-744, Korea

Ho-Young Lee, M.D., Ph.D.
Chief, Nuclear Medicine Department
Borame Hospital, Seoul National University

Jae-Sung Lee, Ph.D.
Department of Nuclear Medicine
Seoul National University School of Medicine
Seoul, Korea

Yun-Sang Lee, Ph.D.
Department of Nuclear Medicine
Seoul National University School of Medicien
Seoul, Korea

Asad Nasir, M.D.
Dept. of Diagnostic and Interventional Radiology
Univ. of Texas Medical School
Houston, Texas 77030

So Won Oh, MD<excellent99@naver.com>
Assistant Professor
Department of Nuclear Medicine
Seoul Metropolitan Government-Seoul National
    University Hospital
Boramae Medical Center

39, Boramae-gil, Dongjak-gu,
Seoul 156-707, Korea

Jin Chul Paeng, MD, PhD <paengjc@snu.ac.kr>
Assistant Professor
Department of Nuclear Medicine
Seoul National University Hospital
101 Daehang-ro, Jongno-gu,
Seoul 110-744, Korea

Hirofumi Shibata, M.D.
Department of Radiology
Yokohama University School of Medicine
Yokohama, Japan

Ukihide Tateishi, M.D., Ph.D. <u_tateishi@yahoo.co.jp>
Associate Professor of Radiology
Yokohama University School of Medicine
Yokohama, Japan

David Q. Wan, M.D.
Assist. Prof. of Nuclear Medicine
Univ. of Texas Medical School
Houston, Texas 77030

Franklin C.L. Wong, MD, PhD, JD <fwong@mdanderson.org>
Professor
Departments of Nuclear Medicine and Neurooncology
The University of Texas MD Anderson Cancer Center
Houston, Texas 77030, USA

Contents

Chapter 10.   Nuclear Imaging of Esophageal, Gastric,
and Pancreatic Cancers   243

Hirofumi Shibata, Ukihide Tateishi and Tomio Inoue

Chapter 11. Nuclear Urology   267

Ukihide Tateishi and E. Edmund Kim

Chapter 15. Tumor Imaging 353

Ukihide Tateishi and E. Edmund Kim

Chapter 16. Receptor-Binding Peptide Imaging 369

E. Edmund Kim and Richard Baum

PART I
Basic Sciences

Chapter 1
Basic Nuclear Physics and Instrumentation

Jae Sung Lee

1.1. Basic Nuclear Physics

1.1.1. *Atom*

The atom is the basic unit of matter and consists of a nucleus surrounded by negatively charged electrons (Fig. 1.1). The atomic nucleus comprises positively charged protons and electrically neutral neutrons. The protons and neutrons are much more massive than electrons. Atomic number (Z) refers to the number of protons in the nucleus, and mass number (A) is the total number of protons and neutrons (N). The chemical properties of an atom are determined by the number of orbital electrons, which is the same as the atomic number in the electrically neutral atom.

Notation

The notation to summarize the atomic and nuclear composition is:

$$^A_Z X_N,$$

where X is the atomic or chemical symbol. Because X is determined by Z and N can be obtained by A-Z, the following shortened notation is also frequently used:

$$^A X$$

Nuclear families

The nuclide is a species of atoms characterized by the number of protons, neutrons, and the energy status of the atomic nucleus. The nuclear species

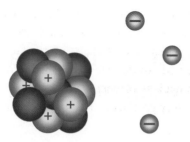

Fig. 1.1. Structure of atom that consists of nucleus and electrons. The nucleus contains protons and neutrons.

Table 1.1.   Nuclear families.

Family	Same quantity	Example
Isotopes	Atomic number (Z)	^{125}I, ^{127}I, ^{131}I
Isobars	Mass number (A)	^{131}I, ^{131}Xe, ^{131}Cs
Isotones	Neutron number (N)	^{131}I$_{78}$, ^{132}Xe$_{78}$, ^{133}Cs$_{78}$

can be grouped into families having certain common properties, as summarized in Table 1.1.

1.1.2. *Radiation and radionuclide*

Radiation

In general, radiation refers to the energy that travels through a medium or space. Radiation can be categorized into two distinct types (ionizing and non-ionizing radiation). The term *radiation* is commonly used in reference to the ionizing radiation that has sufficient energy to ionize an atom.

Radiation can also be categorized into particulate and electromagnetic radiation. Particulate radiation is composed of atomic or subatomic particles and carries energy in the form of kinetic energy of mass in motion; this category includes alpha, proton, electron (β^-), positron (β^+), and neutron particles. Electromagnetic (EM) radiation carries energy in the form of oscillating electrical and magnetic fields. EM radiation has no mass, is not affected by electrical or magnetic fields, and has a constant speed in a given medium. The EM radiation commonly used in nuclear medicine imaging includes gamma (γ) and X-rays. The γ-rays are emitted from the nuclei of radioactive atoms and X-rays are produced in the electron shells.

There are two methods to describe EM radiation (waves and photons [particle-like discrete packets of energy]). The energy (E) of electromagnetic radiation is inversely proportional to the wavelength (λ), as shown in following equation:

$$E = \frac{hc}{\lambda},$$

where h is Planck's constant and c is the velocity of light.

Radionuclide

A radionuclide (also often referred to as a radioisotope) is an atom with an unstable nucleus which is characterized by excess energy. The radionuclide undergoes radioactive decay to be a more stable atom. In radioactive decay, the unstable radionuclide is called the *parent* and the more stable product is the *daughter*.

1.1.3. *Radioactive decay*

Radioactive decay is a process in which an unstable radionuclide transforms into a more stable radionuclide by spontaneously emitting particles and/or photons. Several types of radioactive decay exist.

Alpha decay

An alpha (α) particle is emitted from the nucleus in this decay mode, which occurs primarily among very heavy elements. The α particles are helium nuclei ($A = 4$, $Z = 2$). Alpha particles deposit large amounts of energy ($4 \sim 8$ MeV) within a very short range in body tissues due to the large mass involved. The atomic mass of nuclei is decreased by a factor of four after decay, as shown in the following general equation of α decay:

$$^{A}_{Z}X \rightarrow \, ^{A-4}_{Z-2}Y + \, ^{4}_{2}\alpha + Energy$$

5

Beta minus decay

Beta particles (β^-) are negatively charged electrons emitted from radionuclides that have an excess number of neutrons (*neutron rich*) compared to the number of protons. In this decay mode, a neutron is converted into a proton with the simultaneous ejection of a β^- and an anti-neutrino ($\bar{\nu}$). Consequently, the number of protons is increased by one and the atom is transformed into a different element, as shown by the following equation:

$$^A_Z X \rightarrow {}^{\,\,A}_{Z+1} Y + \beta^- + \bar{\nu} + Energy$$

The emitted β^- particles have a continuous kinetic energy spectrum, ranging from 0 to the maximum energy (E_{max}). The average energy of β^- is approximately 1/3 E_{max}.

Positron decay

Positron decay occurs with *neutron poor* radionuclides. A proton in a nuclide is converted into a neutron with the simultaneous ejection of a positron (β^+) and a neutrino (ν). The positron is the anti-matter conjugate of the electron emitted in β^- decay (β^+ and β^- have the same physical characteristics, with the exception of electric polarity). The number of protons is decreased as the consequence of the positron decay, as follows:

$$^A_Z X \rightarrow {}^{\,\,A}_{Z+1} Y + \beta^+ + \nu + Energy$$

After ejection from the nucleus, a positron loses its kinetic energy in collisions with atoms of the surrounding matter and comes to rest within approximately 10^{-9} sec. The positron then combines with an ordinary electron in an annihilation reaction, in which the entire rest mass of both particles is instantaneously converted to energy and emitted as two oppositely directed 511 keV γ-ray photons. Positron emission tomography (PET) is a nuclear medicine imaging technique which produce the images of positron-emitting radionuclides by measuring the annihilated γ-rays.

Electron capture

Electron capture is an alternative way for positron decay involving *neutron poor* radionuclides. In this mode, an unstable nucleus captures an orbital electron, with the conversion of a proton into a neutron and the simultaneous ejection of a neutrino as described by the following equation:

$$_Z^A X + \beta^- \rightarrow {}_{Z+1}^A Y + \nu + Energy$$

Additional characteristic X-rays are generated when the vacancy in the electron shell created by electron capture is filled by an electron from a higher-energy shell. ^{201}Tl is a well-known radionuclide undergoing electron capture and emitting characteristic X-rays. The electron capture decay frequently results in a daughter nucleus that is in an excited or metastable state. Thus, γ-rays (or conversion electrons) may also be emitted.

Isomeric transition

Often, during radioactive decay, a daughter is formed in an excited (unstable) state. Most excited states transit nearly instantaneously to lower energy states with emission of γ-rays. However, some excited states persist for longer periods, with half-lives ranging from approximately 10^{-12} sec to more than 600 years. These excited states are called metastable or isomeric states and are denoted by the letter *m* after the mass number. ^{99m}Tc, which is the most commonly used radionuclide in nuclear medicine imaging, undergoes this isomeric transition. In the ^{99}Mo/^{99m}Tc generator, ^{99}Mo decays to ^{99m}Tc that remains in the metastable states before decaying to stable ^{99}Tc with a half-life of 6.02 h, as shown in the following equations:

$$^{99}\text{Mo} \rightarrow {}^{99m}\text{Tc} + \beta^- + 1.37\,\text{MeV}$$
$$^{99m}\text{Tc} \rightarrow {}^{99}\text{Tc} + \gamma(0.14\,\text{MeV})$$

1.1.4. *Radioactivity and Half-life*

Radioactivity

The activity (A) is the quantity of radioactive material and is defined as the number of radioactive atoms undergoing radioactive decay per unit time (t). Therefore, the activity is equal to the change (dN) in the total number of radioactive atoms (N) in a given period (dt):

$$A = -\frac{dN}{dt}$$

The SI unit of activity is the becquerel (Bq), which is named after Henri Becquerel, who discovered radioactivity in 1896. One Bq is defined as one disintegration per second (dps). Because a Bq is a very tiny amount of activity, the curie (Ci; the historical unit of activity) is more frequently used in nuclear medicine. One curie is the activity of 1 g of pure ^{226}Ra. Ci and Bq have the following relationship:

$$1 \, \text{Ci} = 3.7 \times 10^{10} \, \text{Bq}$$
$$1 \, \text{mCi} = 37 \, \text{MBq}$$

Decay constant and half-life

The radioactivity (A_t) of a radioactive atom after a time t is given by

$$A_t = A_0 e^{-\lambda t},$$

where A_0 is the initial activity and λ is the decay constant. The decay constant is the unique characteristic of each radionuclide and has the following relationship with the physical half-life ($T_{1/2}$), which is the time required for the activity to decrease by one-half, as follows:

$$T_{1/2} = \frac{\ln(2)}{\lambda} = \frac{0.693}{\lambda}$$

For example, after 10 half-lives, the radioactivity of a sample is reduced by approximately 10^{-3}. The half-lives of typical radionuclides used in nuclear medicine are given in Table 1.2.

Table 1.2. The half-lives of typical radionuclides.

Radionuclide	$T_{1/2}$	Radionuclide	$T_{1/2}$
^{99m}Tc	6.02 h	^{11}C	20.4 min
^{123}I	13 h	^{13}N	9.96 min
^{99}Mo	2.79 d	^{15}O	2.03 min
^{111}In	2.82 d	^{18}F	109.8 min
^{201}Tl	3.08 d	^{68}Ga	68.3 min
^{67}Ga	3.25 d	^{82}Rb	1.25 min
^{131}I	8.05 d	^{124}I	4.18 d
^{125}I	60.2 d	^{64}Cu	12.7 h

1.1.5. *Interaction of radiation with matter*

Particle interactions

High-energy charged particles, such as α and β particles, interact with matter by electrical forces and lead to the excitation and ionization of atoms. The particles predominantly interact with orbital electrons of an atom. The ejected electrons sometimes have sufficient energy to yield secondary interactions with neighboring atoms. These electrons are called delta (δ) rays. The charged particles deposit a large amount of energy in a short distance of travel relative to the photons.

Photon interactions

High-energy photons interact with matter through several different mechanisms, depending on the energy, and include Rayleigh (coherent) scattering, Compton scattering, photoelectric effect, and pair production. The dominant mechanisms in nuclear medicine imaging are photoelectric effect and Compton scattering (Fig. 1.2).

In photoelectric effect, all of the energy in incident photons is transferred into an orbital electron in an atom, and some of the energy is used to overcome binding energy of the electron to be ejected from the atom. The photoelectric effect dominates in human tissues at photon energies $<\sim 100$ keV. In contrast, Compton scattering is a dominant interaction mechanism for photons with $>\sim 100$ keV energy and $<\sim 2$ MeV. In this interaction, loosely

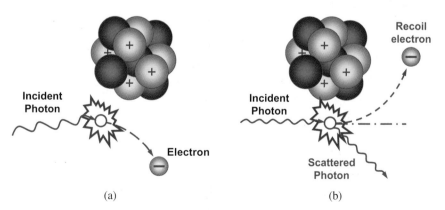

(a)   (b)

Fig. 1.2.   Interaction of photons with matter: (a) Photoelectric effect and (b) Compton scattering.

bound orbital electrons are ejected by absorbing part of the energy of the incident photons. After the interaction, the photon with the reduced energy changes its direction. Attenuation of photons is the removal of photons from a beam of X- or γ-rays as the photons pass through matter. The attenuation is mostly caused by absorption and scattering of the primary photons in nuclear medicine.

1.2. Instrumentation

1.2.1. *Imaging procedures*

The most important role of nuclear medicine imaging modalities is the quantitative measurement of physiologic and biochemical characteristics by the *in vivo* imaging of radioactive substances to investigate biochemical and pathologic phenomena, diagnosis of diseases, and determination of prognosis after treatment. In the typical nuclear imaging procedure, we first inject the radiotracer that tracks a particular biochemical process in our body, and using a gamma (γ) camera or PET scanner, we measure the radiation emitted from the tracer to produce a picture of the body showing where the tracer has accumulated.

Types of nuclear imaging methods

There are two types of nuclear imaging methods (single-photon imaging and PET). The distinction between these two imaging modalities is based on the physical properties of the radioisotopes used for imaging. In single-photon imaging, single-photon emitters are used. These radioisotopes emit single γ-ray photons with each radioactive decay. The most widely used single-photon emitters include ^{99m}Tc, ^{201}Tl, and ^{123}I. In contrast to single-photon imaging, PET uses the radioisotopes that finally emit two γ-ray photons simultaneously.

1.2.2. *Gamma camera*

A γ-camera is a single-photon imaging device, also called a scintillation camera or Anger camera, and comprises a collimator, a scintillation (or semiconductor) detector, and readout electronics (Fig. 1.3).

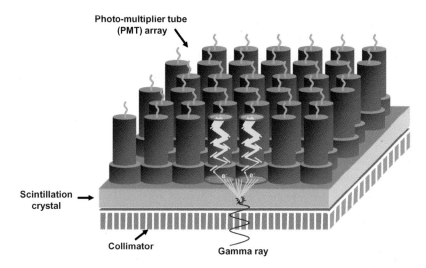

Fig. 1.3. Components inside a γ-camera. (*Reproduced from* Lee JS. "Nuclear medicine physics," In: Chung J-K, Lee MC, eds., *Nuclear Medicine*, Korea Medical Book Publisher, 2008; with permission.)

Collimator

In γ-cameras, the most unique component is a mechanical collimator. This mechanical collimator is made of heavy materials, such as lead or tungsten, to select only the γ-rays traveling in a specific direction. Because these heavy materials absorb radiation energy easily, γ-rays with an oblique direction to the collimator septa are blocked, and only the γ-rays traveling parallel with the collimator septa (except for the pinhole collimator) can be detected by the scintillation detector. Without the collimation, the γ-rays will be detected by the camera in all possible random directions without any information about the incident direction, thus leading to severe blurring of the projection images.

Scintillation detector

The scintillation detector, another component of a γ-camera, is located behind the γ-camera. Most γ-camera systems are based on a scintillation detector that consists of a scintillation crystal (mostly NaI (Tl) in γ-cameras) and photosensors. The scintillation crystal emits visible light following interaction with radiation. Thus, the energy of the γ-ray is absorbed by the scintillation crystal and part of this energy is converted into visible light photons. Therefore, photosensors are required to measure these visible photons. The most common photosensor used in a γ-camera is the photomultiplier tube (PMT), in which the visible light photons are converted into an electrical signal at the photocathode that is amplified by the strong electric potential between the cascading dynodes arranged in this device.

Semiconductor radiation detector

There are increasing attempts to use semiconductor detectors for direct radiation measurement (i.e., Cd-Zn-Te [CZT]) in γ-cameras. The semiconductor detectors provide much better energy resolution than scintillation detectors. The better energy resolution provides improved performance in the rejection of cross-talk photons in dual or multiple isotopes imaging (i.e., simultaneous scans of ^{99m}Tc and ^{123}I). In addition, because the CZT can also be operated in a magnetic field, the SPECT/MRI system based on this device holds promise for simultaneous SPECT/MRI acquisition.

1.2.3. SPECT

Principles and types

Similar to X-ray computed tomography (CT), tomographic imaging is also possible with γ-cameras. This imaging technology is called single-photon emission computed tomography (SPECT). During SPECT, the γ-camera collects projection data by means of rotating around the objects. A dual-head γ-camera is most commonly used for SPECT imaging. A triple-head γ-camera is also available (Fig. 1.4). Currently, the use of SPECT/CT, which is a hybrid imaging system to acquire functional and anatomic information altogether, is on the increase. The major SPECT applications include perfusion imaging in the heart and brain.

Pinhole SPECT

For small animal imaging, pinhole collimators are usually used to achieve high spatial resolution. In the pinhole collimation system, with the smaller aperture diameter, we can obtain images with higher spatial resolution. The cost to obtain high spatial resolution is the loss of sensitivity because the sensitivity of the pinhole collimator is inversely proportional to the diameter

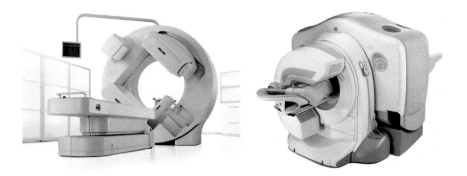

Fig. 1.4. Clinical SPECT(/CT) systems. (*Courtesy*: Philips and GE.)

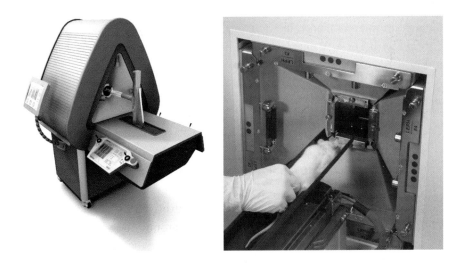

Fig. 1.5. Small animal SPECT(/CT) systems. (*Courtesy*: MILab and Bioscan.)

of the aperture. Therefore, to compensate for this sensitivity loss with the smaller aperture, most small animal SPECT systems now use multi-pinhole collimators in which the multiple pinhole apertures collect the projection data simultaneously (Fig. 1.5).

Multi-pinhole collimator technology has been translated into the clinical SPECT systems as well. A stationary multi-pinhole collimator is used in a cardiac-specific SPECT, in which the each pinhole aperture is focused on the myocardium and provides angular data sufficient for the stationary data acquisition without camera rotation.

1.2.4. *PET*

Basic principles

The radioisotopes used in PET have a fewer number of neutrons than stable isotopes (e.g., ^{11}C has only five neutrons, although the stable isotope, ^{12}C, has six neutrons) and undergo positron decay. As previously described, one of the protons in this unstable isotope is changed into a neutron by emitting the positron to become a stable atom. When the positron is emitted from the nucleus, the positron travels a short distance (the so-called positron range), and finally meets an electron. The positron and electrons that meet each other lose their mass, which is changed into the energy in the form of γ-rays.

In this conversion of particles into the γ-rays, three physical quantities (energy, momentum, and electrical charge) should be preserved. Therefore, 2 γ-rays with 511-keV energy are annihilated in opposite direction, as shown in Fig. 1.6.

PET scanner

The PET scanner detects these two γ-rays to determine the line of response (LOR), which gives us the information about the location where the γ-rays were emitted and the direction of the γ-ray flight. Because LOR provides

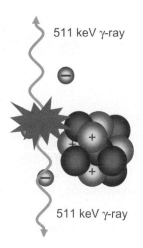

Fig. 1.6. PET principle: mutual annihilation.

the information regarding both the position and direction of the incident photons, PET scanners do not require the mechanical collimator in contrast to the γ-camera. This is the reason why PET has a better sensitivity than a γ-camera in which most of the γ-rays are absorbed by the collimator. To generate the sinogram (raw data for image reconstruction) from the LOR data, the γ-rays are sorted according to the direction of incidence and distance from the center during or after the PET scan. Iterative reconstruction algorithms, such as the OSEM algorithm, are commonly used to obtain the reconstructed PET data.

The elementary module in most PET scanners is a block detector. In the block detector, the scintillation crystal array is coupled with the array of photosensors. Sharing of visible light by multiple photosensors to determine the position of γ-ray interaction is a common method used in the PET block detector. However, the direct coupling of each crystal element with each photosensor is also a possible way. The block detectors compose a PET detector ring, and axial field-of-view of PET scanners can be extended by the combination of multiple rings of detector blocks. General-purpose human PET scanner has a ring diameter between 80 and 90 cm and the axial field-of-view between 15 and 20 cm. Currently, combined PET/CT scanners, in which a PET gantry is in tandem with a CT gantry, are predominantly used (Fig. 1.7).

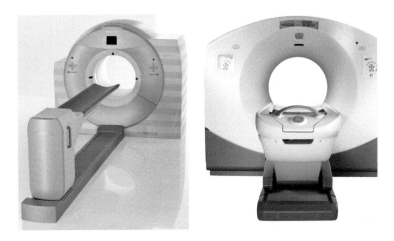

Fig. 1.7. Clinical PET/CT systems.

Time of flight–PET

If we measure the difference in arrival times of two γ-rays (time-of-flight [TOF] information) exactly, we can pinpoint the annihilation position. In this ideal situation, we no longer need the image reconstruction algorithm based on the back-projection technique. However, in the practical situation, there is always uncertainty in the timing measurement. Although the timing resolution of the current PET systems equates to a positional uncertainty of ~9 cm, TOF information is still useful for the back-projection–based image reconstruction to reduce the background noise.

In conventional non–TOF-PET, the probability of annihilation position is equally distributed to all voxels along the LOR for image reconstruction. However, in TOF-PET, the probability can be limited within the segment of response using TOF information (Fig. 1.8). Therefore, TOF information is useful for localizing the source position and reducing the propagation of noise along the LOR.

Small animal PET

Small animal–dedicated PET scanners basically have the same configuration as the clinical PET scanners for human or large animal studies. However, smaller scintillation crystals are employed to achieve better spatial resolution. In addition, a 10- to 20-cm diameter is common in small animal

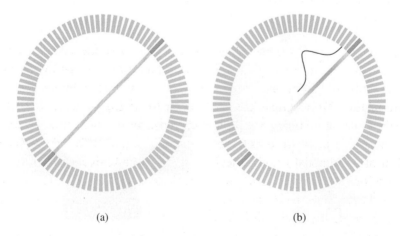

(a)   (b)

Fig. 1.8. Principle of TOF-PET: (a) Non–TOF-PET; (b) TOF-PET. (*Reproduced from* Lee JS, Technical advances in current PET and hybrid imaging systems, *Open Nucl Med J* **2**:192–208, 2010.)

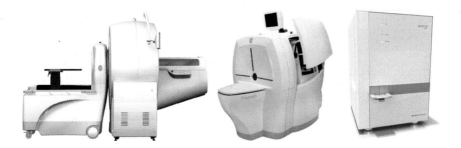

Fig. 1.9. Small animal PET(/CT) systems. (*Courtesy*: Siemens, GE, and Sofie Biosciences.)

PET scanners and the relatively long axial field-of-view and scintillation crystal elements compared to ring diameter ensures better sensitivity than human scanners (Fig. 1.9).

Many advanced detector technologies, such as depth-of-interaction (DOI) measurement, are used in small animal PET scanners for high spatial resolution and sensitivity. The relatively small diameter and long crystal elements in small animal PET cause a parallax error at the periphery of the transverse field-of-view, which is produced by the penetration of oblique γ-rays. If the DOI position in the PET detector is measured, the parallax error can be much reduced.

1.2.5. *Hybrid systems*

PET/CT and SPECT/CT

The combination of the nuclear medicine images with the anatomic imaging modalities, such as CT or MRI, can enhance the clinical information from both modalities and bring on the synergetic effects by merging the information. For example, the accurate anatomic localization, correlative studies, partial volume correction, and statistical reconstruction based on the anatomic prior are possible by the combination. Before the development of multimodal imaging devices, software co-registration and fusion technologies were available. However, these technologies were used for limited clinical purposes because it is time-consuming, non–user-friendly, and unsuccessful outside the brain.

PET/CT and SPECT/CT are the integrated hardware systems in which both modalities are combined in a single gantry. The PET/CT or SPECT/CT images provide accurate anatomic localization of abnormal lesions in PET and SPECT. CT also provides information on photon attenuation. CT-based attenuation correction has several advantages as follows: CT-based attenuation reduces the whole-body PET scan time by up to 40% and provides essentially noiseless attenuation correction factors.

PET/MRI

Although there are many benefits of PET/CT over the stand-alone PET (*vide supra*), several limitations of PET/CT have also been identified. Physiologic or voluntary motion of body and organs between the CT and PET scans often cause artifacts in the fused images because they are not simultaneously acquired. In addition, radiation exposure during the PET/CT examination is twice that of the standalone PET or CT. Therefore, if the PET/MRI is available, it will be especially useful in pediatric studies and repeated scans for treatment monitoring. Another advantage of PET/MRI is the higher soft tissue contrast in MRI. Therefore, PET/MRI is expected to yield superior diagnostic accuracy, particularly in brain studies, to PET/CT. In addition, it would also be useful in local tumor assessment and whole-body staging in which higher soft tissue contrast of MRI is beneficial.

However, simultaneous PET/MR imaging is technically challenging because PMT, the working horse in conventional PET scanners, is very sensitive to the magnetic field. Among the many approaches to overcome this challenge, two approaches currently adopted by major vendors include separation of conventional PMT-based PET scanners away from the MRI

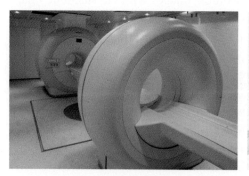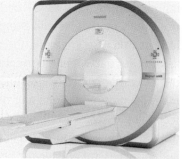

Fig. 1.10. Clinical PET/MRI (left: tandem type, right: integrated type). (*Courtesy*: Philips and Siemens.)

machine (tandem type) and use of semiconductor photosensors in PET that is not influenced by the magnetic field (integrated type) (Fig. 1.10).

Bibliography

Bushberg JT, Seibert JA, Leidholdt EM, Boone JM. (2002) *The Essential Physics of Medical Imaging*. Lippincott Williams & Wilkins, Philadelphia.

Cherry SR, Sorenson JA, Phelps ME. (2003) *Physics in Nuclear Medicine*. Elsevier Science, Philadelphia.

Karp JS, Surti S, Daube-Witherspoon ME, Muehllehner G. (2008) Benefit of time-of-flight in PET: Experimental and clinical results. *J Nucl Med* **49**: 462–470.

Lee JS. (2008) Nuclear medicine physics. In: Chung J-K, Lee MC (eds), *Nuclear Medicine*, Korea Medical Book Publisher.

Lee JS. (2010) Technical advances in current PET and hybrid imaging systems. *Open Nucl Med J* **2**: 192–208.

Lee JS, Hong SJ. (2010) Geiger-mode avalanche photodiodes for PET/MRI. In: Iniewski K (eds), *Electronic Circuits for Radiation Detection*, CRC Press LLC, 179–200.

Lee JS. Kang KW. (2011) PET/MRI. In: Kim EE, Lee MC, Inoue T, Wong W-H (eds), *Clinical PET and PET/CT: Principles and Applications*, Springer, 2011.

Pichler BJ, Wehrl HF, Judenhofer MS. (2008) Latest advances in molecular imaging instrumentation. *J Nucl Med* **49**: 5S–23S.

Prince JL, Links JM. (2006) *Medical Imaging Signals and Systems*. Pearson Prentice Hall, Upper Saddle River.

Townsend DW, Carney JP, Yap JT, Hall NC. (2004) PET/CT today and tomorrow. *J Nucl Med* **45**: 4S–14S.

Vale PE, Bailey DL, Townsend DW, Maisey MN. (2003) *Positron Emission Tomography, Basic Science and Clinical Practice*. Springer, London.

Wernick MN, Aarsvold JN. (2004) *Emission Tomography: The Fundamentals of PET and SPECT*. Elsevier Academic Press, San Diego.

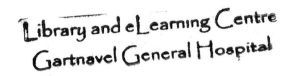

Chapter 2
Radiopharmaceutical Chemistry

Yun-Sang Lee

2.1. Introduction

Radiopharmaceutical chemistry is a basic research area in nuclear medicine and deals with not only the chemistry of radionuclides or radiopharmaceuticals but also the whole process of radiopharmaceuticals production, including chemical synthesis, radionuclide production, the operation of machines for radiolabeling, purification, and sterilization procedures, and even legal issues.

2.2. The Use of Radiopharmaceuticals

Radiopharmaceuticals are radioactive compounds used for the diagnosis and therapeutic treatment of human diseases. Almost 90% of all radiopharmaceuticals are used for diagnostic purposes, while the rest are used for therapeutic treatment. Diagnostic radiopharmaceuticals are administered and localized to the specific organ or tissue by a specific mechanism, after which the required information from radiopharmaceuticals is collected and reconstructed by an imaging instrument. Finally, radiopharmaceuticals also provide information about the disease localization and the specific biological process.

Therapeutic radiopharmaceuticals are used for the treatment of tumor or disease by internal radiation, which can cause tissue or cell damage. Radiation from the diagnostic radiopharmaceutical should be of low toxicity and have good penetration power; on the other hand, the radiation from the therapeutic radiopharmaceutical should have high energy and low penetration power to avoid the damage of normal tissue or cells. Therefore, gamma (γ)

21

or beta (β^+) emitters are used in diagnostic radiopharmaceuticals, and α and β^- emitters are used in therapeutic radiopharmaceuticals. The penetration ratio of γ-rays depends on its energy; higher energy implies higher penetration ratio in the body. However, a very high γ-ray energy can reduce the delectability or the resolution of the detector, therefore, moderate-energy (100 keV~200 keV) γ-ray is good for γ-camera or single-photon emission computed tomography (SPECT) imaging.

Positrons (β^+) can produce two γ-ray (511 keV) photons by annihilation reaction and is used for positron emission tomography (PET) imaging. The positron has a specific kinetic energy, which influences the positron range and reduces the resolution of PET imaging. Therefore, the lower kinetic energy of positron shows better imaging quality. Radiation from the therapeutic radiopharmaceuticals should have a short penetration range. The range of β^- particle is relatively long, from microns to millimeters, and they are effective for solid tumors and large tumor burdens. An important implication of the long range of each β^- particle is the production of the cross-fire effect, a circumstance that negates the need to target every cell within the tumor. However, the cross-fire effect may also result in significant irradiation of normal neighboring tissues.

The range of α particles is from 50 to 100 μm, which is only a few cell diameters. Thus, they are effective in treating circulating malignant cells and micrometastases. The physiological half-life is also an important factor for radiopharmaceuticals, and the half-life of the therapeutic radionuclide is generally longer than that of a diagnostic radionuclide, because some time is needed for treatment effect. Radiopharmaceuticals usually have minimal pharmacologic effect, because in most cases their doses are less than 100 μg. As they are administered to humans, they should be sterile and pyrogen-free and should undergo all required quality control measures.

2.3. Production of Radionuclides

A radiopharmaceutical is composed of two components: a radionuclide and a pharmaceutical, the former acting as a beacon and the later as a tracker. Therefore, radionuclide production forms a major part of radiopharmaceutical chemistry. Most of the radionuclides used in nuclear medicine are artificial. They are primarily produced in a cyclotron or a reactor. The type of radionuclide produced in a cyclotron or a reactor depends on the irradiating particle, its energy, and the target nuclei. These facilities are expensive and limited; therefore, radionuclides are supplied to remote facilities that do not possess such equipment. Because short-lived radionuclides decay rapidly, they are available only in the institutions that have cyclotron or reactor facilities; they cannot be supplied to remote institutions or hospitals. However, there is a secondary source of radionuclides, particularly short-lived ones, which is called a radionuclide generator.

The purification of the crude radionuclide products to get a pure radionuclide with high specific activity (SA) is also important. Since various isotopes of different elements may be produced in a particular irradiating system, it is necessary to isolate isotopes of a single element; this can be accomplished by appropriate chemical methods such as solvent extraction, precipitation, ion exchange, and distillation. We should choose the adequate purification method for consideration of the chemical characteristic of each radionuclide.

2.3.1. *Cyclotron-produced radionuclides*

A medical cyclotron is a round particle accelerator, modified from the linear accelerator for the reduction of the size, and proposed by Ernest O. Lawrence in 1929.[1] In a cyclotron, charged particles such as protons, deuterons, α particles, and ^{3}He particles, are accelerated in circular paths in dees under vacuum by means of an electromagnetic field (Fig. 2.1). Because charged particles move along the circular paths under the magnetic field with gradually increasing energy, the larger the radius of the particle trajectory, the higher the energy of the particle. Particles can possess a few keV to several hundred MeV of energy, depending on the design and type of the cyclotron. In general, a medical cyclotron has less than 30 MeV accelerating capacity for particles.

Cyclotron-produced radionuclides are usually neutron deficient and therefore decay by β^+ emission or electron capture and have a relatively higher SA than reactor-produced radionuclides. Several choices of cyclotron-produced radionuclides with emission of γ or β^+ are listed in

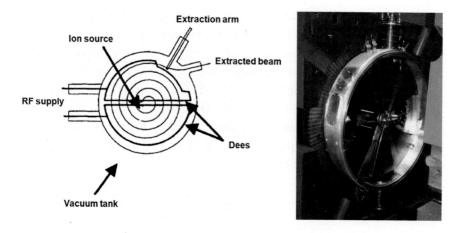

Fig. 2.1. Schematic diagram of a cyclotron.

Table 2.1. ^{67}Ga, ^{123}I, ^{111}In, and ^{201}Tl are used for γ-camera or SPECT, and ^{11}C, ^{13}N, ^{15}O, ^{18}F, ^{64}Cu, and ^{124}I are used for PET imaging. ^{18}F, ^{64}Cu, ^{67}Ga, ^{123}I, ^{124}I, ^{111}In, and ^{201}Tl have half-lives relatively long enough to purchase from commercial suppliers, if available, whereas ^{11}C, ^{13}N, and ^{15}O have to be used on production site only, because they have half-lives of less than 20 min.

2.3.2. *Reactor-produced radionuclides*

A large number of radionuclides are produced in nuclear reactors. However, the relatively low SA obstructs the use of reactor-produced radionuclides, except ^{131}I or several other radionuclides of the generator, which have well-established purification methods. A nuclear reactor is operated with fuel rods made of fissile materials such as enriched ^{235}U and ^{239}Pu. These fuel nuclei undergo spontaneous fission; fission is defined as the breakup of a heavy nucleus into two fragments of approximately equal mass, accompanied by the emission of two to three neutrons with mean energies of about 1.5 MeV. Neutrons emitted in one fission reaction can cause further fission of other fissionable nuclei in the fuel rod, provided the right conditions exist, and initiate a nuclear chain reaction. This chain reaction must be controlled, which is accomplished by the design of the fuel materials. The high-energy neutrons, so-called fast neutrons, are slowed down to

Table 2.1.   Commonly used cyclotron-produced radionuclides.

Radioisotopes	Physical Half-life	Decay Mode (%)	γ-Ray Energy (MeV)	Abundance (%)
^{11}C	20.4 min	β^+ (100)	0.511	200
^{13}N	9.96 min	β^+ (100)	0.511	200
^{15}O	2.03 min	β^+ (100)	0.511	200
^{18}F	109.8 min	β^+ (97)	0.511	194
^{64}Cu	12.8 h	β^+ (19) or β^-(40), EC[a] (41)	0.511	38.6
^{67}Ga	3.3 days	EC(100)	0.093, 0.184, 0.300	40, 20, 17
^{111}In	2.8 days	EC(100)	0.171, 0.245	90, 94
^{123}I	13.2 hr	EC(100)	0.159	83
^{124}I	4.2 days	β^+ (23), EC(77)	0.511	
^{201}Tl	73 h	EC(100)	0.035	9.4

[a]EC; electron capture

form thermal neutrons by interaction with the moderator, such as water, heavy water, or graphite, which is distributed in the spaces between the fuel rods.

Two types of interaction with thermal neutrons can be considered for the production of various useful radionuclides: fission (n, f) reaction of heavy elements and neutron capture (n, γ) reaction. From the fission reaction of ^{235}U, clinically useful radionuclides such as ^{131}I and ^{99}Mo are produced. Many other nuclides are also produced from the fission of ^{235}U, and the crude fission product should be purified with the appropriate purification method. The fission products are usually neutron rich and decay by β^- emission. From neutron capture reaction, the target nucleus captures one thermal neutron and emits γ-rays to produce an isotope of the same element. The radionuclide from neutron capture reaction has a relatively low SA, and so this method is not practical for production of clinically useful radionuclides. Therefore, neutron capture reaction is used for the trace metal analysis with neutron activation analysis. The (n, p) or (n, α) reaction in the reactor is also useful for the production of ^{14}C, ^{32}P or ^{3}H.

2.3.3. *Generator-produced radionuclides*

The first generator for clinical application was designed and used by Failla in 1926.[2] The use of radionuclide generator has grown considerably because it is more convenient and considerably cheaper than cyclotron- or reactor-produced radionuclide. This increase has led to the development of radionuclide generators that serve as convenient sources of radionuclide production. In a generator, a long-lived parent nuclide is basically allowed to decay to its short-lived daughter nuclide and the latter is then chemically separated.

The structure of a radionuclide generator is quite simple and consists of a column and a shielded container (Fig. 2.2). The column is filled with adsorbent material such as cation- or anion-exchange resin, aluminum oxide, titanium oxide or tin oxide, onto which the parent nuclide is adsorbed. The daughter radionuclide grows as a result of the decay of the parent until either a transient or a secular equilibrium is reached within several half-lives of the daughter. Because there are differences between the mother and the daughter radionuclides in chemical properties, the daughter activity is eluted in a carrier-free state with an appropriate solvent, leaving the parent on the column. After one elution, the daughter activity starts to grow again in the column until an equilibrium is reached in the daughter appears to decay

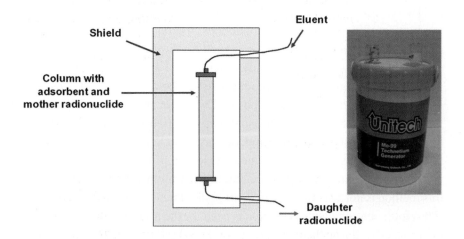

Fig. 2.2. Schematic diagram of a generator.

Table 2.2. Commonly used radionuclide generator systems.

System	Parent Half-Life	Daughter Half-Life	Decay Mode (%)	γ-Energy (keV)	Eluent
^{99}M-^{99m}Tc	66 h	6 h	IT	140	0.9% NaCl
^{68}Ge-^{68}Ga	271 days	68 min	β^+	511	0.1 M HCl
^{82}Sr-^{82}Rb	25.5 days	75 sec	β^+	511	0.9% NaCl
^{188}W-^{188}Re	69.4 days	17 h	β(2.1 MeV), γ	155	0.9% NaCl

^{a} IT; isomeric transition

with the same half-life as the parent. Therefore, the elution of activity can be made repeatedly.

A radionuclide generator must be sterile and pyrogen-free and an ideal radionuclide generator should be simple, convenient, easy to use, and give a high yield of the daughter nuclide repeatedly and reproducibly. A large number of radionuclide generator systems have been developed and tried for routine use in nuclear medicine. Only a few of generators are of importance; they are the ^{99}Mo–^{99m}Tc, ^{68}Ge–^{68}Ga, ^{82}Sr–^{82}Rb, and ^{188}W–^{188}Re systems, and are listed in Table 2.2 along with their properties.

The ^{99}Mo–^{99m}Tc generator is the first successful and most common generator system, because of the excellent radiation characteristics of ^{99m}Tc; its 6-h half-life, very little electron emission, and a high yield of 140 keV γ-rays (90%), which are nearly ideal for imaging devices in nuclear medicine. ^{68}Ge–^{68}Ga and ^{82}Sr–^{82}Rb generator system are used for PET radiopharmaceuticals, and ^{188}W–^{188}Re is for therapeutic application of ^{188}Re radiopharmaceuticals.

2.4. Radiolabeling Chemistry

A radiopharmaceutical is prepared by the reaction of the precursor and a radionuclide using a certain chemical reaction, which is called radiolabeling. Radiolabeling chemistry is based on organic, inorganic, or organometallic chemistry, and its mechanism is not entirely different from original synthetic chemistry.

Each radionuclide has its own chemical property, which is same with naturally abundant isotope, for example, ^{11}C has the same chemical property with ^{12}C. Therefore, one can expect that ^{11}C chemistry is as same as ^{12}C chemistry. However, in radiolabeling procedure, the amount of radionuclide is generally from pico- to nano-molar level, while that of the precursor is milli-molar level. This stoichiometry difference, sometimes more than a million times, between the radionuclide and the precursor can have unexpected results in radiolabeling procedures. Therefore, one should keep this stoichiometry difference in mind in every radiolabeling procedure.

Nowadays, almost all the radiolabeling procedures, including chemical synthesis, purification, and sterilization steps, are done by the automatic synthesis module, which is controlled by a personal computer outside of the hot-cell. However, the radiochemist still manually sets up the new synthetic procedure for new radiopharmaceutical or solving problems from the automated module.

In a radiolabeled compound, one atom of a molecule is substituted by a similar or different radioactive atom. In any labeling process, a variety of physicochemical conditions can be employed to achieve a specific kind of labeling. There are several methods employed in the preparation of labeled compounds for clinical use, including a simple isotope exchange, a foreign isotope labeling, and a labeling with bifunctional chelating agent.

From the point of view of chemistry, there are three major reaction mechanisms in radiolabeling chemistry: (1) the nucleophilic substitution reaction for ^{11}C or ^{18}F; (2) the electrophilic substitution reaction for ^{75}Br, ^{76}Br, ^{123}I, ^{124}I, ^{125}I, and ^{131}I; and (3) coordination chemistry for metallic radionuclide, such as ^{68}Ga, ^{64}Cu, ^{82}Rb, ^{89}Zr, or ^{44}Sc.

Each radionuclide and various factors affecting radiolabeling procedures are discussed below.

2.4.1. ^{11}C Chemistry

The ^{11}C-labeled compound is ideal for development as a radiotracer, because ^{11}C labeling radiopharmaceuticals can have the exact same chemical structure as ^{12}C non-radioactive compounds, thus our body cannot identify between ^{11}C and ^{12}C compounds. [^{11}C]CO$_2$ or [^{11}C]CH$_4$ is produced from a cyclotron by ^{14}N(p, α)^{11}C reaction, and the first precursor for

28

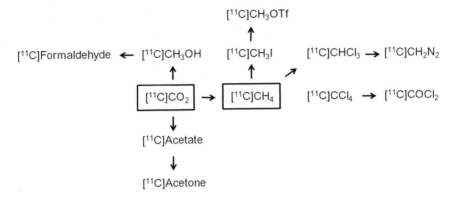

Fig. 2.3. ^{11}C chemical species for radiolabeling.

^{11}C radiolabeling procedure. [^{11}C]CH$_4$ is produced inside of the target in a cyclotron or made from [^{11}C]CO$_2$ by the reduction reaction using Ni catalyst.

In the liquid phase reaction for ^{11}C labeling, [^{11}C]CO$_2$ is converted to [^{11}C]CH$_3$I by the reduction using LiAlH$_4$.

In contrast, [^{11}C]CH$_3$I is produced from [^{11}C]CH$_4$ by radical reaction using iodine. [^{11}C]CH$_3$I is used directly for the *O*- or *N*-methylation reaction to make ^{11}C-labeled compound or more reactive chemical species, such as [^{11}C]CH$_3$OTf ([^{11}C]methyl triflate) (Fig. 2.3).

2.4.2. ^{18}F Chemistry

The hydroxyl (OH$^-$) group is substituted by ^{18}F with minimal chemical structure change to make a radiopharmaceutical. The [^{18}F]F$^-$ is produced by ^{18}O(p,n)^{18}F, and itself has less nucleophilicity, thus it needs a specific phase transfer catalyst to increase the nucleophilicity for the nucleophilic substitution reaction, such as Kryptofix 222 or tetrabutylammonium (TBA) salt (Fig. 2.4). Generally, the solvent for the nucleophilic substitution reaction of [^{18}F]F$^-$ is the polar organic solvent, such as CH$_3$CN, dimathylformamide (DMF), tetrahydrofuran (THF) or dimethylsulfoxide (DMSO).

For the radiolabeling of ^{18}F, a reaction precursor is needed with a good leaving group, such as a mesylate (-OMs), tosylate (-OTs), or triflate (-OTf). The ^{18}F can be directly labeled to thermally stable compounds, such

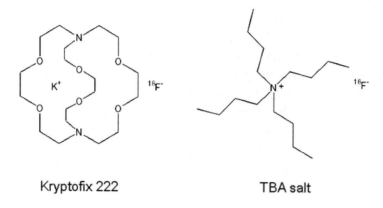

Kryptofix 222   **TBA salt**

Fig. 2.4. Chemical structures of Kryptofix 222 and tetrabutylammonium (TBA) salt.

as small molecules or peptides using an appropriate precursor. However, thermally unstable compounds, including long chain peptide, protein, or antibody, should be labeled with ^{18}F by the indirect method. First, ^{18}F is labeled to an adequate small molecule, then the ^{18}F-labeled small molecule is conjugated to the thermally unstable compound with the mild condition.[3]

2.4.3. ^{99m}Tc Chemistry

^{99m}Tc is one of the most practical radionuclides because it is produced by a generator system and it has the suitable energy for γ camera or SPECT imaging and a moderate half-life. ^{99m}Tc is a transition metal and belongs to group 7 (VIIB; Mn, Tc, and Re) and has the atomic number 43. ^{99m}Tc decays to ^{99}Tc by isomeric transition with half-life of 6 h and emits 140 keV of γ-ray, and no stable isotope of technetium exists in nature. The electronic configuration of the technetium atom is $1s^2 2s^2 2p^6 3s^2 3p^6 3d^{10} 4s^2 4p^6 4d^6 5s^1$, and technetium can be ionized by the loss of a given number of electrons from the 4d and 5s orbitals or gain of one electron to the 4d orbital. Therefore, theoretically technetium atom can be ionized and exist in eight oxidation states from 1− to 7+, Charge states of 7+ and 4+ are most stable, however 1+, 5+ or 7+ is useful for practical ^{99m}Tc radiopharmaceuticals. ^{99m}Tc can form a stable complex with ligands or chelating agents, and stable coordination numbers of ^{99m}Tc-complexes are 4, 5, and 6.

The chemical form of ^{99m}Tc, freshly eluted from a ^{99}M-^{99m}Tc generator, is pertechnetate ion (^{99m}TcO$_4^-$), and it is highly stable in the aqueous solution, thus it should be reduced for forming complex with ligands or chelating agents. Among various reducing agents, including stannous chloride (SnCl$_2$•2H$_2$O), stannous citrate, stannous tartrate, concentrated HCl, sodium borohydride (NaBH$_4$), dithionite, and ferrous sulfate, stannous chloride is the most commonly used reducing agent in most preparations of ^{99m}Tc-labeled radiopharmaceuticals.

^{99m}Tc prefers chemical groups of oxygen, nitrogen, and sulfur electron donors, and commonly used chelating agents that contain these donors for ^{99m}Tc radiopharmaceutical preparations are DTPA (diethylenetriaminepentaacetic acid), glucoheptonic acid, methylenediphosphonic acid (MDP), hydroxymethylenediphosphonic acid (HMDP), diamercaptosuccinic acid (DMSA), mercaptoacetylglycylglycylglycine (MAG$_3$), diaminodithiols (N$_2$S$_2$), L,L-ethylcysteinate dimer (ECD), and HMPAO (hexamethylpropyleneamine oxime). Generally, ^{99m}Tc radiopharmaceuticals are prepared in the clinical routine by the simple mixing of ^{99m}TcO$_4^-$ and the specific kit, which contains the reducing agent, antioxidants, and pH buffer. The kits have a long shelf life and can be purchased and stored well ahead of daily preparation.

2.4.4. *Metallic radionuclide chemistry*

Recently, as metallic radionuclide-labeled radiopharmaceuticals have been used more frequently in clinical routine for diagnostic or therapeutic purposes, the chemistry of metallic radionuclide is getting more important. Commonly used metallic radionuclides for radiopharmaceuticals are ^{68}Ga, ^{64}Cu, ^{67}Cu, ^{82}Rb, ^{89}Zr, ^{111}In, ^{177}Lu, and ^{188}Re. The ^{82}Rb isotope is used for myocardial PET imaging; the other isotopes need specific bifunctional chelating agents (BFCs). However, there is no one BCA that is suitable for all radionuclides. The selection of a suitable chelating agent or BCA for a specific radionuclide depends on numerous factors, which should be considered for its design and its actual use, including the coordination number of the metal ion, the matching cavity size of chelating agent or BCA with the ionic radius of the ion, oxidation state of the metal ion, the hardness or softness of the ion, providing the appropriate chelate density or number of donor-binding groups, and the rate of complex formation and dissociation.[4] Consequently, the ideal goal for selection of chelating agent or BCA for the specific radionuclide is instant radionuclide complex formation with infinite *in vitro* or *in vivo* stability or no dissociation.

There are several types of chelating agent or BCA are reported to be labeled with metallic radionuclides including acyclic and macrocyclic compounds (Fig. 2.5). Ethylenediaminetetraacetic acid (EDTA) derivatives were initially reported for labeling with ^{111}In, and their stability problem forced a move to develop diethylenetriaminepentaacetic acid (DTPA) derivatives that would provide a more appropriate coordination number and the complex stability.[5,6] A widely used chemical, 1,4,7,10-tetraazacyclododacane-1,4,7,10 -tetraacetic acid (DOTA), is used for metallic radionuclide complexation and good for ^{68}Ga, ^{64}Cu, or [89]Zr. The chemical 1,4,7-triazacyclononane-1,4,7-triacetic acid (NOTA) is especially a better choice for ^{68}Ga, because the ^{68}Ga-NOTA complex shows

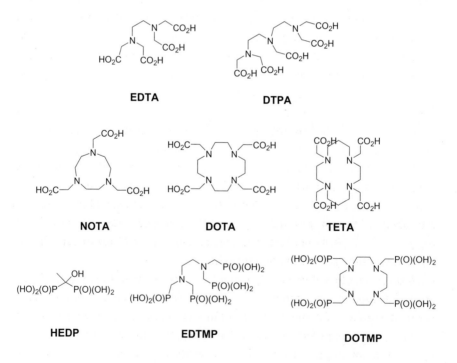

Fig. 2.5. Chemical structures of several bifunctional chelating agents.

extremely higher stability than the ^{68}Ga-DOTA complex. For the same reason, 1,4,8,11-tetraazacyclotetradecane-1,4,8,11-tetraacetic acid (TETA) is better for ^{64}Cu.

2.4.5. *Radioiodine chemistry*

Iodine is a metallic element and belongs to the halogen group 17 (VIIA; F, Cl, Br and I). A number of iodine radioisotopes are commonly used for diagnostic imaging and therapy. ^{123}I is most suitable for *in vivo* diagnostic procedures because it has a convenient half-life (13.2 h) and γ energy (159 keV), and gives a low radiation dose to the patient. ^{125}I is commonly used for *in vitro* procedures and has the advantage of a long half-life (60 days), and ^{131}I, the β- emitter, is for thyroid cancer therapy. Recently, the practical preparation of ^{124}I by the commercially available solid target system of a cyclotron and the use of ^{124}I has been increasing for PET imaging.

Radioiodination is performed by the electrophilic substitution reaction with proton of the aromatic ring of a substrate molecule, such as a peptide, a protein, or an antibody. Tyrosine (Tyr) is the most useful moiety for radioiodination, because its hydroxyl group can activate the electrophilic substitution reaction by the electron donating effect with the ortho-position. Radioiodine is produced or supplied in the form of an I^- (iodide) ion and it should be activated by the specific chemical to form a reactive iodine species, which then labels the compound.

Chloramine-T (sodium salt of N-monochloro-p-toluenesulfonamide) is a mild oxidizing agent which oxidizes iodide ion to a reactive iodine species. Compounds with high SA can be obtained by chloramine-T method and the labeling efficiency is very high ($\sim$90%). However, chloramine-T is a highly reactive substance and can cause denaturation of chemically labile molecules, such as proteins or antibodies.

Iodogen or chloramide (1, 3, 4, 6-tetrachloro-3a, 6a-diphenylglycoluril) is used for labeling of proteins or cell membranes. Iodogen is precoated inside the tube, and the radioiodide and proteins are mixed for 10 to 15 min. The unreacted iodide is separated by column chromatography of the sephadex gel. From the iodogen method, the labeling yield is from 70% to 80%, and the denaturation of protein is minimal. Iodo-bead, which consists of the oxidant *N*-chlorobenzenesulfonamide immobilized on 2.8-mm diameter nonporous polystyrene sphere, is used for various peptides and proteins. This method is very successful with little denaturation of the protein, and the labeling yield is almost 99%.

2.5. PET Radiopharmaceuticals

The PET radiopharmaceutical contains a positron-emitting radionuclide and is used for diagnostic imaging by administration in tracer amount. Commonly used radionuclides for PET radiopharmaceuticals are ^{11}C, ^{13}N, ^{15}O, ^{18}F, ^{44}Sc, ^{64}Cu, ^{68}Ga, ^{82}Rb, ^{89}Zr, ^{75}Br, ^{76}Br and ^{124}I. ^{11}C, ^{13}N or ^{15}O belong to organic nuclides, ^{68}Ga, ^{64}Cu, ^{82}Rb, ^{89}Zr, and ^{44}Sc to metallic nuclides, and ^{18}F, ^{75}Br, ^{76}Br and ^{124}I to the halogen group. For each radionuclide, specific radiolabeling chemistry is needed, and there are three major reaction mechanisms in radiolabeling chemistry: the nucleophilic substitution reaction for ^{11}C or ^{18}F; the electrophilic substitution reaction for ^{75}Br, ^{76}Br; and ^{124}I and coordination chemistry for metallic radionuclide, such as ^{68}Ga, ^{64}Cu, ^{82}Rb, ^{89}Zr, or ^{44}Sc.

^{18}F is the most commonly used PET radionuclide because of 2-[^{18}F] fluoro-2-deoxy-D-glucose ([^{18}F]FDG).[7] [^{18}F]FDG was first introduced in 1978, and within four decades, the use of [^{18}F]FDG has been dramatically increasing throughout the world. Since [^{18}F]FDG, a large number of PET radiopharmaceuticals have been introduced, are used in various research fields and the clinical routine, and have been newly developed.

Here we will discuss about several PET radiopharmaceuticals used for imaging of brain, heart, or cancer and their chemistry-related problems.

2.5.1. *PET radiopharmaceuticals for brain imaging*

PET radiopharmaceutical and imaging can visualize the problems of brain function or changes related to mental activity, brain perfusion, and metabolism, the uptake capability of biologically active substances, and various neurotransmitters with non-invasive and real-time three-dimensional images.

PET radiopharmaceuticals for brain imaging have the moderate molecular weight (less than 1,000 Da) and lipophilicity with a range of 0.5 to

2.0 (Log P; Log value of the partition coefficient of octanol and water distribution) for penetration of blood-brain barrier.[8] Several PET radiopharmaceuticals with targeting mechanisms and biological processes are summarized and listed in Table 2.3.

2.5.1.1. *Brain perfusion and metabolism*

$[^{15}O]CO$ or $[^{11}C]CO$ is used for the evaluation of the blood volume of the brain, and $[^{15}O]H_2O$, $[^{15}O]CO_2$, $[^{13}N]NH_3$, $[^{15}O]$butanol, $[^{11}C]$butanol, or $[^{18}F]$fluoromethane is used for the quantification of the brain perfusion. $[^{15}O]O_2$ is used for brain oxygen metabolism, and $[^{11}C]$glucose or $[^{18}F]FDG$ is for brain glucose metabolism.

2.5.1.2. *Brain neurotransmitter systems*

In the brain neurotransmitter system, there are various neurotransmitters, receptors, and transporters (reuptake sites). Specific receptors can uptake the neurotransmitter and produce the downstream signal, and transporters can uptake and transport the neurotransmitter to the presynapse. Major neurotransmitter systems are dopamine, serotonin, choline, opiate systems, and benzodiazepine receptor family.

Dopamine is a typical neurotransmitter, which is related to action, cognition, and motivation, and is secreted from dopaminergic neurons in the substantial nigra, ventral tegmental region, and retrorubral area of the mid brain. The dopaminergic system has been widely investigated in clinical brain science and PET research field since the first human imaging of the dopamine synthesis using 6-$[^{18}F]$fluoro-3,4-dihydroxyphenylalanine ($[^{18}F]FDOPA$) in 1983.[9] The imaging studies for dopaminergic system are focused on the dopamine synthesis, metabolism, receptor, and transporter. $[^{18}F]FDOPA$ is a representative PET radiopharmaceutical for the imaging of the dopaminergic system function and used for the synthesis and metabolism of the dopamine. Clinically, the uptake of $[^{18}F]FDOPA$ is decreased in striatum area with advancing years in hemiparkinsonism patient. $[^{18}F]$fluorotyrosine is used for the evaluation of the dopamine function of pre-synapse.

Dopamine receptors are classified as the D_1 and D_2 types, and D_5, D_3, and D_4 subtypes by the pharmacological aspect. Dopamine

Table 2.3. PET radiopharmaceuticals for brain imaging.

Biological Process	Target	Radiopharmaceuticals
Blood volume		[^{15}O]CO, [^{11}C]CO
Blood flow		[^{15}O]H$_2$O, [^{15}O]CO$_2$, [^{13}N]NH$_3$, [^{15}O]butanol, [^{11}C]butanol, [^{18}F]fluoromethane
O$_2$ metabolism		[^{15}O]O$_2$
Glucose metabolism	Hexokinase	
	Glucose transporter	[^{11}C]Glucose, [^{18}F]FDG
Neurotransmitter system		
Dopamine system	Metabolism	[^{18}F]FDOPA, [^{18}F]Fluorotyrosine
	D$_1$ receptor	[^{11}C]SCH 23390, [^{11}C]NNC-112
	D$_2$ receptor	[^{11}C]N-Methylspiperone, [^{11}C]FLB-457 [^{11}C]Raclopride, [^{18}F]Fallypride
	Transporter (DAT)	N-[^{11}C]Methyl]-(-)-cocaine, [^{11}C]CFT([11C]WIN 35,428), [^{18}F]FP-CIT, [^{18}F]FE-CNT
	Vesicular amine transporter (VMAT)	[^{11}C]DTBZ, [^{18}F]DTBZ
Serotonin system	Metabolism	[^{11}C]5-HTP, [^{11}C]α-methyl-L-tryptophan, [^{11}C]α-methylhydroxy-tryptophan
	5-HT$_{1A}$ receptor	[^{11}C]DWAY, [^{18}F]MPPF

(Continued)

Table 2.3.   (*Continued*)

Biological Process	Target	Radiopharmaceuticals
	5-HT$_{2A}$ receptor	[^{18}F]Septoperone, [^{18}F]Altanserin
	Transporter (SERT)	[^{11}C](+)McN5652, [^{11}C]DASB, [^{11}C]AFM
Cholinergic system	Muscarinic receptor	[^{18}F]FP-TZTP
	Nicotinic receptor	[^{11}C]Nicotine, [^{18}F]NFEP, [^{18}F]Fluoro-A-85380
	Acetylcholinesterase (AChE)	[^{11}C]MP4A, [^{11}C]MP4P
Opiate system	Receptor	[^{11}C]Carfentanil (μ), [^{11}C]Naltrindole (δ), [^{11}C]GR89696(κ)
Benzodiazepine system	Receptor-central type	[^{18}F]Flumazenil, [^{11}C]Flumazenil, [^{18}F]Fluoroflumazenil
	Receptor-peripheral type	[^{11}C]PK11195, [^{11}C]DPA-713, [^{11}C]PBR28,
Dementia	Amyloid plaque	[^{11}C]PIB, [^{18}F]FDDNP, [^{18}F]AV-1, [^{18}F]AV-45, [^{18}F]GE-067

receptor imaging can be used for the neuropsychiatric disorders, such as schizophrenia, bipolar disorder, Parkinsonism, and Huntington's disease. [^{11}C]SCH 23390 or [^{11}C]NNC-112 is used for D1 receptor, and [^{11}C]N-methylspiperone, [^{11}C]FLB-457 [^{11}C]raclopride or [^{18}F]fallypride is for D2 receptor. For the imaging of dopamine transporters, the cocaine derivatives are used as PET radiotracers, such as [N-[^{11}C]methyl]-(–)-cocaine, [^{11}C]CFT([^{11}C]WIN 35,428), [^{18}F]FP-CIT, and [^{18}F]FE-CNT. Especially, [^{11}C]CFT and [^{18}F]FP-CIT have higher affinity to dopamine transporters and show lower non-specific binding than cocaine. Dopamine is stored in a vesicle inside the cell by the vesicular amine transporter (VMAT). [^{11}C]DTBZ and 9-[^{18}F]fluoropropyl-DTBZ ([^{18}F]AV-133) are used for VMAT imaging. Serotonin (5-hydroxytryptamine; 5-HT) is related to depression or schizophrenia and distributed at the enterochromaffin cells in the intestinal tract and pineal gland. The imaging studies for serotonin system are focused on serotonin synthesis, metabolism, receptor, and transporter. Serotonin is synthesized by the hydroxylation and decarboxylation of the amino acid tryptophan inside the body. Therefore, ^{11}C-labeled tryptophan derivatives, such as [^{11}C]5-hydroxytrytophan ([^{11}C]5-HTP), [^{11}C]α-methyl-L-tryptophan, and [^{11}C]α-methylhydroxytryptophan can be used for the imaging of serotonin synthesis and metabolism.

Serotonin receptor has five subtypes, 5-HT$_1$, 5-HT$_2$, 5-HT$_3$, 5-HT$_4$, and 5-HT$_5$. [^{11}C-carbonyl]WAY 100635 ([^{11}C]DWAY) or [^{18}F]MPPF is used for 5-HT$_{1A}$, and [^{18}F]septoperone or [^{18}F]altanserin is used for 5-HT$_{2A}$.

Serotonin transporter (SERT) is the serotonin reuptake site in the pre-synapse, and [^{11}C](+)McN5652, [^{18}F]paroxetine, [^{11}C]DASB, or [^{11}C]AFM is used for serotonin transporter imaging. Acetylcholine (Ach) is related to learning, memory, cognition, or dementia, and major areas for PET imaging are acetylcholine receptor and acetylcholine metabolism. Acetylcholine receptors are classified muscarinic (mAChR) and nicotinic receptor (nAChR). Acetylcholine system usually consists of muscarinic receptor in the post-synapse, and muscarinic receptor is [^{11}C]scopolamine, [^{11}C]tropanylbenzilate, [^{11}C]N-methyl-4-piperidylbenzilate, and [^{18}F]FP-TZTP are used for muscarinic receptor imaging.

Nicotinic receptors are widely distributed in the central nervous system, peripheral nervous system, and adrenal gland. [^{11}C]Nicotine, [^{18}F]norchlorofluoroepibatidine ([^{18}F]NFEP), or [^{18}F]fluoro-A-85380 is used for this receptor. Acetylcholinesterase (AChE) hydrolyzes acetylcholine to control the concentration of acetylcholine in the synapse. [^{11}C]MP4A and [^{11}C]MP4P have been reported that those can specifically bind to acetylcholinesterase.[10,11] The opiate system can be imaged by the [^{11}C]carfentanil(μ), [^{11}C]diprenorphine(δ), or [^{11}C]GR89696(κ). Benzodiazepine receptor has two types, the central and peripheral, the former is related to epilepsy or anxiety and the latter is to inflammation. [^{18}F]flumazenil, [^{11}C]flumazenil, or [^{18}F]fluoroflumazenil is used for the central type receptor and [^{11}C]PK11195, [^{11}C]DPA-713, or [^{11}C]PBR28 is for the peripheral type.

2.5.1.3. *β-Amyloid plaques imaging*

Accumulation of plaques and beta-amyloid in the brain is a histopathologic hallmark for the diagnosis of Alzheimer's disease. The use of ^{11}C-labeled Pittsburgh compound B (PIB) has enabled accurate classification of patients with versus without Alzheimer's disease and other neurodegenerative diseases.[12] [^{18}F]FDDNP has been reported to visualize not only amyloid plaques but also tau tangles. Recently, ^{18}F-labeled plaque imaging agents, such as [^{18}F]AV-1, [^{18}F]AV-45, [^{18}F]GE-067, have been reported and are now under clinical trials.

2.5.2. *PET radiopharmaceuticals for heart imaging*

Heart imaging in nuclear medicine has been used for the diagnosis and prognosis for the disease of cardiovascular system from information of biological process and metabolism. The evaluation of myocardial function using radiopharmaceuticals is mainly focused on blood flow, perfusion, and metabolism; moreover, an autonomic nervous system in non-invasive ways. Regional myocardial blood flow or perfusion is related to various heart functions and controlled by the regional myocardial metabolism and oxygen consumption.

PET radiopharmaceuticals for the evaluation of regional myocardial perfusion are [^{13}N]NH$_3$, [^{15}O]H$_2$O and [^{82}Rb]Rb$^+$.[13,14] Recently, ^{62}Cu-labeled lipophilic compound, ^{62}Cu-PTSM, and ^{18}F-labeled [^{18}F]fluorobenzyltriphenylphosphonium ([^{18}F]BMS-747158-02) have been reported for myocardial blood flow imaging. [^{82}Rb]Rb$^+$ is the same family of K^+ in the periodic table and a promising radionuclide for myocardial perfusion imaging. $[^{82}Rb]Rb^+$, itself radiopharmaceutical, is continuously produced by the $^{82}Sr–^{82}Rb$ generator within 10 min and the repeated image scan is possible because it has a very short half-life of 75 sec, which is compromised to radiation safety point.

The metabolism of myocardial cells is controlled by the concentration of specific molecules and hormones in an artery. Major energy sources for myocardial metabolism are glucose and fatty acids, thus $[^{18}F]FDG$ and radiolabeled fatty acids are used for imaging of myocardial metabolism. Oxidation metabolism in myocardial cells can be measured by $[^{11}C]$acetate or $[^{15}O]O_2$. ^{11}C-labeled *meta*-hydroxyephedrine (HED) can be used for the sympathetic nerve in heart, and $[^{11}C]CGP$-12177 has been reported to show high affinity to adrenaline receptors in sympathetic nerve system.

2.5.3. *PET radiopharmaceuticals for tumor imaging*

Tumor imaging has begun from the trial of imaging for the specific phenomenon in tumor cells or tissues. Generally in tumor cells or tissues, various molecular and functional changes, including the increase of the metabolism, the specific receptor expression, neovascularization, or hypoxia, are observed. Tumor imaging can be used for the discrimination of tumor malignancy, localization, metastasis, stage, recurrent and prognosis, and divided into two major categories, metabolism and receptor imaging.

Several PET radiopharmaceuticals used for tumor imaging are listed with uptake-accumulation mechanisms and biological processes in Table 2.4. The metabolism of tumor cells is increased in blood flow, glucose uptake and consumption, amino acid transport, protein synthesis, DNA synthesis, and lipid synthesis of membrane. Glucose metabolism of tumor cell or tissue is directly visualized by $[^{18}F]FDG$, which is widely used as a practical PET pharmaceutical in nuclear medicine. $[^{18}F]FDG$ is the analogue of glucose, and same as glucose, accumulated in the cell through the glucose transporters (GLUT) and hexokinase. Therefore $[^{18}F]FDG$ can directly visualize GLUT and hexokinase activities through the measurement of the uptake of $[^{18}F]FDG$ in to the cell (Fig. 2.6).

Bone primary tumor and metastasis can be evaluated by $Na[^{18}F]F$ PET. $[^{18}F]F^-$ is accumulated to the bone formation increased site by the

Table 2.4. PET radiopharmaceuticals for tumor imaging.

Biological Process	Uptake and Localization Mechanism	Radiopharmaceuticals
Metabolism		
Glucose	GLUT, hexokinase substrate	[^{18}F]FDG
Bone	Conjugation with hydroxyapatite of bone	Na[^{18}F]F
Cell membrane lipid synthesis	Choline kinase substrate	[^{11}C]Choline, [^{18}F]Fluorocholine, [^{11}C]Acetate, [^{18}F]Fluoroacetate
Amino acid transport & Protein synthesis	Acetyl-CoA precursor Amino acid & protein substrate	L-[methyl-^{11}C]Methionine, [^{18}F]FMT, [^{18}F]FET, [^{18}F]FACBC
DNA synthesis	Thymidine kinase substrate	[^{18}F]Fluorouridine, [^{11}C]FMAU, [^{18}F]FLT
Neovascularization	Specific binding to $\alpha_v\beta_3$-integrin	^{18}F-Galacto-RGD, ^{68}Ga-NOTA-RGD
Hypoxia Receptor	Reduction inside of cells	[^{18}F]FMISO, [^{18}F]FAZA, ^{64}Cu(II)-ATSM
Peptide receptor	Specific binding to Somatostatin receptor (SSTR)	^{68}Ga-DOTA-TOC, ^{68}Ga-DOTA-NOC
Steroid receptor	Specific binding to estrogen receptor	[^{18}F]FES

adsorption to hydroxyapatite of enamel or dentine materials. Na[^{18}F]F PET can give better resolution images than traditional γ-camera images of ^{99m}Tc-MDP or ^{99m}Tc-HEDP. Phospholipid is the major component of cell membrane and synthesized from the choline. Therefore, radiolabeled choline derivatives, [^{11}C]choline and [^{18}F]fluorocholine, are used for tumor imaging by the incensement of phospholipid synthesis. Acetyl-CoA is used for

Plasma   Cell

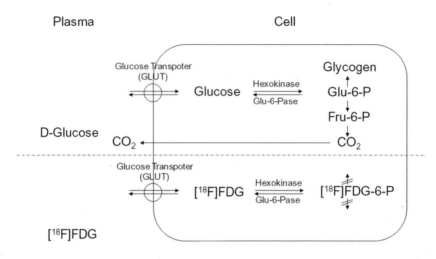

Fig. 2.6. [^{18}F]FDG uptake and accumulation mechanism.

synthesis of cholesterol or fatty acid in tumor cells. Therefore, [^{11}C]acetate and [^{18}F]fluoroacetate are used for cholesterol or fatty acid synthesis in tumor cells or tissues. Radiolabeled amino acid derivatives can directly visualize the level of amino acid transport and protein synthesis *in vivo*. Moreover, because the uptake and accumulation of radiolabeled amino acid to normal cell is less than [^{18}F]FDG, the image contrast from radiolabeled amino acid is better than that of [^{18}F]FDG. Therefore, radiolabeled amino acid image is especially useful for brain tumors. L-[methyl-^{11}C]methionine, [^{18}F]FMT, [^{18}F]FET or [^{18}F]FACBC is used for this purpose in tumor imaging.

DNA synthesis imaging is obtained by using of ^{11}C- or ^{18}F-labeled thymidine analogs, [^{18}F]fluorouridine, [^{11}C]FMAU or [^{18}F]FLT.[15] Angiogenesis is an important process on which tumors depend to maintain growth and is subjected to regulation by growth factors, such as vascular epithelial growth factor (VEGF), inhibitors, and integrins. For imaging of angiogenesis, ^{68}Ga-NOTA-RGD and ^{18}F-galacto-RGD PET imaging of $\alpha_v\beta_3$ integrin have been studied to exploit their binding to RGD containing components on extracellular matrix which are upregulated in the tumor vasculature (Fig. 2.7).[16,17]

Tumor hypoxia is assessed by ^{18}F-labeled misonidazole ([^{18}F]FMISO) PET imaging, which is useful for effective external beam radiation

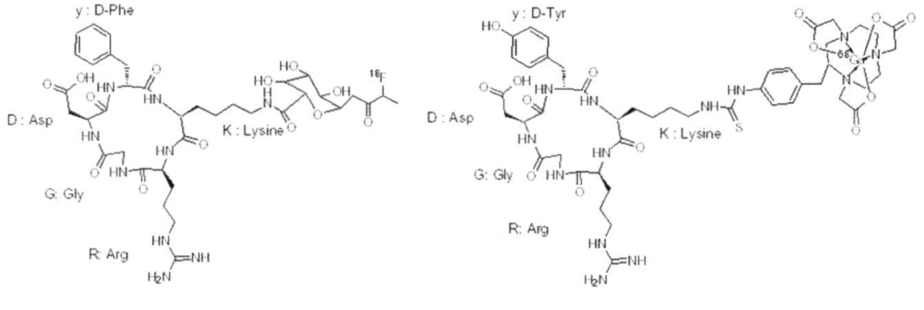

Fig. 2.7. PET angiogenesis imaging agents; ^{18}F-Galacto-RGD and ^{68}Ga-NOTA-RGD.

therapy.[18] ^{18}F-fluoroazomycin arabinoside ([^{18}F]FAZA) and ^{64}Cu-diacetyl-bis(N^4-methylthiosemicarbazone (^{64}Cu-ATSM) are also used for imaging of tumor hypoxia.[19,20]

Tumor-related specific receptors, such as somatostatin or estrogen receptor (SSTR or ER), can be imaged by ^{18}F-labeled estradiol and radiolabeled octreotide derivatives.[21,22] ^{68}Ga-DOTA-Tyr[3]-octreotide (^{68}Ga-DOTA-TOC) is used for direct imaging of SSTR, and evaluates the therapeutic effect of the peptide receptor radiotherapy (PRRT) of neuroendocrine tumors with [90]Y- or ^{177}Lu-DOTA-Tyr[3]-Thr[8]-octreotide ([90]Y- or ^{177}Lu-DOTA-TATE).[23]

2.6. ^{99m}Tc-labeled Radiopharmaceuticals

[99m]Tc-labeled radiopharmaceuticals are the most frequently used radiopharmaceuticals in nuclear medicine and used for the imaging of tumor and the evaluation of the function of brain, heart, kidney, liver, or other organs. In most cases, kits for ^{99m}Tc-labeled radiopharmaceuticals are commercially available for routine clinical use. These kits contain the chelating agent of substrate and the reducing agent in appropriate quantities, and suitable stabilizers are added. Almost all ^{99m}Tc-labeled radiopharmaceuticals have the expiration time of 6 h, which is equal to the physical half-life of [99m]Tc. The following is a description of the characteristics of the routinely used ^{99m}Tc-labeled radiopharmaceuticals.

2.6.1. ^{99m}Tc-labeled radiopharmaceuticals for bone imaging

^{99m}Tc-labeled phosphonate and phosphate compounds localize in bone and, therefore, are suitable for bone imaging. Phosphonate compounds are more stable *in vivo* than phosphate compounds, for this reason, diphosphonate complexes labeled with ^{99m}Tc are now commonly used for bone imaging. The three extensively studied diphosphonates are 1-hydroxyethylidene diphosphonate (HEDP), methylene diphosphonate (MDP), and hydroxymethylene diphosphonate (HDP), of which MDP and HDP are most commonly used in nuclear medicine (Fig. 2.8). ^{99m}Tc-MDP and ^{99m}Tc-HDP are used for bone imaging, whereas ^{99m}Tc-pyrophosphate (^{99m}Tc-PYP) is used for myocardial infarct imaging.

2.6.2. ^{99m}Tc-labeled radiopharmaceuticals for brain imaging

^{99m}Tc-HMPAO is the lipophilic radiopharmaceutical for brain perfusion imaging. HMPAO is a lipophilic substance that forms a neutral complex with ^{99m}Tc and exists in two stereoisomers: *d,l*-HMPAO and meso-HMPAO. The cerebral uptake of *d,l*- isomer is much higher than that of meso-HMPAO.

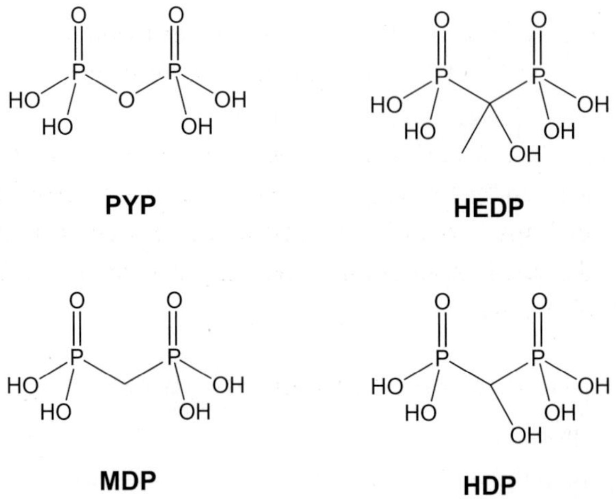

Fig. 2.8. Chemical structures of precursors of ^{99m}Tc bone imaging agents.

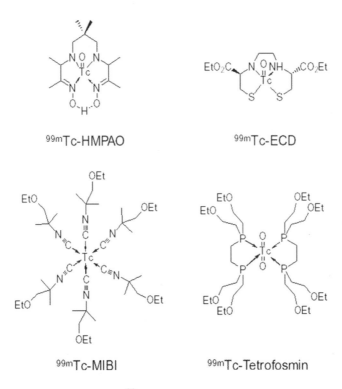

Fig. 2.9. Chemical structures of ^{99m}Tc radiopharmaceuticals for brain or heart imaging.

The primary use of ^{99m}Tc-HMPAO is in brain perfusion imaging.[24] Since it is lipophilic, it is used for labeling of leukocytes, substituting for ^{111}In-oxine.

^{99m}Tc-ECD is also used for brain perfusion imaging. ECD exists in two stereoisomers, *l,l*-ECD and *d,d*-ECD. Both isomers of ^{99m}Tc-labeled ECDs diffuse into the brain by crossing the blood–brain barrier (BBB), but [99m]Tc-*l,l*-ECD is metabolized only by an enzymatic process to a polar species that is trapped in the human brain. Thus, only purified *l,l*-ECD is used for ^{99m}Tc-ECD. (Fig. 2.9)

2.6.3. *[99m]Tc-labeled radiopharmaceuticals for heart imaging*

[99m]Tc-methoxyisobutylisonitrile (^{99m}Tc-MIBI) is a lipophilic cationic complex used as a substitute for ^{201}Tl for myocardial perfusion imaging. MIBI is supplied in a kit containing a lyophilized mixture of the chelating agent

in the form of a copper (I) salt of tetrakis(2-MIBI)tetrafluoroborate, and the MIBI chemical structure contains methoxy group. ^{99m}Tc-MIBI is used primarily for detection of myocardial perfusion abnormalities in patients, particularly for detection of myocardial ischemia and infarcts.[25] Another major myocardial perfusion imaging agent is ^{99m}Tc-6,9-bis(2-ethoxyethyl)-3,12-dioxa-6,9-diphospha-tetradecane (^{99m}Tc-tetrofosmin), which is a lipophilic cationic complex. The oxidation state of ^{99m}Tc in the structure of ^{99m}Tc-MIBI is 1+, while that of ^{99m}Tc-tetrofosmin is 5+.

2.6.4. ^{99m}Tc-labeled radiopharmaceuticals for kidney imaging

The primary use of ^{99m}Tc-DTPA is for renal flow study, glomerular filtration rate (GFR) measurement, and aerosol preparation in lung ventilation studies. DTPA is commonly used for the complex formation of various metallic radionuclides.[26] The chemical structure of ^{99m}Tc-DTPA is uncertain, but it has been reported to be negatively charge. Because of the stability problem of ^{99m}Tc-DTPA, it should be used within 1 h after preparation.

^{99m}Tc-mercaptoacetylglycylglycylglycine (^{99m}Tc-MAG$_3$) is used routinely for assessment of renal function, particularly in renal transplants. MAG$_3$ kit contains benzoyl-protected thiol group, thus to deprotection of thiol group, the labeling temperature should be at 100°C. In the structure of ^{99m}Tc-MAG$_3$, ^{99m}Tc has a coordination number of 5 and the complex has a negative charge of 1−.

2.6.5. ^{99m}Tc labeled radiopharmaceuticals for liver imaging

The ^{99m}Tc-labeled iminodiacetic acid (IDA) derivatives are commonly used as hepatobiliary agents to evaluate hepatic function, biliary duct patency, and mainly in cholescintigraphy. Of all ^{99m}Tc-IDA complexes, diisopropyliminodiacetic acid (DISIDA) and mebrofenin (bromotrimethyliminodiacetic acid) are claimed to be the hepatobiliary agents of choice.

2.6.6. ^{99m}Tc-labeled radiopharmaceuticals for blood flow

^{99m}Tc-red blood cells (^{99m}Tc-RBC) are mainly used for assessment of blood flow and useful in gastrointestinal blood loss and gated blood pool studies. There are three methods currently employed in the labeling of RBCs with ^{99m}Tc: the *in vitro* method, the *in vivo* method, and the modified *in vivo* method. Each method has its own merits and disadvantages.

2.7. Miscellaneous Radiopharmaceuticals

^{131}I, which is a β^--emitter, has been used for the treatment of thyroid disease such as thyroid carcinoma and hyperthyroidism for more than 60 years and is separated from the products of uranium fission or neutron irradiation of tellurium. ^{131}I is available in no-carrier-added (NCA) state. ^{123}I is used most commonly for the measurement of thyroid uptake and imaging, and is much better than ^{131}I because ^{123}I has a photon energy of 159 keV and does not emit any β radiations. Radioiodinated metaiodobenzylguanidine (MIBG) primarily localizes in the medulla of the adrenal gland. Therefore, ^{123}I-MIBG is primarily used for the detection of pheochromocytoma and localization of the myocardial regions depleted of catecholamine stores due to infarction. ^{131}I-MIBG has also been used in the treatment of neuroblastoma.

^{111}In-DTPA is primarily used for cisternography and infrequently in liquid meal for gastric emptying studies. ^{201}Tl is used for myocardial perfusion imaging in order to delineate between ischemic and infarcted myocardium. ^{201}Tl is produced by the cyclotron and is supplied in the form of NCA TlCl in isotonic saline solution at pH 4.5 to 7.0 for intravenous administration. ^{67}Ga-citrate is used primarily for detecting malignant diseases such as Hodgkin's disease, lymphomas, and bronchogenic carcinoma, and also used for localizing acute inflammatory diseases and infections. ^{90}Y is one of most frequently used therapeutic radionuclide in clinical practice, because of its high energy pure β emission and routine availability as a high SA sterile pyrogen-free product. ^{90}Y-ibritumomab tiuxetan (Zevalin) has recently been approved by the US Food and Drug Administration (FDA) as a therapeutic modality for B-cell non-Hodgkin's lymphoma.

^{90}Y-labeled octreotide derivatives as somatostatin receptor targeting peptides have been extensively used for neuroendocrine tumor treatment in current clinical practice.[27] The generator-produced ^{188}Re is a promising therapeutic radionuclide and has been used and reported for intracoronary radiation therapy using ^{188}Re-DTPA–filled balloon, radiation synovectomy using ^{188}Re-sulfur colloid, or ^{188}Re-tin colloid, radioembolization using ^{188}Re-glass microspheres or ^{188}Re-HDD/lipiodol solution, skin cancer therapy using radiolabeled filter paper coated by ^{188}Re-tin colloid or ^{188}Re-microspheres, bone palliation therapy using ^{188}Re-HEDP, radioimmunotherapy using ^{188}Re labeled mAbs, and peptide receptor radionuclide therapy using ^{188}Re labeled SST receptor binding peptides, respectively.[28–34]

2.8. Quality Control of Radiopharmaceuticals

Radiopharmaceuticals intended for human use should be sterile, pyrogen-free, safe, and efficacious for specific indications. Therefore, quality control procedures, including physicochemical, radiochemical, or biological test, should be carried out for each radiopharmaceutical after synthesis. Various *in vitro* physicochemical tests are essential for the determination of the purity and integrity of a radiopharmaceutical. Physicochemical tests consist of physical characteristics, pH, ionic strength, radionuclidic purity, radiochemical purity, and chemical purity.[35] Some of these tests are unique for radiopharmaceuticals because they contain radionuclides. SA is a unique feature of radiopharmaceuticals and is defined as the amount of radioactivity per unit mass of an element, molecule, or compound, which implies that the mass represents the combined mass of radioactive species and the non-radioactive counterpart. The SA units are expressed as Ci/g, Ci/mol, or Gbq/mol, and the SA of radiopharmaceuticals is very important since it is a measure of the number of radioactive probe molecules bound to the target system, and that can give a radioactive signal in a given mass of radiopharmaceuticals. Therefore, a low SA radiopharmaceutical, which contains a larger amount of non-radioactive species than radioactive species, is not proper for receptor or gene imaging because the number or concentration of target molecules is limited and an extremely smaller amount of radioactive species than non-radioactive species may not occupy the binding site of the target systems.

Biological tests are carried out essentially to examine the sterility, apyrogenicity, and toxicity of radiopharmaceuticals. Almost all procedures for biological test can be done after human administration, because radiopharmaceuticals have a relatively short physical half-life in nuclear medicine. In a radiopharmaceutical preparation, record keeping is needed for legal reasons as well as for tracing any faulty preparation in the case of a poor-quality scan. These records help trace the history of a particular radiopharmaceutical should any untoward effect take place in a patient due to its administration.

References

1. Walch MJ, Redvanly CS. (2003) *Handbook of Radiopharmaceuticals Radiochemistry and Applications*. John Wiley & Sons Ltd, West Sussex.
2. Sampson CB. (1999) *Textbook of Radiopharmacy: Theory and Practice*. OPA, Amsterdam.
3. Chang YS, Jeong JM, Lee YS, *et al.* (2005) Preparation of F-18-human serum albumin: A simple and efficient protein labeling method with F-18 using a hydrazone-formation method. *Bioconjugate Chem* **16**: 1329–1333.
4. Packard AB, Kronauge JF, Brechbiel MW. (1999) Metalloradiopharmaceuticals. In: Clarke MJ, Sadler PJ (eds), *A Metalloradiopharmaceuticals II, Diagnosis and Therapy*. pp. 45–116. Springer-Verlag, New York.
5. Meares CF, Wensel TG. (1984) Metal-chelates as probes of biological-systems. *Accounts Chem Res* **17**: 202–209.
6. Brechbiel MW, Gansow OA, Atcher RW, *et al.* (1986) Synthesis of 1-(para-isothiocyanatobenzyl) derivatives of dtpa and edta — antibody labeling and tumor-imaging studies. *Inorganic Chemistry* **25**: 2772–2781.
7. Reivich M, Kuhl D, Wolf A, *et al.* (1979) The [^{18}F]fluorodeoxyglucose method for the measurement of local cerebral glucose utilization in man. *Circ Res*; **44**: 127–137.
8. Waterhouse RN. (2003) Determination of lipophilicity and its use as a predictor of blood-brain barrier penetration of molecular imaging agents. *Mol Imaging Biol* **5**: 376–389.
9. Garnett ES, Firnau G, Nahmias C. (1983) Dopamine visualized in the basal ganglia of living man. *Nature* **305**: 137–138.
10. Iyo M, Namba H, Fukushi K, *et al.* (1997) Measurement of acetylcholinesterase by positron emission tomography in the brains of healthy controls and patients with Alzheimer's disease. *Lancet* **349**: 1805–1809.
11. Sato K, Fukushi K, Shinotoh H, *et al.* (2004) Evaluation of simplified kinetic analyses for measurement of brain acetylcholinesterase. Activity using N-[C-11]methyl-piperidin-4-yl propionate and positron emission tomography. *J Cerebr Blood F Met* **24**: 600–611.
12. Mathis CA, Wang Y, Holt DP, Huang GF, Debnath ML, Klunk WE. (2003) Synthesis and evaluation of ^{11}C-labeled 6-substituted 2-arylbenzothiazoles as amyloid imaging agents. *J Med Chem* **46**: 2740–2754.
13. Budinger TF, Yano Y, Hoop B. (1975) A comparison of ^{82}Rb$^+$ and ^{13}NH$_3$ for myocardial positron scintigraphy. *J Nucl Med* **16**: 429–431.

14. Walsh WF, Fill HR, Harper PV. (1977) Nitrogen-13-labeled ammonia for myocardial imaging. *Semin Nucl Med* **7**: 59–66.
15. Been LB, Suurmeijer AJ, Cobben DC, Jager PL, Hoekstra HJ, Elsinga PH (2004). [18F]FLT-PET in oncology: Current status and opportunities. *Eur J Nucl Med Mol Imaging* **31**: 1659–1672.
16. Jeong JM, Hong MK, Chang YS, *et al.* (2008) Preparation of a promising angiogenesis PET imaging agent: 68Ga-labeled c(RGDyK)-isothiocyanatobenzyl-1,4,7-triazacyclononane-1,4,7-triacetic acid and feasibility studies in mice. *J Nucl Med* **49**: 830–836.
17. Haubner R, Wester HJ, Weber WA, *et al.* (2001) Noninvasive imaging of alpha(v)beta3 integrin expression using 18F-labeled RGD-containing glycopeptide and positron emission tomography. *Cancer Res* **61**: 1781–1785.
18. Jerabek PA, Patrick TB, Kilbourn MR, Dischino DD, Welch MJ. (1986) Synthesis and biodistribution of 18F-labeled fluoronitroimidazoles: Potential *in vivo* markers of hypoxic tissue. *Int J Rad Appl Instrum A* **37**: 599–605.
19. Piert M, Machulla HJ, Picchio M, *et al.* (2005) Hypoxia-specific tumor imaging with 18F-fluoroazomycin arabinoside. *J Nucl Med* **46**: 106–113.
20. Lewis JS, McCarthy DW, McCarthy TJ, Fujibayashi Y, Welch MJ. (1999) Evaluation of 64Cu-ATSM *in vitro* and *in vivo* in a hypoxic tumor model. *J Nucl Med* **40**: 177–183.
21. Brodack JW, Kilbourn MR, Welch MJ, Katzenellenbogen JA. (1986) NCA 16 alpha-[18F]fluoroestradiol-17 beta: The effect of reaction vessel on fluorine-18 resolubilization, product yield, and effective specific activity. *Int J Rad Appl Instrum A* **37**: 217–221.
22. Henze M, Schuhmacher J, Hipp P, *et al.* (2001) PET imaging of somatostatin receptors using [68GA]DOTA-D-Phe1-Tyr3-octreotide: First results in patients with meningiomas. *J Nucl Med* **42**: 1053–1056.
23. Li S, Beheshti M. (2005) The radionuclide molecular imaging and therapy of neuroendocrine tumors. *Curr Cancer Drug Targets* **5**: 139–148.
24. Holmes RA, Chaplin SB, Royston KG, *et al.* (1985) Cerebral uptake and retention of 99Tcm-hexamethylpropyleneamine oxime (99Tcm-HM-PAO). *Nucl Med Commun* **6**: 443–447.
25. Sands H, Delano ML, Gallagher BM. (1986) Uptake of hexakis(t-butylisonitrile) technetium (I) and hexakis(isopropylisonitrile) technetium (I) by neonatal rat myocytes and human erythrocytes. *J Nucl Med* **27**: 404–448.
26. Nielsen SP, Moller ML, Trap-Jensen J. (1977) 99mTc-DTPA scintillation-camera renography: A new method for estimation of single-kidney function. *J Nucl Med* **18**: 112–117.
27. Bodei L, Handkiewicz-Junak D, Grana C, *et al.* (2004) Receptor radionuclide therapy with Y-90-DOTATOC in patients with medullary thyroid carcinomas. *Cancer Biother Radio* **19**: 65–71.
28. Lin WY, Lin CP, Yeh SJ, *et al.* (1997) Rhenium-188 hydroxyethylidene diphosphonate: A new generator-produced radiotherapeutic drug of potential value for the treatment of bone metastases. *Eur J Nucl Med* **24**: 590–595.
29. Lee YS, Jeong JM, Kim YJ, *et al.* (2002) Synthesis of 188Re-labelled long chain alkyl diaminedithiol for therapy of liver cancer. *Nucl Med Commun* **23**: 237–242.
30. Hafeli UO, Casillas S, Dietz DW, *et al.* (1999) Hepatic tumor radioembolization in a rat model using radioactive rhenium (186Re/188Re) glass microspheres. *Int J Radiat Oncol Biol Phys* **44**: 189–199.

31. Lee J, Lee DS, Kim KM, *et al.* (2000) Dosimetry of rhenium-188 diethylene triamine penta-acetic acid for endovascular intra-balloon brachytherapy after coronary angioplasty. *European Journal of Nuclear Medicine* **27**: 76–82.

32. Jeong JM, Lee YJ, Kim YJ, *et al.* (2000) Preparation of rhenium-188-tin colloid as a radiation synovectomy agent and comparison with rhenium-188-sulfur colloid. *Appl Radiat Isotopes* **52**: 851–855.

33. Wang SJ, Lin WY, Hsieh BT, *et al.* (1995) Re-188 Sulfur colloid as a radiation synovectomy agent. *European Journal of Nuclear Medicine* **22**: 505–507.

34. Cyr JE, Pearson DA, Wilson DM, *et al.* (2007) Somatostatin receptor-binding peptides suitable for tumor radiotherapy with Re-188 or Re-186. Chemistry and initial biological studies. *Journal of Medicinal Chemistry* **50**: 1354–1364.

35. Vallabhajosula S. (2009) *Molecular Imaging: Radiopharmaceuticals for PET and SPECT*. Springer, New York.

PART II
Clinical Applications

Chapter 3

Unexpected Nuclear Scan Findings Due to Radiopharmaceutical, Technical, or Patient-Related Factors

Usha A. Joseph, David Q. Wan, Asad Nasir,
David Brandon, Isis W. Gayed and Bruce J. Barron

3.1. Introduction

Diagnostic functional or molecular imaging requires a gamma- or positron-emitting radionuclide (RN) formulated with organ-specific biologic or chemical agent based on the specific organ function to form a radiopharmaceutical (RP), which is then administered orally or most commonly intravenously to the patient. Rarely, the RN is administered as such, for example, technetium pertechnetate intravenously or iodine orally. Functional imaging involves many complicated steps, from manufacture of the radiopharmaceutical or formulation at the local nuclear pharmacy to the final end user, the patient. Appropriate quality control analysis is performed at several points from production to final use in the patient. Problems or breakdowns in these steps result in suboptimal or unexpected nuclear scan findings, which are perplexing, surprising, challenging, and many times require a repeat scan. The RN or RP after manufacture is securely transported to the local radio pharmacy and then reaches the Nuclear Medicine department in unit or bulk dose for individual patient use. Organ function imaging requires a specific RP, formulated under sterile, pyrogen-free conditions using a specific RN, and a chemical/biologic molecule specific to the organ function, along with stabilizer and buffer; the resulting

RP is dispensed like a drug by an authorized physician user for patient administration.

Intradepartmental quality control measures are performed periodically on a daily, weekly, monthly, and annual basis for the optimal operation of the gamma or positron emission tomography (PET) camera, thyroid probe and dose calibrator, to ensure everything is in peak working condition. These quality checks include regular field uniformity, intrinsic and extrinsic flood to evaluate the integrity of the photomultiplier tubes, and application of corrective measures if needed to produce uniformity of flood; quality check for the intrinsic and extrinsic spatial resolution and linearity using bar phantoms. Dose calibrators have to be accurate to ensure accuracy of each administered dose. Prior to each scan, the window and energy settings on the gamma camera are adjusted by the technologist for optimum imaging at the peak energy and correct window setting for the particular RN. Each dose is assayed before administration to ensure it is the right dose amount for administration to the right patient, right RP for the ordered test. Pregnancy is excluded prior to RP administration in women of child-bearing age by documenting the date of last menstrual cycle and, if indicated, urine test or serum beta human chorionic gonadotropin pregnancy test is performed.

The present day gamma and PET cameras are complex electronic devices, with multihead or ringed detectors, designed to move up and down, along the horizontal plane and 360 degrees around the patient. The delicate, complex electronic machinery can break down or malfunction from daily repeated use and multiple users due to their complex electronic circuitry. In addition to the general radiation safety precautions observed in all radiology departments, the Nuclear Medicine department follows additional unique stringent quality control and radiation safety guidelines for patients, visitors, and laboratory personnel to ensure the safe and efficient running of the department. Nuclear Medicine departments have to comply with the strict federal and state requirements for handling RN, RP, and body fluids and maintain up-to-date inventory logs for the different RN and RP received and administered. The radiation waste generated is monitored till it is radiation safety wise safe for disposal.

The factors resulting in unexpected or non-diagnostic scan findings are many and the most common and somewhat preventable ones involve human error, for example, administering the wrong RN or RP to a patient, wrong dose, dose infiltration at the injection site, rare inadvertent intraarterial injection, or the scan is performed off peak or at the wrong window setting, inadvertent RP administration to a patient who recently underwent another scan or therapy using a RN with a longer half-life (due to inadequate patient history), and increased background activity.

The complicated process of RP formulation, transportation, radioassay to the final administration to the patient involve many steps and different personnel, with potential for unanticipated and unidentified missteps along the way. However, this becomes apparent only after the patient receives the RP or on viewing the final images, which is too late to correct in a particular patient. This outcome causes the Nuclear Medicine physicians or radiologist to go into an overdrive and start investigating what, when, where, and how the problem occurred and finding a possible solution. This search for answers leads to loss of time and energy, increased anxiety and stress for the patients, their families, and the Nuclear medicine department personnel, and unnecessary radiation exposure to the patient and can delay diagnosis or therapy in the patient. The system works smoothly most of the time, but the few unanticipated and unexpected scan findings are time consuming, stressful for all, and frequently require a repeat scan due to a non-diagnostic or suboptimal study.

This chapter includes a wide variety of nuclear images of unexpected or unusual scan findings compiled over a 10-year period from the Nuclear Medicine department of a large tertiary care hospital, another university-affiliated teaching hospital, a medical school–affiliated county hospital, and several PET imaging centers representing a good mix of inpatients and out-patients comprising adults and children. Some of the cases were previously reported as case reports by one of the authors, with many additional cases added to this list of cases.[1] The scan findings have been categorized under several broad categories of RP production and formulation problems, human error and patient-related factors. Even routine scans in nuclear medicine can have unexpected outcomes, for example, poor activity observed on thyroid scan in a patient with inadequate withdrawal of thyroid hormone replacement therapy, anti-thyroid drugs, or a recent X-ray contrast study. A well-informed patient with a good medical history, a scan request with pertinent medical history from the referring physician, and a vigilant technologist are crucial to ordering and performing the appropriate tests. Unlike anatomic imaging, awareness of the half-lives of different isotopes plays a key role in effective and optimal scheduling of different scans in the same patient, for example, a bone scan done after recent gallium scan or recent ^{131}I therapy will result in suboptimal or non-diagnostic images due to interfering background activity from residual gallium or ^{131}I therapy. Nuclear physicians are more directly involved with patient-scheduling issues than physicians in the other imaging modalities due to the different radiopharmaceuticals, numerous patient factors, some unique to a particular patient, and the functional nature of nuclear imaging. Although these unexpected errors cannot be entirely eliminated, knowledge and awareness can reduce their occurrence; hence this chapter provides an extensive list of varied unexpected nuclear scans we have encountered in our nuclear practice in more than a decade.

A useful algorithm in evaluating unusual or unexplained scan findings involves asking the following questions: Did the patient have another recent study with residual activity causing confusion? Did any other patient that day have a similar finding, either at site or other sites using the same radiopharmacy? Was the camera QC good? Is the patient on any medication or has any unusual medical condition that can interfere with the nuclear study? This evaluation can help narrow the search to identify whether it is RP, technical, or patient-related problem.

3.2. Unexpected Nuclear Scan Findings From Radiopharmaceutical, Technical, or Patient Related Factors

3.2.1. *Discussion*

The multiple and varied scan examples illustrated in this chapter show us that unexpected nuclear scan findings, although infrequent, can and do occur since many variables, multiple steps, and numerous factors are involved from the manufacture of the radiopharmaceutical, to patient administration to the final end product, the nuclear scan. Fortunately, in the diagnostic setting these findings are generally not life threatening but more of an inconvenience, resulting in delay, additional cost in time and resources from repeat scanning, and unnecessary radiation exposure to the patient.

A mix up in injecting labeled cells from one patient to another can have serious repercussions and increased morbidity and worrisome lifelong consequences in the setting of communicable diseases like human immunodeficiency virus and Hepatitis B and C, which fortunately is extremely rare due to the many safety controls in place, stricter patient identification and labeling methods, and increased vigilance by the technologists and other personnel in the nuclear medicine department. The patient factors resulting from medication or disease states are beyond our control in most cases; a good patient history can avoid or minimize some of these problems. Although manufacturer error very rarely occurs due to strict quality control assays at RP production, it can occur as shown with the sticky [^{18}F] FDG-PET scan (case 1); technical errors resulting from sloppy handling of different RP are infrequent but can occur as shown with the case of cross-contamination of different RP vials.

Many problems can be reduced significantly with technologist training and awareness, well-maintained equipment, adequate and readily available patient history, an informed patient, and strict adherence to the standard protocols already in place in a properly operating nuclear medicine department. Many illustrative cases are useful as a ready reference guide when unexpected scan findings are encountered, and knowledge and awareness can result in the prompt institution of corrective and remedial solutions and sometimes additional safeguards may need to be instituted to improve patient care and avoid future such mistakes. Nuclear medicine is unique in that many factors are involved in the making of a scan, both intrinsic and extrinsic to the patient, hence missteps are possible. Generally there is more interaction between the nuclear medicine physician and the technologist regarding nuclear studies; sometimes the referring physician will need to be contacted to further clarify a particular patient issue. Sometimes we will need to customize a particular nuclear study to suit a patient's specific medical problem. There is also more interaction between the patient and the nuclear physician, especially for studies like thyroid scans. In ^{131}I therapy for hyperthyroidism, many details have to be sorted out, starting with a therapy request from the patient's physician, an informed consent from the patient, a negative serum pregnancy test in women of child-bearing age, pertinent medication withdrawal, thyroid function tests, and the patient's ability to follow and comply with the post-treatment radiation safety precautions.

[131]I therapy in thyroid cancer patients after thyroidectomy or samarium, strontium, or yttrium theraspheres treatment for metastases have their own checklist of guidelines to be satisfied before appropriate treatment can be safely given to the patient. Reduced dose requirements in children, pregnant women, and right-to-left shunt require extra vigilance by the technologist and physician. If all the different steps involved in a nuclear scan work smoothly, the resulting image is an optimal diagnostic quality nuclear scan.

Unknown patient factors, radiopharmaceutical or technical errors, and equipment malfunction can result in unexpected scan finding or suboptimal or non-diagnostic scan that, though infrequent, requires thorough investigation to determine the reasonable cause and sometimes may require institution of additional safeguards and precautions to prevent future such occurrence. In nuclear medicine, the key is in the details; a good diagnostic scan is the end product of dedicated nuclear laboratory personnel paying careful attention to the nuclear study including patient details, correctly administered RP, proper maintenance and operation of imaging equipment and dose calibrator, adequate patient history from the referring physician, and an informed patient.

References

1. Joseph U, Barron BJ, Wan D, Rasberry D. (2007) Mysterious radiopharmaceutical localization: A pictorial interactive exhibit. Electronic exhibit at the American Roentgen Ray Society, Orlando, FL.
2. Malone LA, Malone JF, Ennis JT. (1983) Kinetics of technetium 99m labeled macroaggregated albumin in humans. *Br J Radiol* **56**(662): 109–112.
3. Sandler MP, Coleman RE, Patton JA, Wackers FJTH, Gottschalk A. eds. (2003) *A Diagnostic Nuclear Medicine*. 4th ed. p. 107, Lippincott, Williams and Wilkins, Philadelphia.
4. Hung JC, Redfern MG, Mahoney DW, Thorson LM, Wiseman GA. (2000) Evaluation of macroaggregated albumin particle sizes for use in pulmonary shunt patient studies. *J Am Pharm Assoc (Wash)* **40**(1): 46–51.
5. Ikehira H, Kinjo M, Yamamoto Y, Makino H *et al.* (1999) Hot spots observed on pulmonary perfusion imaging: A case report. *J Nucl Med Technol* **27**: 301–302.
6. Ergün EL, Kiratli PO, Günay EC, Erbaş B. (2006) A report on the incidence of intestinal 99mTc-methylene diphosphonate uptake of bone scans and a review of the literature. *Nucl Med Commun* **27**(11): 877–885.
7. Butler EB, Scardino PT, The BS, Uhl BM *et al.* (1997) The Baylor College of Medicine Experience with gold seed implantation. *Semin Surg Oncol* **13**(6): 406–418.

8. Loutfi I, Collier BD, Mohammed AM. (2003) Nonosseous abnormalities on bone scans. *J Nucl Med Technol* **31**(3): 149–153; quiz 154–156. Review.

9. Afzelius P, Henriksen JH. (2008) Extra cardiac activity detected on myocardial perfusion scintigraphy after intra-arterial injection of 99mTc-MIBI. *Clin Physiol Funct Imaging* **28**(5): 285–286.

10. Pickhardt PJ, McDermott M. (1997) Intense uptake of technetium-99m-MDP in primary breast adenocarcinoma with sarcomatoid metaplasia. *J Nucl Med* **38**(4): 528–530.

11. Burnett KR, Lyons KP. Theron-Brown W. (1984) Uptake of osteotropic radionuclides in the breast. *Semin Nucl Med* **14**: 48–49.

12. Worsley DF, Lentie BC. (1993) Uptake of technetium-99m-MDP in primary amyloidosis with a review of the mechanisms of soft-tissue localization of bone-seeking radiopharmaceuticals. *Nucl Med* **34**: 1612–1615.

13. Janssen S, van Rijswijk MH, Piers DA, de Jong GM. (1984) Soft-tissue uptake of 99mTc-diphosphonate in systemic AL amyloidosis. *Eur J Nucl Med* **9**(12): 538–541.

14. Lee VW, Caldarone AG, Falk RH, Rubinow A, Cohen AS. (1983) Amyloidosis of heart and liver: Comparison of Tc-99m pyrophosphate and Tc-99m methylene diphosphonate for detection. *Radiology* **148**(1): 239–242.

15. Sampson CB. (1996) Complications and difficulties in radiolabel ling blood cells: A review. *Nucl Med Commun* **17**(8): 648–658 [review].

16. Salimi Z, Thomasson J, Vas W, Salimi A. (1985) Detection of right-to-left shunt with radionuclide angiocardiography in refractory hypoxemia. *Chest* **88**(5): 784–786.

17. Lu G, Shih WJ, Chou C, Xu JY. (1996) Tc-99m MAA total-body imaging to detect intrapulmonary right-to-left shunts and to evaluate the therapeutic effect in pulmonary arteriovenous shunts. *Clin Nucl Med* **21**(3): 197–202.

18. Lindholm P, Minn H, Leskinen-Kallio S, Bergman J, Ruotsalainen U, Joensuu H. (1993) Influence of the blood glucose concentration on FDG uptake in cancer — a PET study. *J Nucl Med* (1): 1–6.

19. Minn H, Nuutila P, Lindholm P, Ruotsalainen U, Bergman J, Teräs M, Knuuti MJ. (1994) *In vivo* effects of insulin on tumor and skeletal muscle glucose metabolism in patients with lymphoma. *Cancer* **73**(5): 1490–1498.

20. Chilab S, Macias E, Garvie NW. (2004) A patient with back pain and unusual appearances on bone scintigraphy. *Br J Radiol* **77**(921): 801–802.

21. Armijo S, Peña M, Bustos F, Morales B. (2009) The "bat sign" of pectoral rhabdomyolysis. *Clin Nucl Med* (9): 636–637.

22. Lim ST, Sohn MH, Jeong HJ. (2008) Cold exposure-induced rhabdomyolysis demonstrated by bone scintigraphy. *Clin Nucl Med* **33**(5): 349–350.

23. Watanabe N, Inaoka T, Shuke N, Takahashi K, Aburano T, Chisato N, Nochi H, Go K. (2007) Acute rhabdomyolysis of the soleus muscle induced by a lightning strike: Magnetic resonance and scintigraphic findings. *Skeletal Radiol* **36**(7): 671–675.

24. Selimoglu O, Basaran M, Ugurlucan M, Ogus TN. (2009) Rhabdomyolysis following accidental intra-arterial injection of local anesthetic. *Angiology* **60**(1): 120–121.

25. Lin FI, Foster CC, Hagge RJ, Shelton DK. (2009) Extensive FDG uptake in accessory muscles of respiration in a patient with shortness of breath. *Clin Nucl Med* **34**(7): 428–430.

26. Caglar M, Naldöken S. (1993) Increased bone marrow uptake on Tc-99m DMSA scintigraphy in a patient with renal osteodystrophy. *Ann Nucl Med* **7**(4): 281–283.

27. Cerci SS, Suslu H, Cerci C, Yildiz M, Ozbek FM, Balci TA, Yesildag A, Canatan D. (2007) Different findings in Tc-99m MDP bone scintigraphy of patients with sickle cell disease: Report of three cases. *Ann Nucl Med* **21**(5): 311–314.

28. Berk F, Demir H, Hacihanefioglu A, Arslan A, Erdincler O, Isgoren S, Aktolun C. (2002) Hepatic and splenic uptake of Tc-99m HDP in multiple myeloma: Additional findings on Tc-99m MIBI and Tc-99m sulfur colloid images. *Ann Nucl Med* **16**(2): 137–141.

29. Yapar AF, Aydin M, Reyhan M. (2004) Diffuse splenic Tc-99m MDP uptake in hypersplenic patient. *Ann Nucl Med* **18**(8): 703–705.

30. Kawamura E, Kawabe J, Hayashi T, Oe A, Kotani J, Torii K, Habu D, Shiomi S. Splenic accumulation of Tc-99m HMDP in a patient with severe alcoholic cirrhosis of the liver. *Clin Nucl Med* **30**(5): 351–352.

31. Peller PJ, Ho VB, Kransdorf MJ. (1993) Extraosseous Tc-99m MDP uptake: A pathophysiologic approach. *Radiographics* **13**(4): 715–734.

32. Gezici A, van Duijnhoven EM, Bakker SJ, Heidendal GA, van Kroonenburgh MJ. (1996) Lung and gastric uptake in bone scintigraphy of sarcoidosis. *J Nucl Med* **37**(9): 1530–1532.

33. Spicer JA, Slaton CK, Raveill TG, Baxter KG, Preston DF, Hladik WB. (1999) Unexpected stomach uptake of technetium-99m-MDP. *J Nucl Med Technol* **27**(1): 43–44.

34. Meyer MA, McClaughry P. (1995) Reversible Tc-99m diphosphonate uptake in gastric tissue associated with malignancy related hypercalcemia. A comparative study using PET FDG whole body imaging. *Clin Nucl Med* **20**(9): 767–769.

35. Wynchank S, Brendel AJ, Leccia F, Lacoste D, Maire JP, Ducassou D. (1983) Transient intense gastric fixation of 99mTc-MDP. *Eur J Nucl Med* **8**(10): 458–460.

36. Corstens F, Kerremans A, Claessens R. (1986) Resolution of massive technetium-99m methylene diphosphonate uptake in the stomach in vitamin D intoxication. *Nucl Med* **27**(2): 219–222.

37. Capelle J, Leclere J, Kraiem A. (1984) Metastatic calcifications in Burkitt's lymphoma. *J Radiol* **65**(8–9): 593–596.

38. Franco A, Hampton WR, Greenspan BS, Holm AL, O'Mara RE. (1993) Gastric uptake of Tc-99m MDP in a child treated with isotretinoin. *Clin Nucl Med* **18**(6): 510–511.

39. Kanoh T, Uchino H, Yamamoto I, Torizuka K. (1986) Soft-tissue uptake of technetium-99m MDP in multiple myeloma. *Clin Nucl Med* **11**(12): 878–879.

40. Soni S, Leslie WD. (2008) Bone scan findings in metastatic calcification from calciphylaxis. *Clin Nucl Med* **33**(7): 502–524.

41. Indar AA, Beckingham IJ. (2002) Acute cholecystitis. Clinical review. *Bri Med J* **325**(9): 639–643.

42. Fenig E, Mishaeli M, Kalish Y, Lishner M. (2001) Pregnancy and radiation. *Can Treat Rev* **27**(1): 1–7.

43. O'Riordan TG, Smaldone GC. (1994) Regional deposition and regional ventilation during inhalation of pentamidine. *Chest* **105**(2): 396–401.

44. Cabahug CJ, McPeck M, Palmer LB, Cuccia A *et al.* (1996) Utility of Technetium-99m-DTPA in determining regional ventilation. *J Nucl Med* **37**: 239–244.

45. Schwartz M, Swayne LC, Macaulay RD, Schwartz JR. (1996) Lung scan detection of SVC clot with collateral flow to liver. *J Nucl Med* **37**(11): 1826–1827.

46. Makie GC, Thomas A, Greenspan B, Singh A. (2007) Focal hepatic activity during ventilation — perfusion scintigraphy due to systemic-portal shunt due to superior vena cava obstruction from histoplasmosis-induced fibrosing mediastinitis. *Clin Nucl Med* **32**(9): 707–710.

47. van Dongen AJ, van Rijk PP. (2000) Minimizing liver, bowel and gastric activity in myocardial perfusion SPECT. *J Nucl Med* **41**: 1315–1317.

48. Iqbal SM, Khalil ME, Lone BA, Gorski R, Blim S *et al.* (2004) Simple techniques to reduce bowel activity in cardiac SPECT imaging. *Nucl Med Commun* **25**(4): 355–359.

49. Shehab D, Elgazzar AH, Collier D. (2002) Heterotopic ossification. *J Nucl Med* **43**: 346–353.

50. Chalmers J, Gray DH, Rush J. (1975) Observations on the induction of bone in soft tissues. *J Bone Joint Surg Br* **57**: 36–45.

51. Urist MR, Nakagawa M, Nakata N, Nogami H. (1978) Experimental myositis ossificans: Cartilage and bone formation in muscles in response to diffusible bone matrix derived morphogen. *Arch Path Lab Med* **102**: 312–316.

52. Ho SSW, Stern PJ, Bruno LP *et al.* (1988) Pharmacological inhibition of Prostaglandin E 2 in bone and its effect on pathological new bone formation in a rat brain model. *Trans Orthop Res Soc* **13**: 536.

53. Resnick D, Niwayama G. (1988) Soft tissues. In: Resnick D, Niwayama G, eds. *Diagnosis of Bone and Joint Disorders*, 2nd ed. pp. 4171–4294, WB Saunders, Philadelphia, PA.

54. Jensen LL, Halar E, Little J, Brooke MM. (1987) Neurogenic heterotopic ossification. *Am J Phys Med Rehabil* **66**: 351–363.

55. Muhein G, Donath A, Rossier AB. (1973) Serial scintigrams in the course of ectopic bone formation in paraplegic patients. *AJR* **118**: 865–869.

56. Tanaka T, Rossier AB, Hussey RW, Ahnberg DS *et al.* (1977) Quantitative assessment of para-osteo- arthropathy and its maturation on serial radionuclide bone images. *Radiology* **123**: 217–221.

57. Orzel JA, Rudd TG. (1985) Heterotopic bone formation: Clinical, laboratory and imaging correlation. *J Nucl Med* **26**: 125–132.

58. Smith R, Russell RG, Woods CG. (1976) Myositis ossificans progressiva: Clinical features of eight patients and their response to treatment. *J Bone Joint Surg Br* **58**: 48–57.

59. Sastri VR, Yadav SS. (1977) Myositis ossificans progressiva. *Int Surg* **62**: 45–47.

60. Connor JM, Evan DA. (1982) Fibrodysplasia ossificans progressiva: The clinical features and natural history of 34 patients. *J Bone Joint Surg Br* **64**: 76–83.

61. Cremin B, Connor JM, Beighton P. (1982) The radiological spectrum of fibrodysplasia ossificans progressiva. *Clin Radiol* **33**: 499–508.

62. Wei BPC, Somers GR, Castles L. (2003) Dystrophic calcification and amyloidosis in old subcutaneous injection sites. *ANZ J Surg* **73**: 556–558.

63. Walsh JS, Fairley JA. (1995) Calcifying disorders of the skin. *J Am Acad Dermatol* **33**: 693–706.

64. Ullman HR, Dasgupta A, Recht M, Cash JM. (1995) CT of dystrophic calcification in subcutaneous soft tissues secondary to chronic insulin injection. *J Comp Assist Tom* **19**: 657–659.
65. Figueiredo GC, Figueiredo EC. (2000) Dystrophic calcinosis in a child with a thumb sucking habit: Case report. *Rev Hosp Clin Fac Med (Sao Paulo)* **55**(5): 177–180.
66. Jeon SW, Park YK, Chang SG. (2009) Dystrophic calcification and stone formation on the entire bladder neck after potassium-titanyl phosphate laser vaporization for the prostate: A case report. *J Korean Med Sci* **24**(4): 741–743.
67. Lipskeir E, Weizenbluth M. (1989) Calcinosis circumscripta: Indications for surgery. *Bull Hosp Jt Dis Orthop Inst* **49**: 75–84.
68. Tristano AG, Villarroel JL, Rodriguez MA, Millan A. (2006) Calcinosis cutis universalis in a patient with systemic lupus erythematosus. *Clin Rheumatol* **25**: 70–74.
69. Cohade C, Osman M, Pannu HK, Wahl RL. (2003) Uptake in supraclavicular area fat ("USA-Fat"): Description on 18F-FDG PET/CT. *J Nucl Med* **44**(2): 170–176.
70. Williams G, Kolodny GM. (2008) Method for decreasing uptake of 18F-FDG by hypermetabolic brown adipose tissue on PET. *AJR Am J Roentgenol* **190**(5): 1406–1409.
71. Agrawal A, Nair N, Baghel NS. (2009) A novel approach for reduction of brown fat uptake on FDG PET. *Br J Radiol* **82**(980): 626–631.
72. Paidisetty S, Blodgett TM. (2009) Brown fat: Atypical locations and appearances encountered in PET/CT. *AJR Am J Roentgenol* **193**(2): 359–366.
73. Vogel WV, van Dalen JA, Wiering B, Huisman H, Corstens FH, Ruers TJ, Oyen WJ. (2007) Evaluation of image registration in PET/CT of the liver and recommendations for optimized imaging. *J Nucl Med* **48**(6): 910–919.
74. Goerres GW, Burger C, Kamel E, Seifert B, Kaim AH, Buck A, Buehler TC, Von Schulthess GK. (2003) Respiration-induced attenuation artifact at PET/CT: Technical considerations. *Radiology* **226**(3): 906–910.
75. Mansi L, Rambaldi PF, Procaccini E, Gregorio FD, Laprovitera A, Pecori B, Vecchio WD. (1996) Scintimammography with technetium-99m tetrofosmin in the diagnosis of breast cancer and lymph node metastases. *Eur J Nucl Med* **23**(8): 932–939.
76. Kobayashi H, Sakahara H, Hosono M, Shirato M, Endo K, Kotoura Y, Yamamuro T, Konishi J. (1994) Soft-tissue tumors: Diagnosis with Tc-99m (V) dimercaptosuccinic acid scintigraphy. *Radiology* **190**(1): 277–280.
77. Kandula P, Shirazi P. (1995) Localization of Tc-99m sestamibi and TI-201 in an unsuspected calcified intrathoracic mass. *Clin Nucl Med* **20**(11): 1000–1002.
78. Maurer AH, Caroline DF, Jadali FJ, Manzone TA, Maier WP, Au FC, Schnall SF. (1993) Limitations of craniocaudal thallium-201 and technetium-99m-sestamibi mammoscintigraphy. *J Nucl Med* **36**(9): 1696–1700.
79. Low RD, Hicks RJ, Arkles LB, Gill G, Adam W. (1992) Progressive soft tissue uptake of Tc-99m MDP reflecting metastatic microcalcification. *Clin Nucl Med* **17**(8): 658–662.
80. Kim DW, Jeong HJ, Park SA, Kim CG. (2007) Gastric accumulation of bone seeking agent in a patient with advanced gastric cancer. *J Korean Med Sci* **22**(1): 153–155.

RADIOPHARMACEUTICAL PRODUCTION/ FORMULATION PROBLEMS:

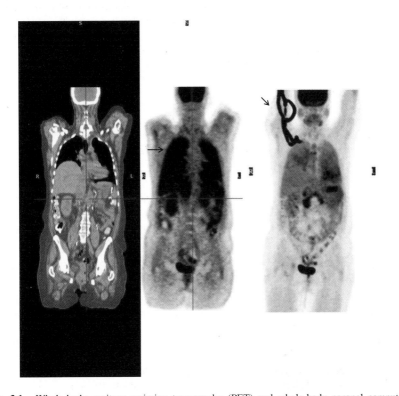

Fig. 3.1. Whole-body positron emission tomography (PET) and whole-body coronal computed tomography (CT) images showing diffuse intense bilateral lung activity and intense tracer uptake in intravenous tubing, resulting from injection of incompletely processed F-18 FDG (Fluoride-18 Fluorodeoxyglucose) into intravenous line (due to poor venous access) CT showed no abnormality in bilateral lungs to account for the unusual PET appearance. This rare PET finding resulted from incomplete production process of F-18 FDG; the resulting product, a "sticky" compound, became apparent only after it was intravenously administered. The intense activity seen in the IV line from injection of FDG into the intravenous line peripheral port is a reason for injecting radioisotopes directly injected into the patient's vein. On further investigation, it was discovered that other PET scans on the same date from the same manufacturer and same lot showed similar lung uptake on PET scan and was an artifact related to the RP resulting in a non-diagnostic PET scan.

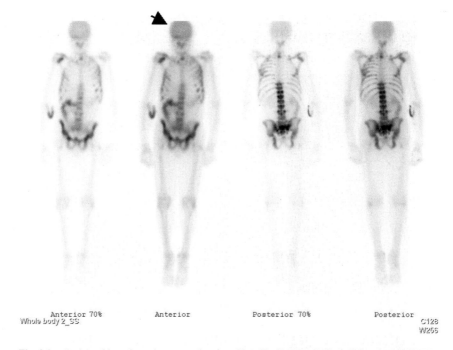

Anterior 70%   Anterior   Posterior 70%   Posterior

C128
W255

Fig. 3.2. Brain and bowel uptake on a technetium 99m (Tc 99m) methylene diphosphonate (MDP) whole-body bone scan may result from a previous study or in this case from technician error using the same syringe to constitute the Tc MDP bone and Tc 99m ethyl cysteinate dimer (ECD) vial resulting in cross-contamination of the two vials. Diffuse decreased tracer activity seen in upper two-thirds of thoracic spine is related to post-radiation changes.

→

Fig. 3.3. (a) and (b) Cross-contamination of Tc 99m sulfur colloid (Tc SC) and Tc MDP in the same vial due to technician error; several bone scans on the same day showed similar finding of diffuse intense liver spleen activity on the anterior and posterior total body bone scan, giving the appearance of "liver and spleen scan on bone scan." Expected physiologic increased tracer uptake is seen in the epiphyseal growth plates in the long bones of the extremities in this child. (c) Free (Tc 99m) effect on bone scan due to poor labeling shows stomach, bowel, and thyroid activity on total body bone scan.

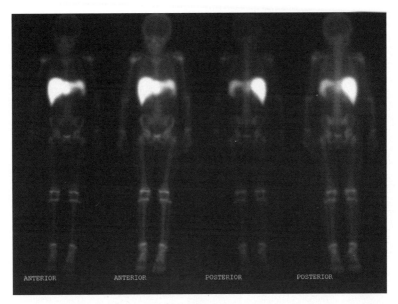

(a)

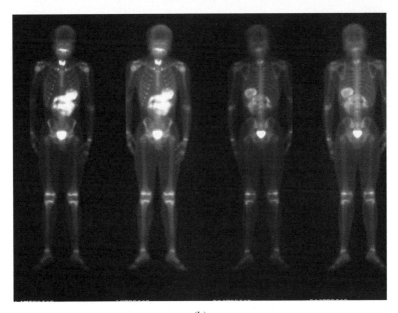

(b)

Fig. 3.3. (*Continued*)

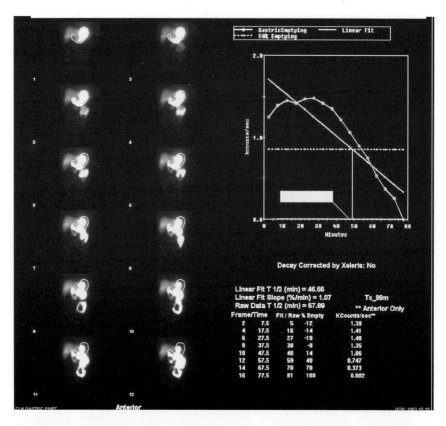

Fig. 3.4. Liver activity is seen on gastric emptying study. The patient had a prior Tc 99m iminodiacetic hepatobiliary scan (HIDA), which can result in inaccuracy in the calculated gastric emptying half time due to the superimposed liver activity. Background subtraction of the average liver activity obtained using an abdominal spot image prior to the gastric emptying scan can provide a more accurate gastric emptying $T_{1/2}$. The easier and better approach in a patient with a prior HIDA scan, if previously known, is after discussing with the referring doctor to postpone the non-emergent gastric emptying study by 24 h or better still 48 h for more optimal imaging.

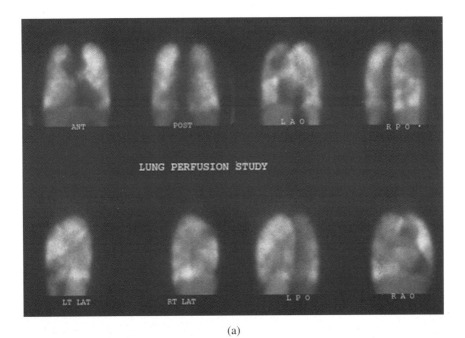

(a)

Fig. 3.5. (a) Perfusion lung scan obtained using Tc 99m macro-aggregated albumin (MAA) showed expected diffuse tracer localization in the lungs. Unexpected radiotracer activity in the liver and spleen is likely due to tag/label breakdown of the MAA into smaller particles and subsequent phagocytosis of the smaller particles by the reticuloendothelial cells. This resulted from using MAA that was more than 8 h after preparation of the MAA.[2] This scan emphasizes the importance of using radiopharmaceuticals within the recommended time after reconstitution so as to prevent radiopharmaceutical breakdown and suboptimal/unexpected scan findings.

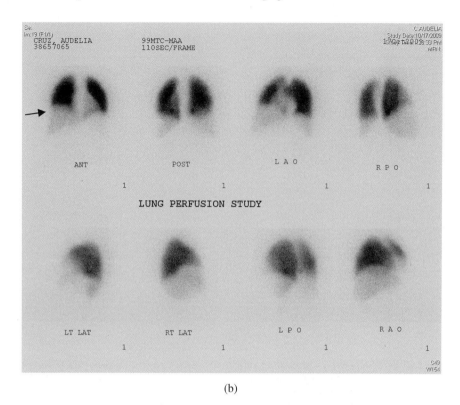

(b)

Fig. 3.5. (*Continued*) (b) Faint diffuse liver-spleen activities on MAA perfusion lung scan is likely from increased numbers of small-sized MAA particles; other lung scans performed on different patients that day using the same MAA vial showed similar findings on lung scan. The MAA was freshly made and used within the recommended time post formulation. MAA average particle size is 10–40 μm (range is 15–90 μm) which lodges in the lung capillary bed (capillary diameter 8.2±1.5 μm). MAA fragmenting into smaller particles, are then taken up in the liver and undergo further proteolytic digestion (2.4). Residual Tc 99m sulfur colloid (SC) activity from a previous day liver spleen scan, cross-contamination of Tc SC in the MAA vial, or tag breakdown from use of MAA beyond the recommended post formulation time did not apply in this patient.

HUMAN ERROR

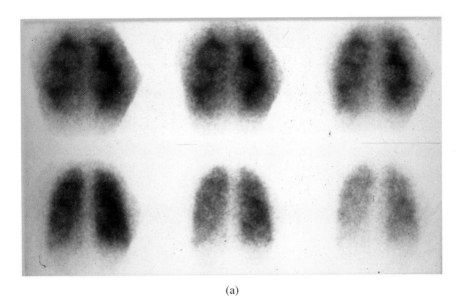

(a)

Fig. 3.6. (a) Wrong window setting for Xenon (Xe) giving a blurry, fuzzy-looking ventilation lung images and faint visualization of photomultiplier tubes on the top row images, a preventable error by the technician. Bottom row shows images were obtained at the correct window setting. (b) Wrong window setting showing suboptimal images with heterogeneous appearance and visualization of photomultiplier tubes giving a polka dot appearance on the Tc 99m MDP bone scan. (c) Multifocal hot spots (increased activity) in both lungs are due to clumping of MAA particles. This can result from MAA formulation problems with incomplete separation of the MAA particles during radiopharmaceutical preparation, poor intravenous access resulting in fine clumping of blood and MAA particles in the injection syringe from prolonged attempt at injection, or faulty injection techniques. This is avoided by gently agitating the MAA vial and injection syringe to break up the protein particles prior to injection, paying careful attention to radiopharmaceutical preparation, and following good injection techniques. These artifacts have been reported with embolization of the MAA particles in the upper extremity venous blood after injection, a patient related factor not under the control of the nuclear technologist.[5] Multiple bilateral lungs septic emboli have to be considered if similar findings are seen on an [111]Indium-labeled white blood cell (In-WBC) scan.

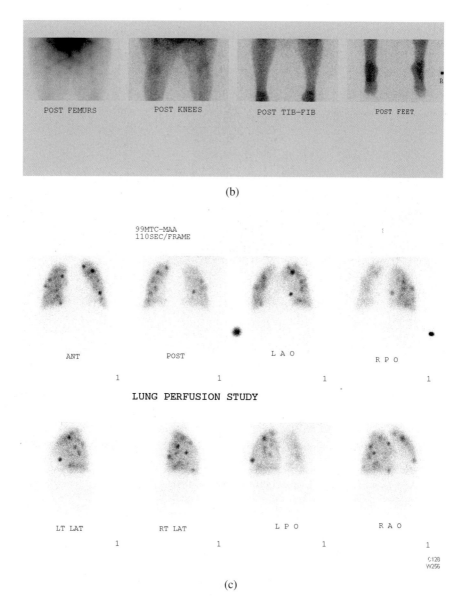

(b)

LUNG PERFUSION STUDY

(c)

Fig. 3.6. (*Continued*)

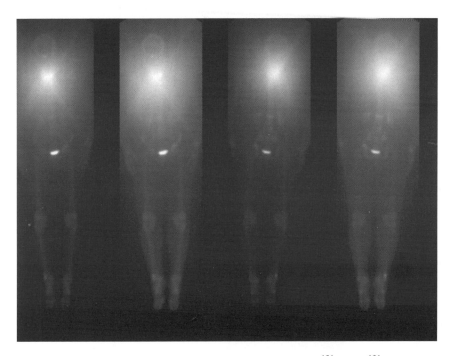

Fig. 3.7. Bone scan in a patient performed within 9 days of 15 mCi of ^{131}Iodine (^{131}I) therapy for hyperthyroidism (Graves). ^{131}I has a longer physical half-life (8 days), a longer biologic half-life, and higher keV photons compared to the 6 h physical $T_{1/2}$ for Tc 99m and 140 keV gamma ray photons. ^{131}I treatment for hyperthyroidism can interfere with performance of nuclear studies using isotopes with lower energies like Tc, Xe, and Thallium 201 chloride (Tl). The intra-thyroidal iodine retention post treatment is influenced by iodine uptake by the thyroids, thyroid gland size, dose of ^{131}I administered, and patient hydration status. This scan illustrates the need for strict radiation safety precautions after treatment so as to minimize unnecessary radiation exposure to others. It also emphasizes the importance of a good patient history and the significance of half-life and photon energies of different radionuclides in scheduling different nuclear studies in a patient.

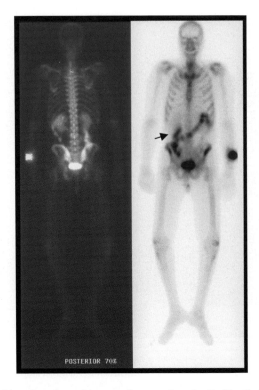

Fig. 3.8. Intestinal bowel uptake on bone scan from previous day Tc 99m Sestamibi (MIBI) scan. Intestinal uptake of MDP is seen in 1% of bone scans as prominent ascending colon or rarely generalized intestinal or thorax activity from Chilaiditi's syndrome, which may be an intermittent process.[6]

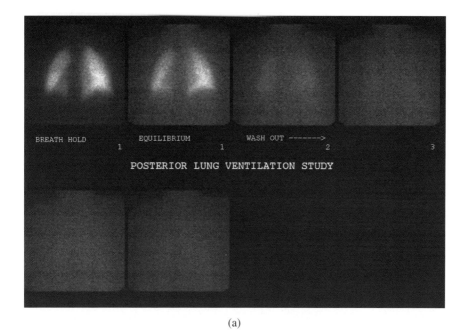

(a)

Fig. 3.9. (a) and (b) Diffuse increased background and mild heart activity (perfusion images) from renal Tc 99m ethylenediaminetetraacetic acid (Tc DTPA) scan done the previous day in a patient with a poorly functioning renal transplant resulting in delayed, decreased clearance of the radiotracer and mildly increased background activity; however, the lung scan was of diagnostic quality. Spot chest image on Xe and Tc setting pre lung scan is helpful to estimate the intensity of interfering background activity if history of a prior nuclear study is known. (c) Residual focal bowel activity from previous day Tc Sestamibi myocardial perfusion scan did not cause interference on the otherwise diagnostic quality lung scan in this patient. A chest spot image in the anterior and posterior projection prior to the lung scan in the Xe (ventilation) and Tc 99m (perfusion) window setting for 1 min and 2–3 min, respectively, are useful to evaluate the extent of interference from residual background activity if prior history of nuclear study is available. An active gastrointestinal bleed is a remote consideration; patient history can help eliminate this differential.

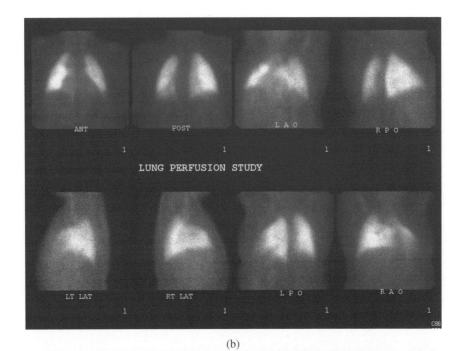

(b)

(c)

Fig. 3.9. (*Continued*)

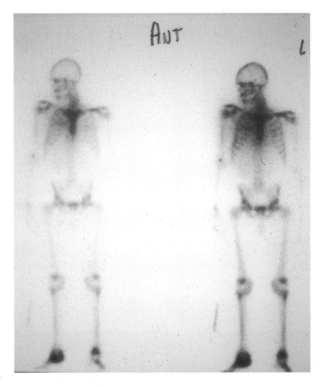

Fig. 3.10. Bone scan demonstrating diffuse increased soft tissue activity in the right chest of a patient with indwelling radioactive gold seeds used in treatment of right lung cancer. This activity can persist for months after treatment due to the long $T_{1/2}$ of radioactive Gold seeds. Diffuse increased activity is seen in right greater than left ankle joints. Gold seeds inserted into the pelvis for prostate and bladder cancer (brachytherapy) can result in a suboptimal scan due to increased scatter pelvic activity on the bone scan, which is dependent on the number of gold seeds inserted and the interval duration between therapy and scan. A good patient history can help avoid or explain the finding on bone scan.[7]

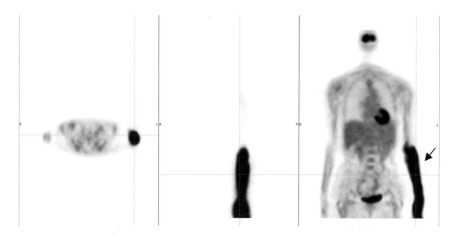

Fig. 3.11. Inadvertent intra-arterial injection of [^{18}F] FDG for PET scan demonstrates diffuse intense activity in the left forearm and hand (downstream to the injection site). This has been reported with Tc 99m MDP injection but can occur with injection of any Radiotracer injection.[8,9]

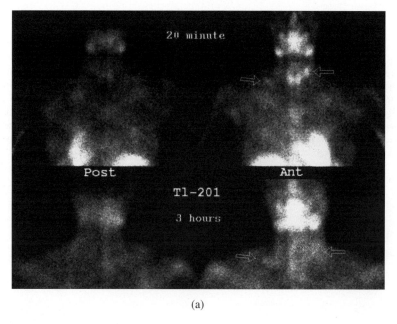

(a)

Fig. 3.12. (a) Wrong window setting on a Tc 99m Sestamibi (MIBI) scan for parathyroid adenoma resulting in a heterogeneous appearance and a suboptimal scan.

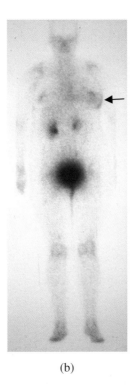

(b)

Fig. 3.12. (*Continued*) (b) In this patient, the wrong RP was given, resulting in poor skeletal visualization with good renal and bladder activity. No activity was missing from the MDP vial to suggest the inadvertent withdrawal of a dose for a bone scan injection; no other bone scan on that day exhibited such scan findings. Diffuse increased soft tissue uptake in left breast was later confirmed to be breast cancer. The mechanism of Tc MDP uptake in soft tissue malignancy or metastasis is unclear but is likely due to multiple factors, including tumor vascularity, inflammation, local pH factors, altered calcium metabolism, hormonal influences, and cell wall damage.[10-12] Most frequently, the uptake of MDP is due to microcalcification or new bone formation within the tumor.

Patient Factors

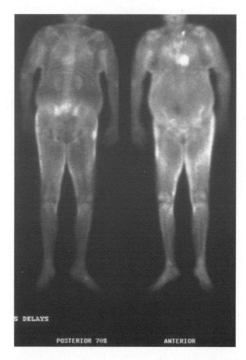

Fig. 3.13. Chronic renal insufficiency, revealing poor skeletal activity on bone scan, diffuse increased soft tissue background activity, especially in the extremities. Increased cardiac activity is suggestive of possible secondary amyloidosis. The decreased renal activity in bilateral small sized kidneys and absent bladder activity is consistent with history of chronic renal insufficiency and end stage renal disease.[13,14]

---→

Fig. 3.14. (a–c) Tc 99m red blood cells (RBCs) labeled multi-gated acquisition (MUGA) scan demonstrating poor heart activity, which is unchanged on a repeat study done two weeks later (not shown). There is free Technetium 99m pertechnetate (Tc 04) present as shown by bilateral salivary gland, thyroid gland and diffuse increased liver and bilateral renal activity seen (Fig. 3.14 (b) and (c)). No history of recent heparin administration (the most common reason for absent heart activity). Red cell labeling can have difficulties during the labeling process due to pharmaceutical factors, insufficient cells in the sample, sedimentation problems or instability of the cell chelator, choice of anticoagulant, level of stannous ion, and oxidation of Technetium 99m, resulting in problems with radiolabeling and RP preparation. Patient-related factors are only manifested after the patient is injected with the labeled cells. Medications such as cyclosporine, nifedipine, verapamil, hydrazaline, propranalol, digoxin and drug combinations of nifedipine, etoposide, idarubicin, and cefataxime cause labeling problems or alter the biodistribution.[15] Teflon catheter use has been implicated in a few cases. This patient had high titers of cold agglutinins which we presumed to be the cause of the abnormal MUGA scan findings.

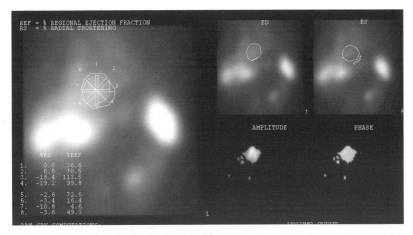

(a)

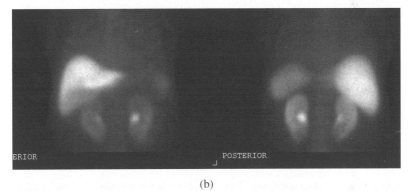

(b)

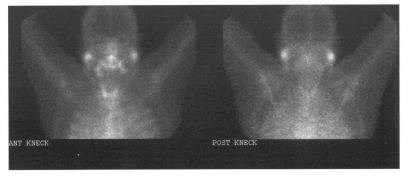

(c)

Fig. 3.14. (*Continued*)

81

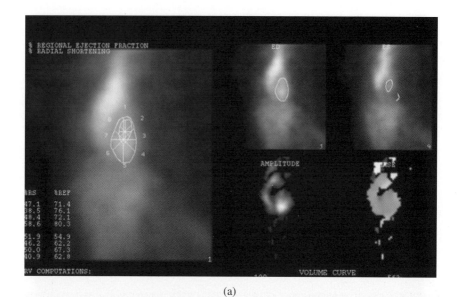

(a)

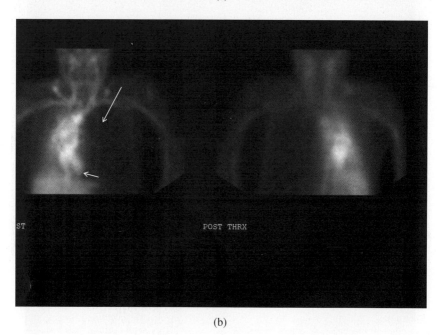

(b)

Fig. 3.15. (a) and (b) MUGA scan using Tc 99m labeled autologous Red blood cells in a patient with metastatic breast cancer shows a centrally located and elongated appearing left ventricle with a large area of photopenia in the entire left chest and rightward mediastinal shift.

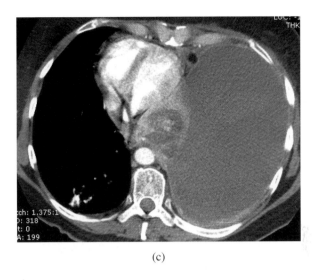

(c)

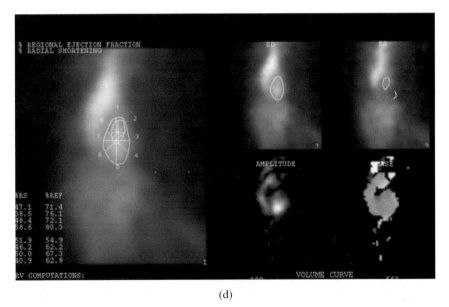

(d)

Fig. 3.15. (*Continued*) (c) CT axial image of chest done at same time showed a new large left pleural effusion, left lung collapse, mediastinal shift to opposite side, and increase in size and number of metastatic right lung nodules. A prior MUGA scan done 6 months previously showed the heart in its usual location in left chest (Fig. 3.15 (d)).

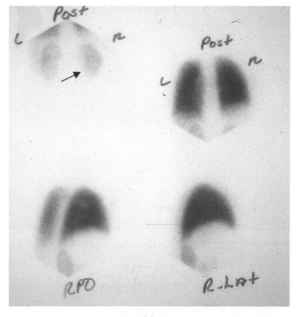

(a)

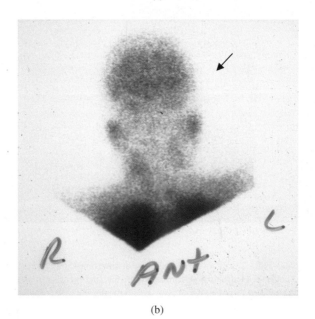

(b)

Fig. 3.16. (*Continued*)

Fig. 3.16. (a) and (b) Right to left shunt on scan is seen as diffuse increased brain and renal activity on Tc 99m MAA perfusion lung scan.[16,17] A reduced dose of Tc 99m MAA is given to patients with history of right to left shunt, pulmonary hypertension, a single lung from congenital or surgical resection, children, and pregnant women to reduce the number of alveolar capillaries that are embolized by the MAA particles and to decrease the number of shunted particles to the brain and kidneys. Patient history plays an important role in dose selection. Free Technetium from poor labeling results in thyroid, salivary gland, choroid plexus, and gastric and renal activity as seen in Fig. 3.3(b), which is different from the pattern seen in right to left shunt.

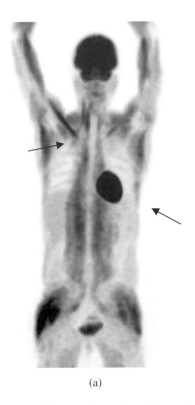

(a)

Fig. 3.17. (a) [18][F] FDG-PET scan shows diffuse muscle and intense heart activity with poor liver activity that resulted from eating a donut prior to the FDG injection. Patient was instructed to eat nothing after midnight on the night prior to PET scan. In this case, the peak insulin surge after eating likely coincided with the time of FDG injection resulting in a "muscle scan." Hyperinsulinemia pushes the glucose into the skeletal muscles and heart, resulting in a suboptimal and many times a non-diagnostic study.[18,19] In young actively exercising patients, heavy exercise days prior to the PET scan can result in increased muscle activity in the well-developed healthy muscles. FDG-PET tracer distribution patterns are very sensitive to baseline glucose levels and level of muscle activity pre- and post-tracer injection, and the patient is instructed not to do heavy physical activity for few days prior to the PET scan and to remain as still as possible post injection.

85

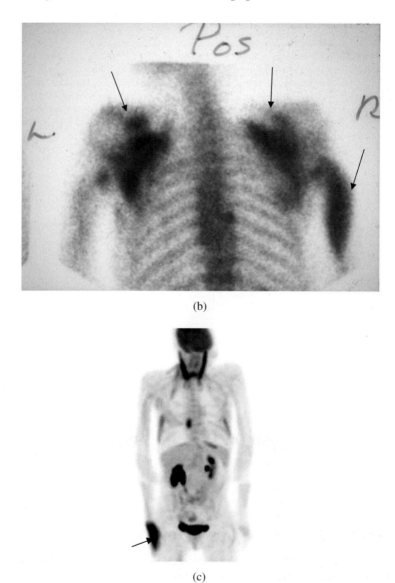

(b)

(c)

Fig. 3.17. (*Continued*) (b) Rhabdomyolysis in this patient is seen as diffuse increased shoulder girdle and arm muscle activity on Tc 99m MDP bone scan. Rhabdomyolysis occurs from significant blunt trauma, prolonged immobilization, excessive muscular activity, myoclonal seizures, ingestion of toxins (ethanol, isopropanolol, drug-like barbiturates, antihistamines, salicylates, hypothermia, Epstein Barr, human immunodeficiency virus (HIV), Influenza A and B, enzyme deficiencies in carbohydrate and lipid metabolism[20−22] or following lighting strikes[23] and after intra-arterial injection of local anaesthetic.[24]

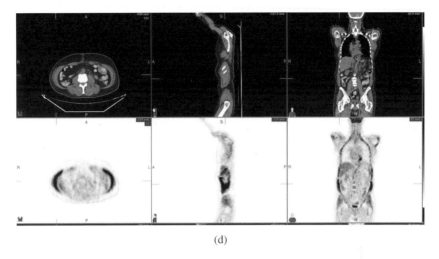

(d)

Fig. 3.17. (*Continued*) (c) Increased muscle activity in neck and chest muscles in a patient with end stage lung disease and chronic use of accessory respiratory muscles for breathing.[25] Incidental dose infiltration is seen at injection site in right wrist. (d) Diffuse increased [^{18}F] FDG activity on PET/CT scan in bilateral abdominal and thoracic muscles from repeated coughing post-tracer injection. Physical activity pre- and post-tracer injection and regular heavy physical exercise prior to PET scan can show generalized increased muscle uptake, which can result in a suboptimal PET scan, a reason for patient having to stay still after the ^{18}[F] FDG is injected so as to not to cause increased muscle uptake on the PET images.

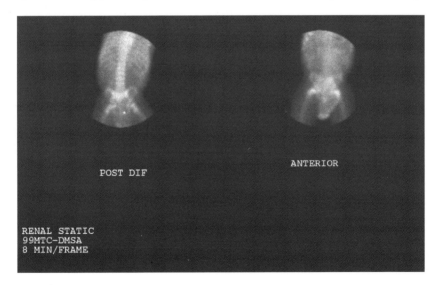

Fig. 3.18. Tc DMSA renal in a child with chronic renal insufficiency on dialysis demonstrating very poor renal activity and increased bone/bone marrow activity, a "DMSA super scan" which although rare should be recognized.[26]

87

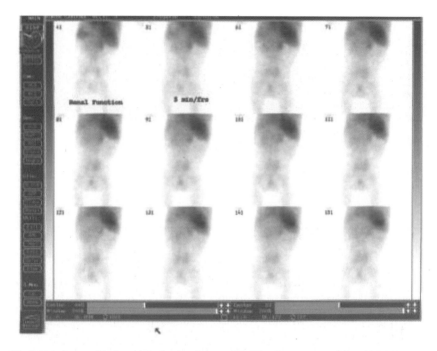

Fig. 3.19. Acute cortical necrosis showing decreased Tc 99m dimercaptosuccinic acid (DMSA) cortical uptake in the bilateral kidneys and relative increased vicarious hepatic extraction of radiotracer is noted.

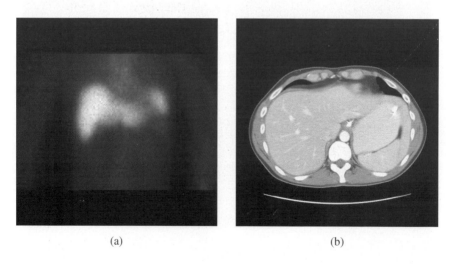

(a)   (b)

Fig. 3.20. (*Continued*)

Fig. 3.20. (a) Diffuse increased activity in left upper quadrant gives appearance of splenic activity on HIDA scan, which in reality is a wraparound left lobe of liver activity (black arrow) as seen on the axial CT abdomen image (Fig. 3.20(b)). HIDA is taken up by the hepatocytes and excreted via the biliary pathway; hence splenic activity is not seen on HIDA scan. In liver- spleen scan utilizing sulfur colloid, Tc 99m sulfur colloid is taken up by the reticuloendothelial cells which are present in the liver, spleen, and bone marrow, resulting in visualization of both liver and spleen activity on the colloid scan. In cirrhotic livers with poor hepatic function, increased bone marrow and at times lung activity can be seen. This case illustrates the value of reviewing other radiology studies to help explain unusual nuclear scan findings, which can be easily and directly compared using the same computer terminal these days when all radiology studies can be accessed using the picture archiving system (PACS). A single-photon emission computed tomography (SPECT), if available, can also help explain the unusual scan findings.

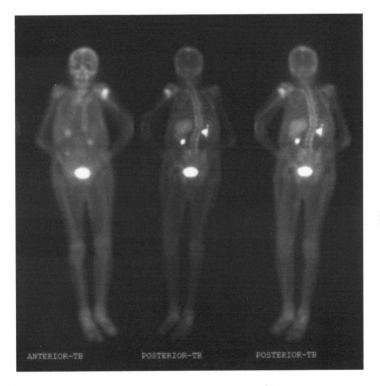

Fig. 3.21. Splenic uptake on bone scan is abnormal and may be related to alumina excess, sickle cell disease with infarctions and calcifications,[27] multiple myeloma,[28] or splenic embolization, hyper-splenism in sickle cell beta + Thalassemia,[29] severe alcoholic cirrhosis of the liver with hematochromatosis resulting from alcohol abuse.[30] The patient hands are over the anterior pelvis, which may limits pelvic evaluation; the arms should optimally be at the patient's side. Kyphoscoliosis of the thoracic and lumbar spine is noted on the bone scan, a patient factor.

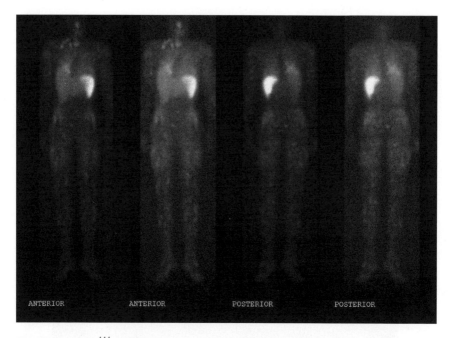

Fig. 3.22. A 24-h ^{111}In WBC anterior and posterior total body images show heterogeneous diffuse increased soft tissue uptake in bilateral thighs and gluteal regions, which may be due to multiple septic emboli in a 17-year-old football player with no history of drug abuse. Clumping of ^{111}In-labeled WBC resulting from poor tag generally results in larger, more intense focal areas of uptake. The persistent bilateral lung uptake on the 24-h images is likely due to adult respiratory distress syndrome. Diffuse bilateral lung uptake on the 4-h scan is a transient finding related to the transient effect of the labeling procedure on the WBC, but is not seen on the 24-h as the WBC has recovered from the trauma of labeling.

---→

Fig. 3.23. (a) Bone scan showing a diffuse band like increased soft tissue activity seen best in the posterior and lateral pelvic walls and lateral aspects of bilateral thighs, left being worse than right. This was shown to be due to a large soft tissue tumor in the posterior pelvic wall on CT (Fig. 3.23(b)) (*Courtesy*: Dr. L M Lamki). The CT scan findings helped make the diagnosis, thus reinforcing the importance of anatomic image correlation to explain unusual nuclear scan findings and the complementary role of anatomic and functional imaging in solving unexpected disease findings. PET/CT is the best example of the fusion of functional and anatomic imaging. SPECT/CT is being increasingly used in nuclear medicine for better anatomic localization in parathyroid imaging; lower extremities bone imaging and prostaScint imaging are examples where SPECT/CT imaging is helpful. Urine contamination artifact is not likely, given the pattern of soft tissue activity in this patient. Dermatomyositis and rhabdomyolysis are in the differential, but history and physical examination helped to exclude them. Mechanisms leading to increased extraosseous Tc-99m MDP uptake include extracellular fluid expansion, enhanced regional vascularity and permeability, and elevated tissue calcium concentration.[31]

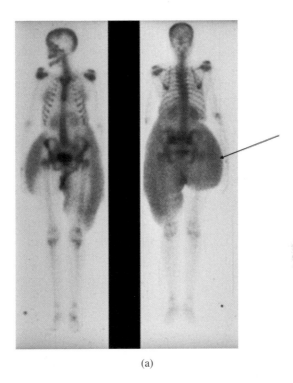

(a)

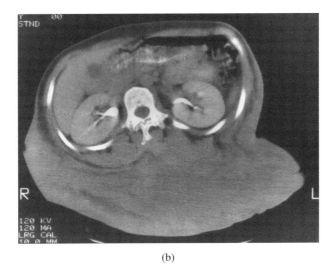

(b)

Fig. 3.23. (*Continued*)

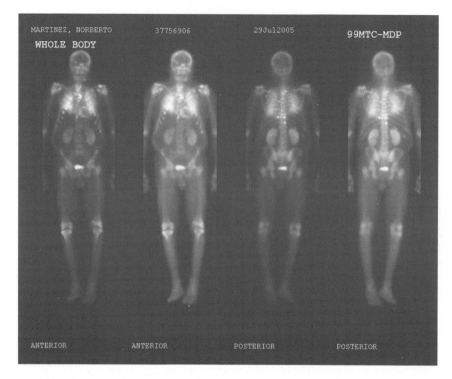

Fig. 3.24. Hypercalcemia resulting in cardiac/pericardial and diffuse lung activity is seen on the bone scan. Myocardial infarction and amyloid or calcific pericarditis is seen as isolated heart activity in the appropriate clinical setting. Diffuse lung and gastric uptake on bone scan in a patient with sarcoidosis from hypercalcemia and soft tissue calcinosis has been reported. Parathyroid adenoma and Vitamin D intoxication are other non-malignant conditions. Hypercalcemia is seen in renal failure and end-stage renal disease. Malignant conditions showing lung and gastric uptake are multiple myeloma, breast cancer, non-Hodgkins lymphoma and bladder cancer.[32,33]

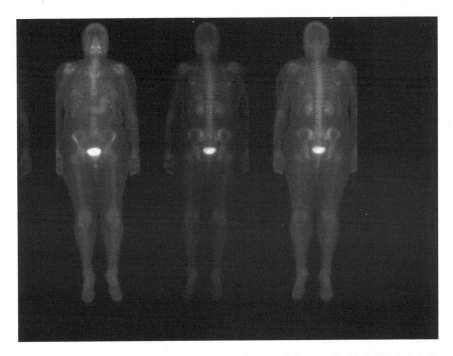

Fig. 3.25.   Diffuse increased stomach activity without thyroid activity on the Tc-99m MDP whole body bone scan is an uncommon finding. Intravenous histamine H2 receptor antagonists causing isolated stomach activity was reported in a case report.[32] Hypercalcemia is associated with malignancy,[31–35] Vitamin D intoxication,[36] and metastatic calcification; stomach and gastric uptake of MDP was reported in Burkitts lymphoma[37]; abnormal gastric uptake on bone scan was reported in a child treated long term with isoretinoin for a dermatologic disorder.[38] Abnormal MDP stomach uptake in a case of multiple myeloma and hypercalcemia was found to have amyloid deposits and metastatic calcification in the gastric mucosa at autopsy.[39] Metastatic calcification and calciphylaxis (calcific uremic arteriolopathy) is characterized by subcutaneous soft tissue calcifications, painful ulcerations, high morbidity and mortality, extensive tracer localization in the superficial subcutaneous tissues, myocardium, lungs, stomach and kidneys.[40] Radiopharmaceutical formulation with presence of free technetium can result in thyroid and choroid plexus and stomach activity was ruled out in this patient. A gastric emptying study within 24 h of bone scan and delayed gastric emptying can be considered but is less likely, given that less than 1 mCi dose of radiotracer is used for the gastric emptying study and some intestinal activity is usually seen.

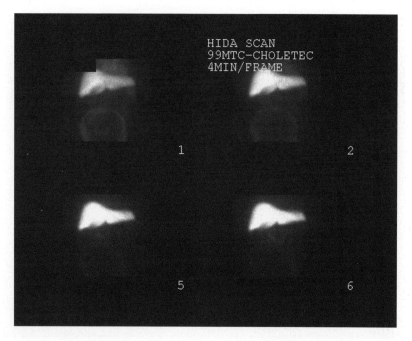

Fig. 3.26. A narrow band of hyperemia corresponding to the complicated/gangrenous acute cholecystitis is seen in addition to the outline of the birth sac in this pregnant woman who underwent an emergency HIDA scan for serious medical problems in the pregnant woman. Biliary tract disorders are the second most common general surgical condition in pregnancy after acute appendicitis; however, the incidence of symptomatic gall stone disease is equal or less than 0.1%. Surgery is delayed until after delivery unless conservative treatment fails or patient's symptoms recur in the same trimester.[41] Nuclear scan in pregnant women is always a concern since shielding of the uterus is not possible after the radiotracer administration. Hence the fetus will be exposed to the radiation, which is dependent on the dose of radiotracer, its excretion, and the stage of patient's pregnancy. Radiation can reach the fetus via the penetrating gamma rays emitted by the radionuclide concentrated in maternal organs and the placenta, or the radionuclide can cross the placenta and be taken up by the fetus. If a radionuclide study is indicated for the mother's health, informed consent is obtained from the patient after explaining the radiation hazards to the fetus and mother, and a reduced dose is given to minimize the radiation exposure to the fetus. Generally, it is advisable to avoid nuclear studies in the first trimester due to the development of the critical organs; thyroid scans after the first trimester causes increased radiation to fetal thyroid, which starts to concentrate radio-iodine at 10–12 weeks of gestation.[42] [131]I therapy is not given to pregnant women, and breast feeding is stopped prior to ^{131}I therapy or gallium and thallium scans as they are secreted in the breast milk.

———————————————————————————————→

Fig. 3.27. Tc-99m Diethylene triamine penta acetic acid (DTPA) aerosol scan shows patchy central deposition of the DTPA aerosol particles due to poor patient inspiration. Regional ventilation can deliver particles to a particular region, but its retention is determined by gravitational sedimentation, inertial impaction and to a lesser extent diffusion.[43] The relative importance of these processes is determined by the density, diameter, diffusion coefficient of the inhaled particle, its residence time in the airway, the anatomy and dimensions of the airway, and the volumetric flow rate of air.[44] There is increasing

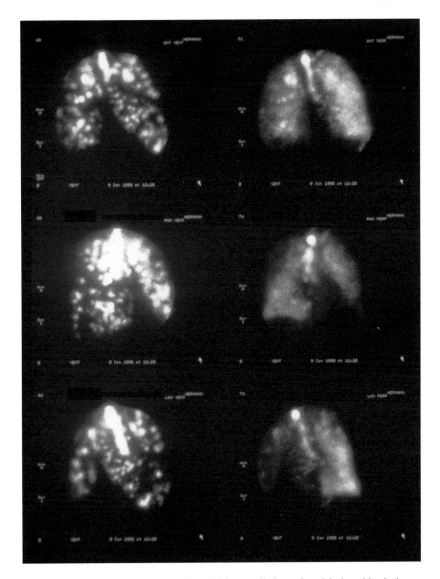

Fig. 3.27. (*Continued*) apex to base gradient, with less ventilation and particle deposition in the upper lobe relative to the lower lobe in the upright position. Regional deposition is significantly affected by gravity through its effects on regional anatomy and changes in distribution related to supine position may be related to factors other than simple changes in regional ventilation.[43] Regional ventilation is dependent on local pulmonary compliance and airway resistance and quantitative regional measurement is best done with radioactive gases rather than radio-aerosols.[43,44] The advantage of radio-aerosol ventilation is that multiple views of both lungs can be obtained similar to the lung perfusion images making for easier, direct comparison of ventilation and perfusion.

95

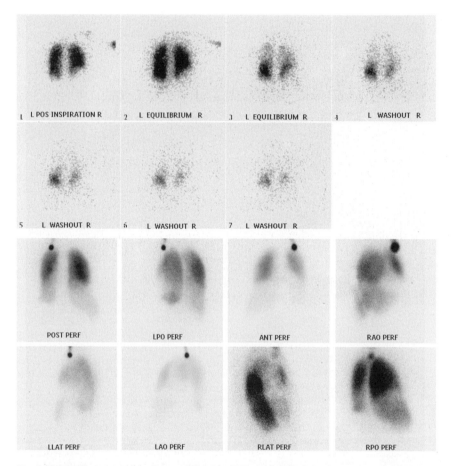

Fig. 3.28. Radiotracer activity is seen diffusely within the liver on a Tc 99m MAA perfusion lung scan. This can result from poor radiopharmaceutical tagging, degradation to submicron particle size of injected particles, right to left cardiac shunts, or shunting of material away from heart after injection due to collateral flow via the portal veins to the liver with uptake usually seen as focal activity in the quadrate lobe of liver.[45,46] A recent HIDA scan with delayed liver clearance or Tc sulfur colloid liver spleen scan did not apply in this patient.

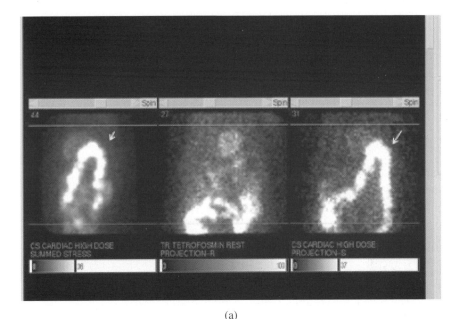

(a)

Fig. 3.29. (a–c) Intense bowel loop activity seen near the lateral wall on the initial Tc-99m tetrofosomin (Myoview) stress SPECT resulted in a non-diagnostic study as the focal bowel activity artifact compromises a true estimation of myocardial perfusion.[47] The bowel activity did not move in spite of repeated delayed stress SPECT imaging the same day after oral intake of cold water. Repeat stress SPECT one week later showed moderate ischemia of the inferior and inferolateral walls, which was difficult to identify on the initial scan due to the intense bowel activity. Tc Myoview, like other labeled myocardial perfusion agents, is cleared by liver and excreted by the biliary system. Abdominal activity at rest may be increased since there is no exercise effect to reduce splanchnic activity. Increased bowel and liver activity can interfere with the visual and quantitative interpretation of the infero-posteroseptal myocardial walls especially on rest imaging. This can be mitigated by having patient drink whole milk and water prior to repeating the scan.[47] Our protocol consists of same day low dose (10 mCi) rest SPECT followed by high dose (30 mCi) gated stress myocardial SPECT using Tc Tetrofosmin (Myoview) for both imaging studies. "Halo" effect is an artifact associated with filtered back projection seen as focal increased activity in otherwise low count surroundings[47]; iterative reconstruction will eliminate the halo artifact but will not diminish scatter so it is important to reduce the scatter effect from liver, bowel and gastric activity.[47] Spillover of activity in the myocardium results from photon scatter associated with activity in the liver, bowel, and stomach and may result in overestimation of activity in this area. Both artifacts are patient dependent and their severity is hard to predict.[47] Use of oral radiographic contrast and water improved the image variability related to bowel activity as the oral contrast in the bowel can absorb the gamma rays emitted from the Tc Myoview in the bowel, thereby reducing scatter and improving the cardiac SPECT images.[48]

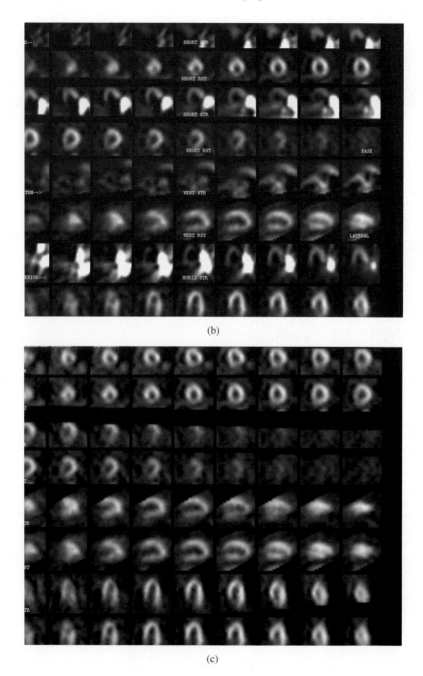

(b)

(c)

Fig. 3.29. (*Continued*)

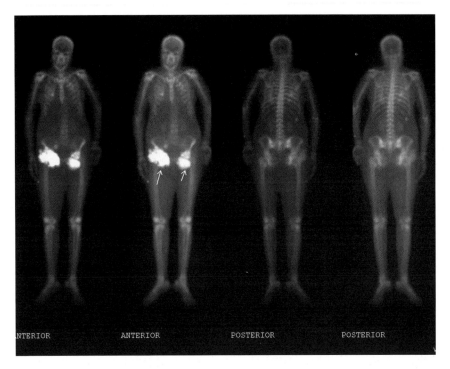

INTERIOR   ANTERIOR   POSTERIOR   POSTERIOR

Fig. 3.30. Heterotopic ossification (HO) on Tc-99m bone scan. HO, also known as heterotopic bone formation or myositis ossificans, is the presence of abnormal bone where bone normally does not exist (e.g., in soft tissues) and results from an initial inflammatory lesion of muscle or soft tissues followed by abnormal bone formation. It must not be confused with metastatic calcification seen in hypercalcemia from various benign or malignant conditions or dystrophic calcification resulting from local tissue injury or abnormality in association with normal serum levels and metabolism of calcium and phosphate. Acquired HO, the most common variety, is usually precipitated by trauma (fracture, direct muscular trauma, and total hip arthroplasty [THA]) with incidence of 0.6% to 90% in THA). It may result from neurogenic causes like spinal cord injury (20%–30%) or central nervous system injury (head injury 10%–20%).[49] Three conditions postulated by Chalmers *et al.*[50] for HO to develop are osteogenic precursor cells, inducing agents, and a permissive environment. A small hydrophobic bone morphogenetic protein has been proposed by Urist *et al.*[51] as a causative agent capable of changing the development of mesenchymal cells in muscle into bone under favorable conditions rather than fibrous tissue. Role of prostaglandin E2 is also suggested as a mediator in the differentiation of progenitor cells.[52] Myositis ossificans and HO show similar distinctive histologic properties of peripheral ossification as an ossified radio-opaque peripheral rim surrounding a non-ossified radiolucent center, in contrast to malignant osteosarcoma with a dense central ossification. The periphery of myositis ossificans shows mature lamellar bone surrounded by a capsule of compressed muscle fibers and fibrous tissue.[53] The development of HO is extra-articular, occurring outside the joint capsule; bone forms in the connective tissue between the muscle planes and not within the muscle itself.[54] A radiolucent cleft is seen radiographically around the myositis ossificans, differentiating it from osteosarcoma which maintains an attachment to normal bone and from osteochondroma which features an open communication with the medullary cavity.[49,51] The proximal joints are typically involved and more than a single

Fig. 3.30. (*Continued*) joint region can be involved; it is often bilateral, for example, hips in a paraplegic patient, also femurs, knees, shoulders, and elbows.[49] Serial three-phase bone scan is the most sensitive imaging modality for early detection of HO. Activity on the delayed bone scan usually peaks a few months after injury and returns to normal at 6–12 months, with most scans returning to baseline within 12 months. Three-phase bone scans are used to evaluate maturity of the HO; when successive bone scan performed after an adequate time interval demonstrate no further increase in extent or shows stable or decreasing intensity of MDP accumulation, it indicates that the process has stabilized or matured and HO surgery can be performed.[55–57] Surgery done prematurely before the maturation/stabilizing process is complete can result in the HO recurring.[49] The autosomal dominant congenital form of HO, myositis ossificans progressiva or fibrodyspalsia ossificans progressive is extremely rare. It is associated with skeletal abnormalities, including malformation of the great toes, shortening of the digits, deafness and baldness, starting generally at age 4 years and progressing to severely impaired joint mobility and ankylosis by early adulthood.[49,58–61]

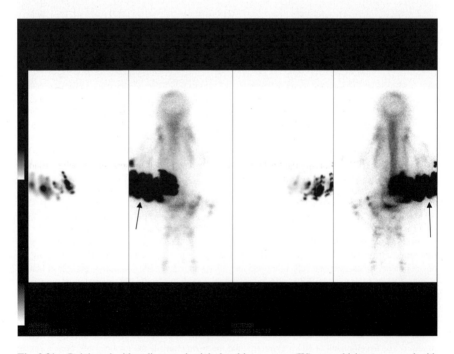

Fig. 3.31. Pt injected with radiotracer in right-hand intravenous (IV) port which was covered with bandages. Patient kept moving his arms, especially the right arm, during the study and was noted to have extensive dose infiltration at the injection area which appears to encroach on the total body images due to arm movement resulting in a degraded non-diagnostic images.

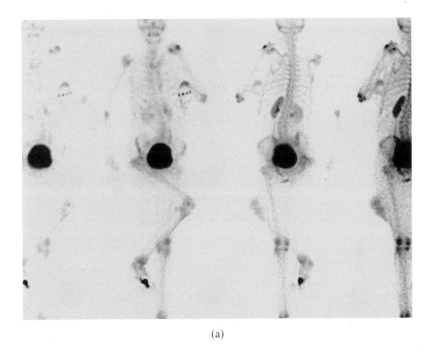

(a)

Fig. 3.32. (a) Huge bladder seen on Tc-99m total body bone scan in a patient who was unable to empty bladder. Contracture deformity of right-lower extremity and findings related to complex regional pain syndrome in the left upper extremity are noted. (b) A large bladder activity seen on whole body ^{18}[F]FDG-PET scan in a patient (top row) remains unchanged on the delayed post void PET spot image of the pelvis as patient had difficulty in emptying the bladder (bottom row). (c) CT pelvis done four days earlier in this patient again showed huge bladder similar to the PET scan findings. Both these patients had difficulty emptying the bladder, resulting in suboptimal imaging of the pelvis. Bladder activity is important in imaging of the pelvis as the presence of a large bladder activity can obscure pelvic pathology; this is the reason why patient is asked to void prior to the bone scan.

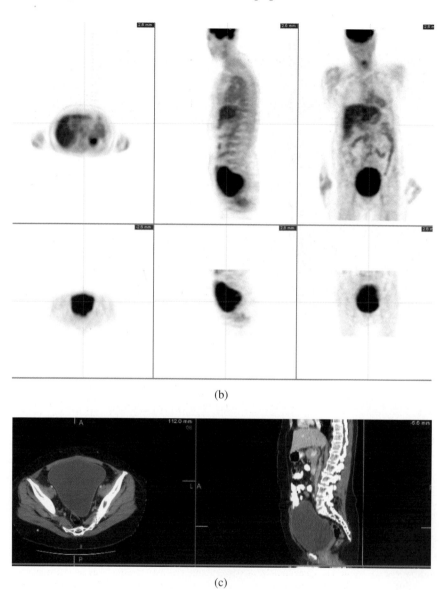

(b)

(c)

Fig. 3.32. (*Continued*)

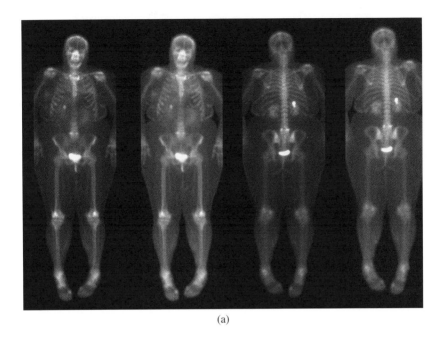

(a)

Fig. 3.33. (a, b) Dystrophic calcification in right kidney noted on CT abdomen demonstrates intense focal MDP uptake on MDP bone scan. Dystrophic calcifications (DCs) occur with local tissue injury or local tissue abnormality and in association with normal metabolism and serum levels of calcium and phosphates.[62] Local tissue abnormality consists of alterations in collagen, elastin, or subcutaneous fat, leading to precipitate calcification. Metastatic calcification occurs when there is abnormal calcium and/or phosphate metabolism resulting in hypercalcemia or hyperphosphatemia resulting in calcification of normal cutaneous, subcutaneous, and deep tissues.[63,64] In dystrophic calcification, the mitochondria serve as the calcifying nidus, demonstrating a high affinity for calcium and phosphate to levels that allow calcium to crystallize. Walsh and Fairley[63] postulated that the high levels of intracellular calcium result from membrane damage leading to increased calcium influx. Cell necrosis may change the internal environment to a more acidic milieu and, in association with the absence of certain calcification inhibitors seen at the site of previous inflammation or damage, can result in dystrophic calcification.[62,65,66] Hydroxyapatite crystals are formed initially within the protective microenvironment of the membrane microspace.[66] DCs are seen in calcinosis (universalis or circumscripta) from childhood dermatomyositis, scleroderma, systemic lupus erythematosis, and after trauma.[65] In rare cases DCs resolve spontaneously. Medical therapy including etidronate disodium, sodium warfarin, diltiazem, aluminium hydroxide, and intralesional corticosteroids are generally first line of treatment.[66] Surgery is indicated for painful masses, local functional impairment, and cosmetic reasons.[67] Metastatic calcification is seen in conditions associated with hypercalcemia-like milk-alkali syndrome, hypervitaminosis D, sarcoidosis, hyperparathyroidism, and renal failure.[68] Metastatic calcification from hyperphosphatemia is seen in tumoral calcinosis, renal failure, hypoparathyroidism, pseudohypoparathyroidism, and cell lysis following chemotherapy for leukemia. The crystal deposition diseases associated with metastatic calcification are gout and calcium pyrophosphate deposition disease.[65] A major category of extraskeletal calcification is related to myositis ossificans from burns, surgery or neurologic injury or fibrodysplasia (myositis) ossificans progressive.[65]

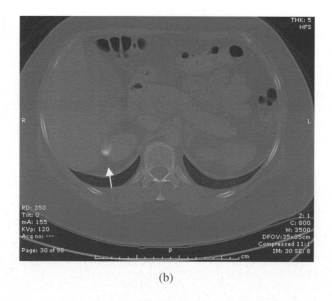

(b)

Fig. 3.33. (*Continued*)

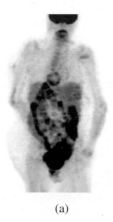

(a)

Fig. 3.34. (a) Whole body ^{18}[F] FDG-PET image shows extensive, intense FDG activity in the large bowel which limits evaluation of the abdomen and pelvis. (b) A 45-min delayed PET spot image of the same patient shows improvement in the bowel activity allowing for better visualization of the abdomen and pelvis on PET. This shows the usefulness of delayed PET image to differentiate physiologic from true abdominal pathology. (c) Urine diaper contamination artifact on anterior and posterior whole body Tc 99m MDP images. (d) Urine diaper contamination artifact on sagittal F18 FDG PET image.

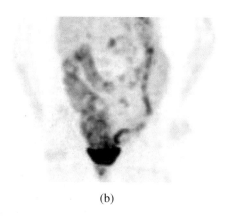

(b)

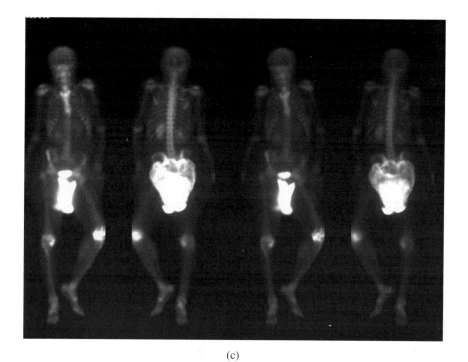

(c)

Fig. 3.34. (*Continued*)

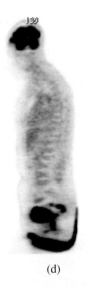

(d)

Fig. 3.34. (*Continued*)

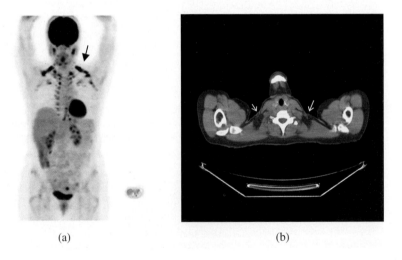

(a)   (b)

Fig. 3.35. (*Continued*)

Fig. 3.35. (a) PET coronal image shows extensive brown fat activity as increased activity in the bilateral neck and multiple bilateral thoracic paraspinal regions. (b) Axial CT of the neck region showing no abnormality in the bilateral neck to correspond to the PET scan uptake in the neck on the PET/CT scan. The benign increased brown fat or increased muscle activity can be mistaken for malignant lymph nodes, abnormal soft tissue activity, and inflammatory or infectious lymph node activity, especially if corresponding CT images are not available, thereby changing the patient's prognosis and leading to unnecessary therapy. Muscle uptake is increased by endogenous or exogenous insulin and recent muscle activity. Muscle relaxants and sedatives have been tried to reduce muscle activity.[69] Brown fat hibernomas have rarely been reported in the supraclavicular region.[69] Brown adipose tissue (BAT) is histologically and physiologically distinct from white adipose tissue; it is highly metabolically active as reflected by the increased FDG activity.[69,70] BAT contains considerable cytoplasm, small lipid droplets, round centrally located nuclei, and abundant mitochondria[70] as opposed to white fat which consists of a scant ring of cytoplasm around a single large lipid droplet, an eccentric flattened nucleus, and essentially no mitochondria.[70] Brown fat is rich in mitochondria and highly vascularized, giving it a "brownish color"[71]; it has the ability to increase its blood flow with nor-epinephrine stimulation, and its main purpose is to generate heat in response to acute cold exposure (non-shivering thermogenesis).[72] It utilizes an uncoupling protein, UCP-1, while the white fat serves as an insulator for energy/heat storage.[69,73] Glucose is not the major energy supply for brown fat but its use increases during cold stimulation or exposure and is accompanied by glucose transporter 4 increase.[69] Fatty acids, the main fuel used to maintain the BAT thermogenic function, are obtained from triglycerides with the help of lipase or from lipoproteins with the help of lipoprotein lipase. Tumor glycolysis is independent of normal control mechanisms and independent fatty acid levels.[70] Brown fat is usually recognized as symmetric areas of curvilinear or focal uptake in the neck and supraclavicular regions, mediastinum, paravertebral spaces, and paranephric area around the upper poles of the kidneys.[70,73] Brown fat is abundant in those for whom generating supplemental body heat is vital, namely new born babies.[73] Consumption of a high-fat, very low carbohydrate, protein-permitted diet 3–5 h prior to FDG injection minimizes FDG uptake by BAT, thus decreasing false-positive findings on FDG-PET and increasing the pool of FDG available for tumor uptake.[70] Other interventions that have been tried to reduce brown fat uptake are keeping the patient warm (safe and least inconvenient for the patient) and administering medications like propranalol, fentanyl, or diazepam.[71,73] Atypical locations of BAT reported are in the posterior neck, axillae, perirenal and retrocrural area, interatrial septum, para-aortic, and upper left paratracheal areas in the mediastinum.[73] It is found in approximately 4% of patients referred for oncologic PET scans.[69]

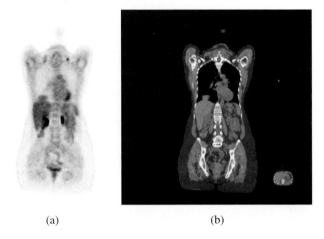

(a)   (b)

Fig. 3.36. (a) Attenuation-corrected FDG-PET coronal whole body image. (b) Corresponding coronal CT image showing upward migration of the liver dome related to respiration creating an isolated nodule like abnormality in the right lower lung. This is an artifact and not focal abnormal lung activity. The companion CT images on a PET/CT study can help identify it as due to a high-riding liver dome related to breathing artifact, as no abnormality is seen in the right lower lung on CT scan. Awareness of this artifact can avoid mistakenly diagnosing the focal FDG activity in the right lower lung as a lung metastasis, especially when only FDG-PET findings are available. Non attenuation-corrected PET images can help resolve this issue on a FDG-PET only study. Supine PET and CT images are acquired without change in position at the same sitting. For the PET and CT image displays and fusion, the anatomic registration of both sets of images should be accurate and the liver should have the same anatomic position and shape during the CT and PET image acquisitions. However, respiratory motion is different for both image acquisitions; in PET, free breathing is mandatory and necessary due to the long time required for PET image acquisition (several minutes per field of view/bed position involving many breathing cycles) which can result in blurring of lower thoracic and upper abdominal areas.[72] CT acquisition using modern CT scanners occurs within a fraction of a breathing cycle; a snapshot freezing an individual respiration point in the attenuation map acquisition is adapted to match this by scanning during free breathing[74] or by timed unforced expiration but neither approach fully eliminates the risk of risk of registration errors between PET and CT. These registration errors introduce artifacts in the hybrid PET/CT since the CT image is used for attenuation correction of the PET images.[72] CT obtained during maximum inspiration cannot be optimally co-registered with PET data as it does not provide an adequate attenuation map for correction of the PET images resulting in severe deterioration of the final image.[74] The resulting artifacts can compromise the clinical interpretation and the quantitative evaluation of PET images.[74] CT scanning during normal expiration yields data that better match the PET emission image than if CT scanning is done during shallow respiration.[74] Hence, a normal breath hold protocol for CT scanning is recommended so that an attenuation map that matches the PET emission image can be obtained without degradation of the final attenuation corrected PET image as long as the patient does not move between the two studies.[74] Anatomic miss-registration errors of the liver in PET/CT may be significant, occurring primarily in the crania-caudal direction, due to breathing differences during the acquisition of PET and CT, with subsequent attenuation corrected artifacts at the diaphragmatic dome. Awareness of this problem and viewing of the non-attenuation corrected images and CT images can help resolve this issue and identify small lesions that may be missed or misplaced on the attenuation-corrected images in the diaphragmatic area of the liver and the lower lung fields.[74]

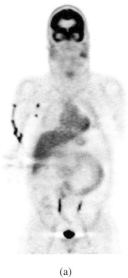

(a)

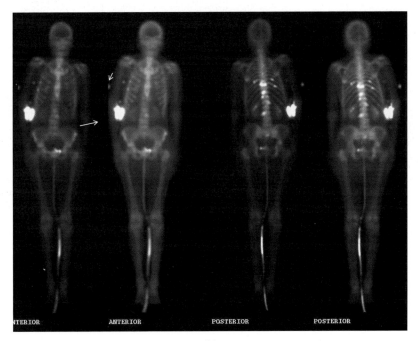

(b)

Fig. 3.37. (*Continued*)

←——

Fig. 3.37. (a) PET scan showing two foci of increased FDG activity in right axilla is likely due to physiologic lymph nodal uptake related to dose infiltration at the injection site due to poor intravenous access. The intense FDG accumulation at the injection site in the right antecubital vein has been blocked by a lead shield although tracer is seen to travel along the lymphatic channel in the right arm. This similar concept is utilized in sentinel lymph node localization in melanoma and breast cancer from subdermal and subcutaneous injection of radiotracer, resulting in movement of radiotracer via the lymphatics into the sentinel nodes. A PET/CT scan can more easily identify the lymph nodal uptake in a physiologic or malignant lymph node. In case of PET-only studies, it can be more easily confused for abnormal lymph nodal activity, especially if one is unfamiliar with this physiologic nodal uptake pattern. In such cases, the non-attenuation corrected PET images can help confirm the physiologic nature of this uptake.
(b) Dose infiltration of Tc-99m MDP at the injection site in right antecubital fosssa on total body bone scan due to poor venous access. However, the bone scan is of diagnostic quality, demonstrating multiple skeletal metastases in spite of the dose infiltration. A small focal area of soft tissue increased activity in the right axilla is presumed to represent physiologic right axillary lymph nodal activity as patient had no history of right axillary lymphadenopathy.

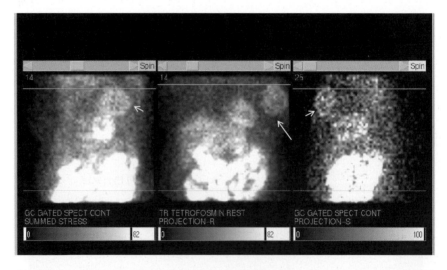

Fig. 3.38. On the stress/rest raw myocardial Tc-99m tetrofosmin same day 10 mCi low-dose/30 mCi high-dose stress myocardial SPECT images shows abnormal soft tissue increased uptake in the patient's known left breast malignancy, resulting in a positive scinti-mammography. This case demonstrates the importance of carefully evaluating the raw images on myocardial SPECT imaging for incidental finding of parathyroid adenoma, breast, lung, and other malignancy or metastasis. Caution should be exercised to avoid mistaking the abnormal breast uptake for left ventricular activity and calling it as a double or piggy-back left ventricle on scan. Although [18F] FDG is the best and most widely used oncologic imaging agent today, various other radionuclides such as Tl 201 Cl, Ga 67citrate, and RP-like Tc 99m DMSA, DTPA, sestamibi, and tetrofosmin, Tc 99m MDP have been reported to concentrate in benign and malignant soft tissue tumors by various mechanisms.[75–80] Tc 99m MIBI breast scinti-mammography can help identify breast malignancy in women with dense breasts and inconclusive mammogram findings, if PET scan is not available.

Chapter 4
Nuclear Medicine in Neurological Disorder

Yu-Keong Kim and Dong-Soo Kim

4.1. Cerebrovascular Disease

Stroke is the third leading cause of death in developed countries. The detection of hemodynamic alteration is important not only in symptomatic patients but also in those with silent stroke and other asympomatic lesions to facilitate patients sub-typing and management. The major role of brain perfusion SPECT in cerebrovascular disease is the assessment of outcome and risk stratification through evaluation of hemodynamic reserve.

4.1.1. Radiopharmaceuticals: Imaging protocol and analysis method

99mTc-labeled hexamethyl propylene amine oxime (HMPAO, Ceretec®) and ethyl cysteinedimer (ECD, Neurolite®) are most widely used as single-photon emission computed tomography (SPECT) agents for imaging of cerebral perfusion. Even though the characteristics of both two compounds are not perfect, they are very close to those for ideal blood flow imaging agents. They easily cross the blood–brain barrier due to lipophilicity and are efficiently extracted by normal brain tissue, and their retention in the brain is long enough to be imaged without significant change after initial regional distribution proportional to regional cerebral blood flow. The kinetic properties of both two compounds are very similar; however, some differences in their uptake and retention mechanism and brain kinetics are characterized in Table 4.1.

For SPECT of the brain, triple- or dual-head gamma cameras equipped with high-resolution collimators (low-energy high-resolution [LEHR] or

Table 4.1. Pharmacokinetics of technetium radiopharmaceuticals for brain perfusion SPECT.

Parameter	^{99m}Tc-HMPAO	^{99m}Tc-ECD
In vitro Characteristics		
Stability	30 min (>4 h with stabilizer)	>6 h
Biologic Characteristics		
Plasma protein binding	Higher extraction	Hydrophilic
First extraction (%)	hydrophilic conversion	conversion by
Retention mechanism	by interaction with glutathion	de-esterification
Brain kinetics		
	2%–3%*	4%–7%
Brain uptake (% I.D)	2 min	2 min
peak brain activity	12%–15% over 15 min	12%–14% the first hour; then
Brain washout		6%/h
	50% liver–gut	15% liver–gut
Excretion (% at 48 h pi)	40% kidneys	75% kidneys
Dosimetry		
	555–1,100 MBq	555–1,100 MBq
injection dose (MBq)	Lachrymal glands	Urinary bladder
Target organs	Gallbladder wall	Gallbladder wall
Imaging		
Recommended imaging time	Upto 4 h p.i.	Up to 2 h p.i.
Ratio of Gray matter to white matter	2–3:1	4:1

low-energy ultrahigh-resolution [LEUHR]) are recommended, which can provide reduced scan time and enhanced image quality. The reconstructed images are usually processed with post-reconstruction filtering and corrected for attenuation.

In most cases of sterno-occlusive cerebrovascular diseases (transient ischemic attack [TIA], stroke, or asymptomatic carotid stenosis) and vascular abnormalities, vasodilatory-challenged perfusion studies are conducted for assessment of vascular perfusion reserve. Acetazolamide (Diamox^{TM}), which is a carboanhydrase inhibitor and leads to an increase in resting cerebral blood flow (rCBF) in normal cerebral vessels dilatation, is commonly used as a vasodilatory stimulator. For assessment of vascular perfusion reserve, two-perfusion SPECT studies (baseline condition and acetazolamide provocation) are required, and the studies can be performed with one-day or two-day protocol according to the condition of each institute (Fig. xx). In a one-day protocol, basal- and acetazolamide-challenged SPECT images are acquired consecutively with the same position using split-dose technique.[1] The acetazolamide stress image can be reconstructed by subtraction from the first scan (basal scan), where the redistribution of ^{99m}Tc-labeled CBF agent in the brain is negligible between the studies. In this case, the positioning error of patient head between the first and the second scan should be prevented, therefore, close cooperation of patient is required for longer imaging time for two consecutive scans. On the other hand, rest and acetazolamide stress images are separately obtained on different day in two-day protocol (Fig. 4.1). This two-day repeat study technique is very simple but has a disadvantage in that patient condition may change.

In the analysis of SPECT images, absolute rCBF measurement has not been fully implemented. Semiquantitative analysis based on the tracer uptake ratios relative to reference region or contralateral hemisphere using region of interest (ROI) is commonly used, which allows an estimation of the relative rCBF distribution. In the calculation of region-to-reference uptake ratios, the selection of the reference region is crucial. The whole brain or the cerebellum is generally used as a reference, however, they do not always represent the best choice because the reference region must have anatomic and functional integrity.

4.1.2. *Normal brain perfusion*

In a normal brain perfusion SPECT, high perfusion is observed in the gray matter including basal ganglia and thalami, and especially in the primary

(a) Two-split day protocol for acetazolamide –challenged brain perfusion SPECT

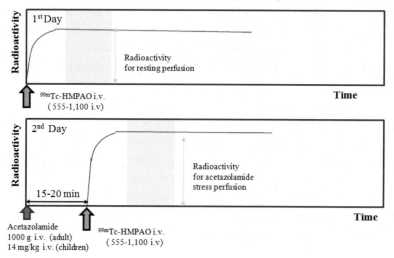

(b) One-day protocol for acetazolamide –challenged brain perfusion SPECT

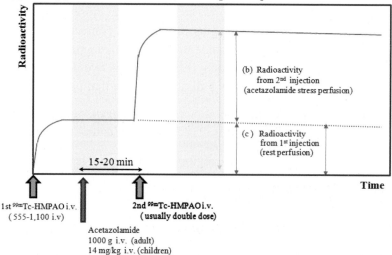

Fig. 4.1. Study protocols for acetazolamide-challenged brain perfusion SPECT.

visual cortex. The global blood flow in an adult is 70–90 mL/min/100 g in the gray matter, and 20–30 mL/min/100 g in the white matter, and around 50–54 mL/min/100 g on average.[2] During development period, absolute cerebral perfusion and regional distribution is changed. Brain perfusion

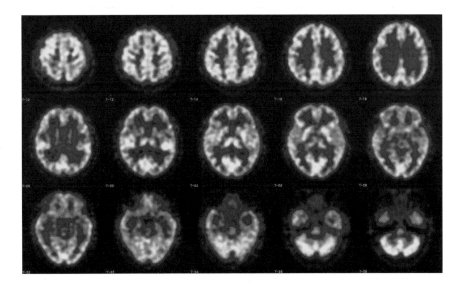

Fig. 4.2. Distribution of normal cerebral blood flow measured by ^{99m}Tc-ECD SPECT.

at birth is globally lower than adulthood and gradually increases to be even higher than that of an adult until the age of 7 years.[3] Afterward, global brain perfusion gradually decreases to be similar to that of an adult at adolescence.[4] Although there are some age-related variations of regional cerebral perfusion, the perfusion patterns are similar between different ages more than 10 years.[5] Meanwhile, it is generally agreed that aging is associated with regional changes in resting blood flow and/or metabolism.[6-8] Most commonly, these changes are a selective reduction of blood flow and metabolism in the frontal and anterior cingulate cortices. Normal brain perfusion SPECT image in an adult is demonstrated in Fig. 4.2.

4.1.3. *Brain perfusion SPECT in cerebrovascular disease*

The anatomic feature of sterno-occlusive carotid artery disease, defined as percent stenosis on angiography, does not always correlate with the hemodynamic significance of the lesion. Cerebrovascular reserve (CVR) or perfusion reserve means the ability of the cerebrovascular system to compensate hemodynamic comprise, in which vasodilation induced by autoregulatory mechanism of cerebral blood vessels as well as collateral circulation all play important roles. When compensation for compromised flow occurs sufficiently, resting rCBF may appear normal or minimally altered even though angiographically evaluated stenosis or obstruction is significant.

Brain perfusion SPECT with acetazolamide may detect perfusion abnormalities that would otherwise be missed even in the presence of a normal baseline perfusion in patients with carotid stenosis. In the early stages of compromised cerebral perfusion, resting CBF is decreases but normalizes after vasodilatory challenge by recruitment of previously mentioned mechanisms. In this stage, the compromised flow is well compensated. When the cerebral hemodynamic status worsens, the decreased CBF either does not change by vasodilatory challenge or is further reduced relative to the area of normal vascularity. In acetazolamide-challenged brain perfusion SPECT, intravenous injection of 1 g acetazolamide produces increases rCBF by 30%–50% above baseline throughout the normally perfused brain within 20–30 min, returning to normal in 2–3 h. In the brain region which is hypoperfused with maximal compensatory vasodilatation, the area shows little or no further vasodilatione to the acetazolamide challenge. Thus, the evaluation of cerebral hemodynamic compromise and rCBV would be beneficial for making treatment decisions regarding medical therapy, surgery, or intervention for revascularization and potentially improve prognosis.

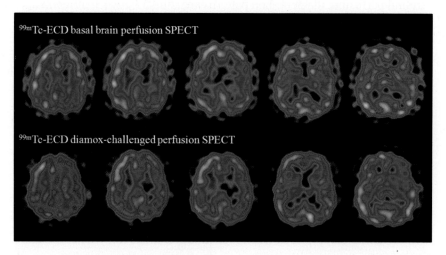

Fig. 4.3. Minimal decreased cerebral perfusion in the left middle cerebral artery territory is observed on basal perfusion SPECT. After diamox challenged, perfusion decrease is profoundly seen.

In acute stroke, rCBF alterations occur earlier and are initially better defined than structural change. Brain SPECT with ^{123}I-iodoamphetamine (^{123}I-IMP), ^{99m}Tc-HMPAO, or ^{99m}Tc-ECD is far superior to anatomic imaging modalities such as CT or MRI in the detection of acute stroke in the first few hours that follow the event. For example, 8 h after infarction, only 20% if CT scans will be positive, while approximately 90% of SPECT rCBF scans will be positive in the same time interval. In particular, SPECT is more sensitive in cortical ischemia or infarction, and the overall sensitivity and specificity are 93%–95% and 98%, respectively.[9,10] False-negative brain SPECT findings in acute stroke may be caused by s or small cortical infarcts. In the sub-acute phase (beyond the first 48 h), SPECT may be even less sensitive because of the presence of spontaneous reperfusion. The early imaging within a few hours after stoke has prognostic implication and is also important for choosing the best candidates for therapy. Acute focal absence of rCBF suggests poor prognosis and unlikely benefit from therapy, decreased but not absent blood flow possibly indicates the best candidates for therapy, and normal or near-normal blood flow indicates patients who do not need.[11] In a study with 458 stroke patients, 97% of those with normal or increased perfusion recovered well, 52% of those with decreased perfusion had a moderate stroke, while, 62% of those with severe perfusion defect had a poor outcome.[12,13]

Usually, perfusion defect on brain SPECT is larger than the lesion that delineated on CT, and they most likely arose from the changes of diaschisis or low flow or as a result of tissue salvage occurring after spontaneous reperfusion. Crossed cerebellar diaschisis (CCD) is frequent in cortical strokes and is caused by disconnection of the cerebellar–corticopontine fibers as a consequence of ischemia or stroke. Diaschisis can also be seen in the overlying cortex in cases of subcortical infarction in the basal ganglia or internal capsule.

Meanwhile, establishment of perfusion status using acetazolamide-challenged perfusion SPECT in chronic sterno-occlusive carotid artery diseases is clinically important. Atherosclerosis and moyamoya disease are the most common cause of chronic sterno-occlusive carotid artery diseases and usually presented as recurrent transient attack or strokes. Usually, the risk of developing acute stroke or recurrent ischemic attack is high in patients with ischemic symptom or a history of transient attack. However, stenosis

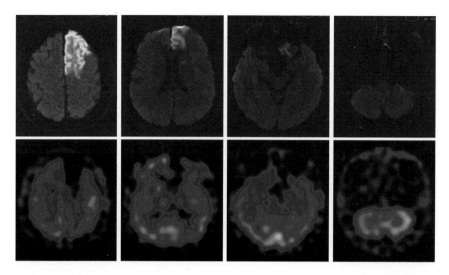

Fig. 4.4. Acute infarction at left medial frontal lobe (ACA territory) and crossed cerebellar dischisis.

can be accidently detected without any symptom of ischemia or infarction. At the time of ischemic attack, a focal or diffuse area of hypoperfusion is typically found. However, after the event of ischemia, resting perfusion may be normal. In some cases, the perfusion defect can persist in the first few days after TIA, which may suggest the high risk of early stroke.[14] The sensitivity of brain SPECT for detection of TIAs is approximately 60% in the first 24 h and declines to approximately 40% in the first week. The sensitivity can be improved significantly with substances that measure CVR using acetazolamide.[1,15]

In Moyamoya disease, as in other chronic steno-occlusive cerebrovascular diseases, the steno-occlusive change in the main cerebral arteries decreases the cerebral perfusion pressure, and collateral circulation maintains CBF, which results in decreases of CBF and CVR in the affected vascular territories. Hemodynamic alteration in symptomatic patients is more severe, and specific symptoms from MMD are related to the specific regions of hemodynamic impairment. Because internal carotid arteries are predominantly affected in moyamoya disease, decreases in rCBF and rCVR are commonly seen in the parietal and frontal cortex and also in the basal ganglia. Sometimes, perfusion defects presenting cerebral infarction in the vascular territory or borderzone areas are demonstrated. Posterior circulation is frequently spared, and hemodynamic alteration in the occipital cortex is usually normal. However, in cases where the posterior circulation is impaired, more severe ischemia is presented due to loss of the source for collateral supply.[16]

In sterno-occlusive cerebrovascular diseases, medical treatment is inappropriate in patients with decreased CBF and CVR, and revascularization surgery or neuroradiologic intervention is recommended.[17] After revascularization, hemodynamic changes can be easily monitored using acetazolamide-challenged brain perfusion SPECT since it easy to perform non-invasively and can be analyzed quantitatively compared with conventional cerebral angiography.[18] Hemodynamic improvement in resting perfusion and CVR can be demonstrated from early after successful revascularization on acetazolamide-stress brain perfusion SPECT. Usually improvement of resting perfusion is more prominent in moyamoya disease than in artherosclerotic occlusive disease. Further improvement of CVR may show up to several months after surgery.[19] Sometimes, transient hyperperfusion in resting perfusion has been shown within several days or a week after revascularization, which usually shows around the site of the anastomosis and returns to normal after a while. Infrequently, transient focal neurological deficit (TND) mimicking ischemic attack may be accompanied without any pathological sign on CT.[20] Preoperative cerebrovascular capacity, severity of ischemia during surgery, and anatomical vascular structures around the site of the anastomosis are known to be related with transient hyperperfusion. Also, patients with more depressed preoperative perfusion and a greater increase in CBF after STA-MCA anastomosis are more prone to suffer from post-bypass TND. Postoperative hemodynamic status measured on acetazolamide-stress SPECT after the completion of the surgery on both hemispheres is closely related to further prognosis. In a study on clinical outcome of MMD patients after revascularization surgery, regional CVR status on postoperative SPECT was the most significant predictor for the symptomatic outcome of patients.[18,21,22] If a patient's CVR was still poor after revascularization surgery, prognosis on symptoms or neurologic deficits was also poor. Therefore, additional surgical intervention is recommended if a patient's hemodynamic status after initial revascularization surgery still shows abnormality.

4.2. SPECT and PET in Epilepsy

Epilepsy is a common chronic neurological disorder that is characterized by recurrent unprovoked seizures and affects approximately 3% of the population during their lifetime.[23] However, significant numbers (20%–30%) of patients with epilepsy continue to have seizure despite treatment with antiepileptic drugs. Epilepsy surgery is considered as a potentially curative option for these patients with medically refractory partial seizures. In pre-surgical evaluation, the most important aspect is to identify a discrete epileptogenic region, which can be resected without causing an unacceptable loss of neurological function and will lead to complete seizure control.

Brain MRI is the best structural imaging study and can well demonstrate epileptogenic lesions. In case of medial temporal lobe epilepsy (mTLE) which is the most common type of epilepsy, hippocampal sclerosis and/or atrophy is well known for pathologic diagnostic criteria, and easily found on MRI. However, despite great progression of imaging technique on MRI, the epileptic focus may not be revealed on MRI in considerable cases (approximately 20%–50% patient with medially refractory epilepsy). Meanwhile, brain perfusion SPECT and FDG-PET, combined with structural MRI and EEG, have been used as diagnostic aids in management of epilepsy. These images suggest epileptic focus by showing functional changes in the brain regions related with epilepsy. These functional abnormalities are frequently accompanied by normal or almost normal CT or MRI scans.

4.2.1. *Brain perfusion SPECT in epilepsy*

Perfusion brain SPECT studies in epilepsy reveal characteristic time-dependent changes in regional cerebral perfusion following a partial seizure. Brain perfusion SPECT is considered as a snapshot of cerebral blood flow at a given time of interest because The Tc-99m–labeled ligands for brain perfusion imaging have a characteristics of rapid extraction and trapping into the neuronal cells in the distribution of blood flow within the first pass after intravenous injection. If the tracer is immediately injected after the start of a seizure, hyperperfusion at the ictal onset zone can be captured, this provides an opportunity to localize an epileptogenic focus. Furthermore, the tracer remains fixed in the brain for several hours, permitting imaging a convenient time after recovery of from ictus. These advantages of are considerable practical value over all other imaging modality.

In earlier studies for ictal perfusion, ^{99m}Tc-ECD had been preferred than ^{99m}Tc-HMPAO because of its advantage of rapid injection at the time of ictus with long shelf stability after labeling. But now, both ^{99m}Tc-HMPAO and ^{99m}Tc-ECD have been most commonly used since after stabilized forms of ^{99m}Tc-HMPAO have become available. And the diagnostic performances of both two compounds are similar in TLE. In cases of neocortical epilepsy, however, ^{99m}Tc-HMPAO ictal SPECT may be superior to ^{99m}Tc-ECD ictal SPECT in sensitivity. And ictal hyperperfusion seems to be greater for ^{99m}Tc-HMPAO SPECT than ^{99m}Tc-ECD SPECT. This difference may result from different tracer kinetics in the brain.

Ictal SPECT studies always require video-EEG monitoring, and the timing of the injection is extremely important. Ictal SPECT has a limited temporal resolution of ictal SPECT considering rapid evolving seizure activities, which often make some difficulties in reliable interpretation of ictal SPECT. Ictal brain perfusion image may reflect not only the hyperperfusion in the ictal onset zone, but also peri-ictal propagation of seizure activity. Successful ictal SPECT study has been considered when the injection is performed within 45 sec of seizure onset on EEG. Injections within less than 20 sec clearly showed a higher rate of correct localization. If the radioligand is injected during the earlier part of a seizure, ictal propagation might be limited to structures surrounding the epileptogenic focus and subsequent ictal hyperperfusion might also be limited to this area. Furthermore, it is important to be aware of propagation patterns when interpreting ictal perfusion brain SPECT studies and thus to have knowledge of the moment of tracer injection relative to the start of the seizure, the type of seizure, and the ictal EEG recording. Generally, it is assumed that the brain regions showing most intense and largest hyperperfusion in ictal SPECT represents the seizure focus (Fig. 4.5). In TLE, ictal SPECT shows striking hyperperfusion in more than 90% of cases.[24] And the pattern of hyperperfusion is also clearly identified, in which propagation of seizure activity to the contralateral temporal lobe and ipsilatera linsula, basal ganglia, and frontal lobe often occurs; propagation to the parieto-occipital region has also been described. In particular, isilateral or bilateral hyperperfusion in the basal ganglia during seizure

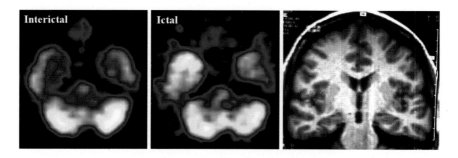

Fig. 4.5. A typical interictal/ictal perfusion SPECT of medial temporal lobe epilepsy.

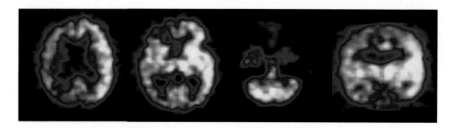

Fig. 4.6. Ictal propagation in left temporal lobe epilepsy. In addition to the ictal hyperperfusion in the epileptogenic temporal lobe, hyperperfusion is extended to the ipsilateral frontal, parietal cortex, and subcortical structures. Also, hyperperfusion in the cerebellum contralateral side of epileptic focus is seen as crossed cerebellar hyperperfusion.

correlates with upper limb dystonia.[25] In the cerebellum, crossed cerebellar hyperperfusion (CCH) in which the cerebellar hemisphere contralateral to the epileptic focus shows increased blood flow during ictal status. CCH can be found to occur in as few as 33% of patients with partial epilepsy or in as many as 100% (Fig. 4.6).

Beyond the temporal lobes (neocortical epilepsy), ictal SPECT has also been reported to be able to localize seizure foci in the frontal, parietal, and occipital lobes (Fig. 4.13, neocortical epilepsy in brain SPECT).[26,27] In cases of neocortical epilepsy, seizure activity is frequently brief and may spread very rapidly, leading to the possibility of ambiguous ictal blood flow changes. In fact, the changes may be misleading if an area of brain remote from the seizure onset zone takes over as the main generator of seizure activity. Delayed injection of the tracer within 2 to 15 min of ictal onset may demonstrate postictal perfusion abnormalties, which has been also used to identify epileptic zones. However, post-ictal perfusion abnormalties can be seen as a long-lasting ictal hyperperfusion.[28]

For localization of epileptic focus, it is generally agreed that ictal SPECT is more sensitive than FDG-PET, which is usually obtained during interictal period. Interictal SPECT is also helpful for detection of epileptic foci, which may provide hypoperfusion at seizure focus. However, interictal SPECT perfusion imaging itself seems to be inefficient in localizing the seizure onset zone. According to the meta-analytic analytic sensitivities from 30 studies in localization of epileptic focus in patients with TLE,[29] the sensitivity of interictal SPECT is only 0.44, whereas the sensitivity of ictal SPECT is 0.97. Therefore, interictal SPECT is commonly used as a baseline perfusion measure in the comparison of ictal perfusion images, and the accuracy of ictal SPECT analysis may be increased when compared with interictal perfusion data.

Detection of focal hyperperfusion change, which may indicate potential sites for ictal on set, has been evaluated by visual assessment of ictal SPECT or side-by-side visual comparison of ictal and interictal SPECT. However, traditional side-by-side visual comparisons of interictal and ictal images may be difficult because of differences in the overall intensities of the two images or differences in slice level and orientation. Recently, computer-aided image analysis techniques, such as subtraction ictal SPECT coregistered to MRI (SISCOM), ictal–interictal SPECT analyzed by SPM (ISAS), or statistical ictal SPECT coregistered to MRI (STATISCOM), are used to improvement the reliability of SPECT findings in seizure focus localization.[30–34] These analytic methods are fast, accurate, and routinely available. Furthermore, these methods are more sensitive and specific in the detection of the epileptic onset zone than visual assessment and provide objective ways to study individual propagation patterns, especially in extratemporal epilepsies and when fast seizure propagation after an early tracer injection is present.

In SISCOM analysis, image digital subtraction of an interictal scan from an ictal scan, and then coregistration to MRI anatomic images. Subtraction techniques allow comparison with the patient's individual baseline pattern of rCBF variability, and subsequently, detection of changes in blood flow which may be reflective not of an absolute increase but of a relative one from an interictal state of focal relative hypoperfusion. Furthermore, with coregistration to MRI, anatomical detail is provided for precise localization that is not possible with relatively low-resolution SPECT.

Further improvement in sensitivity, specificity, and reliable interpretation of ictal perfusion may be achieved by the use of SPM analysis. In early trials of SPM analysis, an ictal SPECT from a patient was compared with a normal brain SPECT atlas using SPM to identify regions of statistically significant alterations in rCBF related to seizure activity. A few studies support SPM analysis of ictal SPECT scans.[35] Further refinement of SPM-ictal SPECT methodology has been shown in a methodological pilot study to identify ictal increases in rCBF from subtraction images.[30,33] In this work, the use of pairs of sequential interictal images from epilepsy patients and controls to define a *standard deviation image* is included so that regional variance between scan pairs could be taken into account to improve sensitivity. More recently, pairs of scans for the controls are included in the analysis, which is allowed to assess interscan variability and has the advantage of subtraction analysis and combined it with the inherent objectivity of SPM analysis. STATISCOM, which is lately developed SPM analysis of ictal–interictal differences combined with SISCOM, permits the localization of increased and decreased rCBF in the patient's anatomy as a result of reverse registration. A recent study shows a great performance of STATISCOM in localization of an abnormal focus in TLE patients with nonlesional MRI, in which correct localization rate are almost twice that of SISCOM (80% versus 47%). Careful quality control of registration (e.g., assessment of acquisition movement artifacts, registration errors) and subtraction is important in using these analytical methods to avoid false-positive and false-negative results. Generally, subtraction methods provide concordant results with superior sensitivity in comparison with visual assessment for localizing of epileptic focus. However, SISCOM may provide false-negative results if the sub-clinical seizure activity existed at the moment of tracer injection of interictal SPECT imaging.[16] EEG monitoring during the interictal injection, therefore, should be routinely performed.

4.2.2. *FDG-PET in epilepsy*

FDG-PET is the most established functional imaging modality in the evaluation of patients with epilepsy. In contrast to perfusion SPECT, FDG-PET

Interictal [99mTc]HMPAO SPECT

Ictal [99mTc]HMPAO SPECT

Ictal-Interictal Subtraction

SPM analysis (comparison with healthy controls)

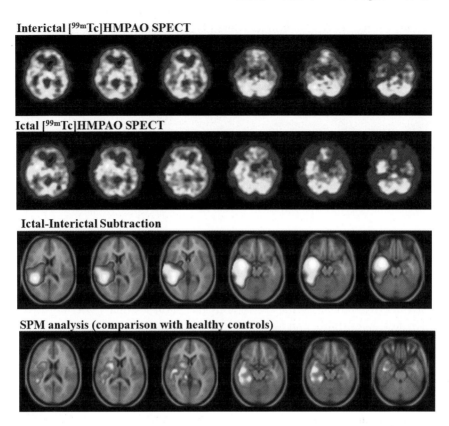

Fig. 4.7. Detection of hyperperfusion as an epileptogenic focus using subration and SPM analysis.

studies during ictal period are not practical because of the long duration for steady-state uptake of FDG, which often leads to scans that contain a difficult-to-interpret mixture of interictal, ictal, and post-ictal states. Thus, pre-surgical epilepsy FDG-PET scans are typically performed in the interictal state with the goal of detecting focal areas of decreased metabolism, relative *hypometabolism,* that are presumed to reflect focal functional disturbances of cerebral activity associated with epileptogenic tissue. FDG-PET may provide localized information independent of that provided by MRI.

The classic pattern for FDG-PET in mTLE (without lesions other than mesial temporal sclerosis) reveals relative hypometabolism in mesial-temporal, temporal-polar, and anterolateral-temporal neocortical regions

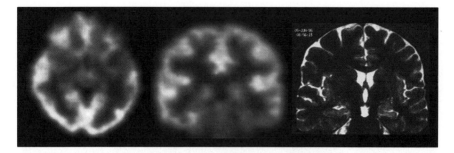

Fig. 4.8. A typical FDG-PET finding of temporal lobe epilepsy. Hypometabolism in the left temporal lobe is examined. On T_2-MRI, hippocampal sclerosis is observed in the left side.

(Fig. 4.8). The typical sensitivity of FDG PET for detecting temporal lobehypometabolism in mesial temporal lobe epilepsy (mTLE) ranges between 80% and 90%.[36-40] If structural lesions are present in brain MRI, the presence of hypometabolism at the lesion is almost 100%. FDG-PET also effectively localizes the epileptic focus in non-lesional (MRI-negative) medial temporal lobe epilepsy.[38,40] When more imaging modalities agree with respect to the seizure focus, an excellent surgical outcome is generally expected. However, in case of non-lesional TLE, good post-surgical outcomes can be also expected if hypometabolism is present in the ipsilateral temporal lobe.[42-45]

However, the functional abnormality, hypometabolism on FDG, is generally larger than the structural lesion. In cases of TLE, hypometabolism is often extended far beyond the temporal lobe, both contiguously in adjacent cortex and to remote subcortical and cortical areas (Fig. 4.9).[46-48] The mechanism of extratemporal hypometabolism remains unclear, although it has been suggested that propagation of seizures beyond the temporal lobe may cause hypometabolism in extratemporal regions. For instance, remote hypometabolism is the most commonly found in the frontal cortex which is the preferential route of seizure propagation in TLE.[49,50] Lateral temporal hypometabolism is thought to result from repeated seizures spreading to the temporal neocortex.[51] Furthermore, the presence of extratemporal hypometabolism as well as severity of hypometabolism in epileptogenic temporal cortex has been thought to be related with seizure duration and the postsurgical seizure outcome {Muzik, 2000 #17}.[44,48,52-54] With longer epilepsy duration, hypometabolism in the epileptogenic temporal

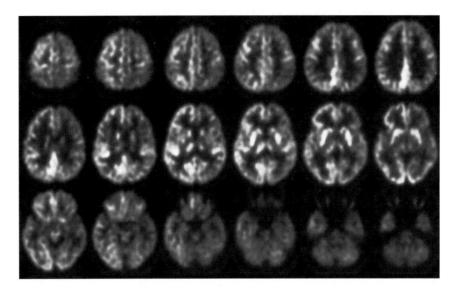

Fig. 4.9. Extratemporal hypometabolism in a patients with left temporal lobe epilepsy. Decreased metabolism in the adjacent temporal area and ipsilateral frontal, parietal cortex is observed.

cortex increases and may extend to the neighboring cortical regions beyond of epileptogenic temporal cortex.[47] The presence of extratemporal hypometabolism in the basal ganglia, thalamus, or remote cortical areas of the ipsilateral frontal, parietal, or contralateral temporal cortices seems to be associated with poor outcome.[54–56] However, this association seems to be contrary in some studies, and the studies could not demonstrated the significant relationship between the extratemporal hypometabolism and surgical outcome.[57–59]

Meanwhile, the alteration of cerebral glucose metabolism in the extratemporal areas is thought to be related to neuropsychological deficits. Based on neuropsychological test studies, it has been suggested that patients with TLE exhibited frontal dysfunction in addition to the dysfunction of temporal epileptogenic zone. Memory deficits seem to be related with the side of seizure focus, and the frontal dysfunction is frequently seen in patients with asymmetric hypometabolism in the frontal lobe.[53] Cognitive outcome, including verbal memory and changes in glucose metabolism, seem to depend on type of surgery. If basal temporal language area is spared with limited resection, improved memory function is usually expected regardless of the resected side, accompanied by metabolic improvement in the adjacent temporal cortex and remote areas.[50,53,60] These results indicate that a decrease in the epileptic activity emanating from the seizure focus in temporal lobe improved the interictal cerebral glucose metabolism in a wide range of projection areas. However, in cases of anterior temporal lobe was resected, regional metabolism in remote areas such as the basal ganglia, thalamus, fusiform gyrus, ligual gyrus, and post insular cortex would be decreased compared with preoperative study. This may be a result of differentiation following the resection of anterior temporal structure.[61,62]

In neocortical epilepsy beyond TLE, the clinical value of FDG-PET in neocortical epilepsy is less clear. The sensitivity of FDG PET in neocortical epilepsy is lower than in TLE, and reported sensitivity is about 30%–60%. Hypometabolic regions are often associated with structural imaging abnormalities including tumors and vascular abnormalities. Advanced MRI technology such as MR spectrometry and diffusion tensor images increase the MR detectabiliy of epileptic focus, thus the role of FDG PET in pre-surgical evaluation may seem to be reduced. However, in most FDG-PET studies in neocortical epilepsy, smaller number of study patients was included, and the etiology and location of the seizure were quite heterogeneous unlike TLE, therefore the localization accuracy of FDG PET may not be rightly justified. Nevertheless, several studies still provide favorable results in the lateralization or localization of epileptic focus in neocortical epilepsy using FDG-PET, which may provide localization information that is independent of that provided by MRI. This is important in patients with a normal MIR in whom the PET findings are critical to allowing that patient precede to surgery. Furthermore, the information of FDG PET is thought to be prognostic of the patient's seizure outcome. Therefore, FDG PET remains an essential imaging modality for presurgical evaluation of refractory neorcortical epilepsies, especially in non-lesional neocortical epilepsy.

In neocortical epilepsy, cortical dysplasia, including microdysgenesis, is one of the common findings during pathologic examination. It has been reported that in patients with focal cortical dysplasia, cortical hypometabolism of the lesion was revealed on FDG-PET in 88% cases, in which the extent of the cortical abnormality was larger on PET than on MRI in 65% cases.[63] In particular, some focal cortical dysplasia undetected on

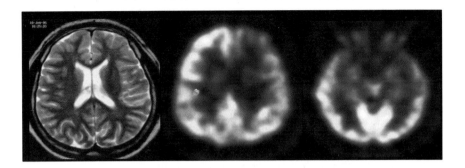

Fig. 4.10. A typical case of cryptogenic frontal lobe epilepsy.

MRI can be detected with FDG-PET. Figure 4.10 shows a representative image of FDG-PET detection of a focal metabolic defect associated with a cryptogenic epileptogenic lesion involved in the left frontal cortex. The detection rate for hypometabolism in the non-lesional neocortical epilepsy with FDG PET is reported as 30%–50%. A study involving 462 cases showed that 32% of normal MRIs were associated with abnormal findings.[64] FDG-PET also indicated hypometabolism in 12 of 13 FLT children with normal MRI who had pathologic diagnoses of microdysgenesis.[64] In a study including 72 patients with non-lesional neocortical epilepsy, FDG-PET localized the epileptic lobe in 29 patients (35%), and the study showed that FDG-PET localization was significantly related to seizure-free surgical outcome.

Generally, multimodal diagnostic approaches and invasive studies are required in pre-surgical evaluation of neocortical epilepsy because any single modality cannot achieve the sufficient diagnostic performance in neocortical cortex. Concordant results among the diagnostic modalities, especially with a visible abnormality on MRI, may lead to an expectation of a good surgical outcome.[65] However, if the results are discordant, or no lesion was found on MRI, presence of localized hypometabolism indicating seizure focus is significantly related to a good surgical outcome regardless of presence of structural lesion on MRI.

Similar to interpretation of ictal SPECT, several analytical methods have been adopted to improve the accuracy of FDG-PET in detection of metabolic abnormalities corresponding to seizure focus. SPM is particularly widely used.[40,44,48,67,68] Added to the SPM analysis, several parcellation techniques providing standard region of interests as structural or functional units allow the quantification of regional metabolism in specific regions and measurement of asymmetry in regional metabolism.[40,68,69] Since bilateral temporal hypometabolism is not uncommon in TLE, evaluation of metabolic asymmetry based on SPM and ROI analysis is also useful in localization of seizure focus in TLE.[39,66] Such analytical methods also provide more subjective information regarding the extent of hypometabolism and patterns of propagation and further perspective analysis related to the prognosis of the patients with epilepsy after surgery. (Fig. 4.11).[44,48,49,69,70]

SPM analysis has been also tried in the localization of the epileptogenic lobe in some patients with neocortical epilepsy (especially frontal lobe epilepsy) whose hypometabolic area is not clearly discernible visually. A study including 29 frontal lobe epilepsy patients (normal MRI in 15 patients) demonstrated that the sensitivity of SPM analysis provided superior in detection of epileptogenic lobe in cases with non-lesional epilepsy compared with visual interpretation.[71] In another study comprising 38 patients with suspected FLT, SPM results provided a better concordance with the results of surface EEG monitoring compared with visual scan analysis.[72] Although not all SPM analyses provide statistically improved

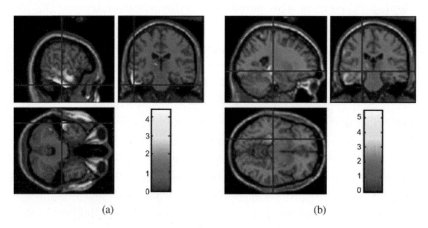

(a)   (b)

Fig. 4.11. Statistical parametric map used to examine the correlation with epilepsy duration independently for mTLE and nTLE subgroups: glucose hypometabolism (shown in red) is seen in the epileptogenic temporal cortex with increasing epilepsy duration in patients with (a) nTLE and (b) mTLE. The number of voxels remained above the threshold, indicating decreased metabolic activity in the epileptogenic temporal cortex. The SPM results are superimposed onto the realigned MRI data to demonstrate temporal lobe hypometabolism.[49]

sensitivity compared with visual analysis, SPM analysis for such a clinical utility offers improvement in accuracy and confidence of diagnostic imaging by eliminating some of the subjectivity and expertise required with visual analysis.[56]

4.3. Dementia

As the prevalence of dementia is expected to increase dramatically, accurate diagnosis is extremely important, particularly at the early and mild stages of dementia when treatment effects would be most effective. Furthermore, increasing attention has been devoted to patients with mild cognitive impairment (MCI), which is considered a prodromal condition to dementia. Use of FDG-PET, which can demonstrate the regional distribution of the rate of glucose metabolism, is increasingly used to support the clinical diagnosis of dementia. The ability to diagnose AD early in its course, non-invasively and reliably with PET, will have significant impact in field of medicine and treatment costs since the magnitude of the health problem resulting from dementing illnesses is great in terms of medical practice, economics, and family hardship.

In management of patients with symptom of dementia, conventional brain imaging using MRI or CT may be useful for identifying unsuspected clinically significant lesions, which can be present in approximately 5% of patients. However, in patients with AD, such scans are typically read as showing normal findings, as demonstrating the non-specific finding of cortical atrophy which overlaps with results seen in normal elderly, or as revealing ischemic changes that are (mis)interpreted as pointing to cerebrovascular disease as the primary or sole cause of the patient's. The ability of FDG-PET to view characteristic changes in metabolic activity in dementia is critical to imaging the disease, since these changes are too microscopic to appear on a structural level. By the time a patient presents with clinical symptoms of dementia, decreases in cerebral glucose metabolism have occurred that are detectable on $[^{18}F]$FDG-PET scans as specific patterns of regional hypometabolism as compared with age-matched healthy elderly individuals.

FDG-PET can be used for three major purposes in management of patients with dementia. First, it is a non-invasive tool to help establish an early diagnosis. Second, it is useful in determining differential diagnoses, for example, distinguishing Alzheimer's disease from other dementia disorders such as vascular dementia and identifying coexisting conditions. Finally, we may use it to evaluate response to therapy — observing whether a patient benefits from a particular medication or treatment.

4.3.1. *Alzheimer's disease and mild cognitive impairment*

Alzheimer's disease (AD) is a leading cause of neurodegenerative dementia and accounts for approximately 60%–70% cases of dementia. AD is characterized by a progressive, global, and irreversible deterioration of cognitive function, which usually begins with memory problems, followed by deficits in language, mathematical, and visuospatial skills, abstract thinking, and planning, as well as personality and behavioral changes.

FDG-PET shows a characteristic pattern of metabolic impairment in AD, which is typically seen in the posterior cingulate cortex and parietotemporal association cortices and often is bilateral (Fig. 1). In addition, the medial temporal lobes, particularly the hippocampus, are also hypometabolic in AD. These characteristic findings of metabolic impairment can be seen even in pre-symptomatic people at high genetic risk for AD as well as MCI.[73–79] FDG-PET with characteristic findings offers an average sensitivity of 95% (range 90%–96%) and specificity of 71% (range 67%–97%) in diagnosis of AD. However, the hypometabolism in the medial temporal lobe seems to be less sensitive in early AD.[80,81] This may be contradictory to that the hippocampal atrophy is a major finding on MRI in AD, and possibly associated with functional compensation for local neurologncal damage or entorhinal disconnection occurring during the early process of AD.[80,81]

The hypometabolism on FDG-PET in patient with AD is progressive and correlated with dementia severity[74] and predict subsequent clinical decline. The areas of cortical involvement with hypometabolism are expand as the disease progresses. In early stage of the disease, regional metabolism in the frontal cortex may be still preserved. In advanced disease, decreased metabolism is found in the frontal cortex, but the primary sensorimotor cortices and primary visual cortex are typically spared from hypometabolism until late stages of the disease, corresponding to the preserved brain functions associated with these regions(Fig. 4.12, FDG-PET in AD). However,

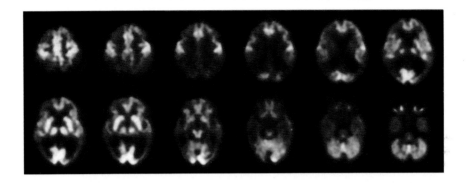

Fig. 4.12. A typical finding of FDG PET in a patient with Alzheimer's disease.

some AD patients occasionally show frontal lobe dysfunctions in the early stage that are known to emerge only at advanced stage, whereas typical AD patients at early stage present memory decline and impairments of language and visuospatial functions.[82] This subtype of AD is called frontal variant of AD. In these patients, hypometabolism in frontal cortex as well as temporoparietal regions may be shown on FDG-PET scans. Visual variant of AD with prominent visual symptoms and metabolic impairment in occipital cortex has also been reported.

Thalamus has been known to be relatively unaffected in FDG PET findings,[84] which is inconsistent with current understandings of AD pathology. Cerebellar metabolism is relatively preserved in mild to moderate AD. In later phase of AD, a significant reduction in cerebellar glucose metabolism without evidence of cerebellar atrophy has been reported.[13] In a recent study of 12-month follow-up with FDG-PET, the brain region showing metabolic declines and spared regions from metabolic declines have been statistically determined from large AD and MCI cohorts. Longitudinal studies showed well-demonstrated patterns of cerebral metabolic changes in disease progression on FDG-PET (Fig. 4.13).[15]

The degree of hypometabolism at the initial diagnosis of AD is associated with several factors such as severity of illness, genetic factors, age, and the level of education. General cognitive ability measured by mini-mental status examination (MMSE) or clinical dementia rating (CDR) is correlated with cerebral metabolism, in particular, in the parietal and temporal association cortex.[87–89] In particular, memory impairment which is most

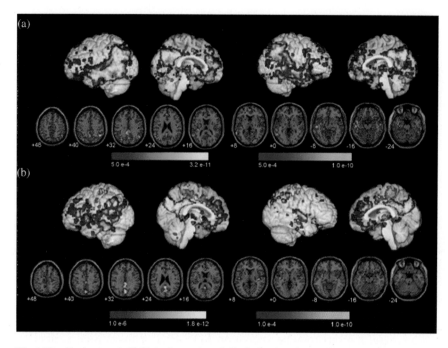

Fig. 4.13. Twelve-month CMRglc change (metabolic decline in red-to-yellow color scale, and spared decline in blue-to-green color scale) in probable AD (a) and MCI patients (b).[86]

commonly complained by patients in early AD is correlated with the degree of metabolic impairment in the limbic cortex as well as parieto-temporal cortex. The epsilon 4(ε4) allele of the apolipoprotein E (ApoE) gene, which is known as a major genetic risk factor for AD, has been demonstrated to have the metabolic interaction in the several FDG PET studies.[90–92] The ε4 allele regionally affects brain metabolism leading to a more generalized metabolic impairment in regions of the posterior cingulate, precuneus, parietotemporal, and frontal regions for AD patients in a dose-dependent fashion. This is the same in cognitively normal ε4 carriers even with at least a single copy of the ε4 allele by showing low metabolism in the same regions as patients with the clinical diagnosis of AD. Age of onset is one of the factors affecting metabolic impairment in AD. Greater metabolic dysfunction in the parietotemporal and posterior cingulate areas is generally observed in early onset AD relatively to late onset AD.[88] Furthermore, additional metabolic impairment in the thalamus can be found in early AD, where the metabolism is usually unaffected in early AD.[93] Meanwhile, it has been demonstrated that higher education is associated with more severe metabolic impairment in patients with Alzheimer's disease on FDG-PET, controlling for age and disease severity. The differences in the degree of metabolic impairment at the time of initial presentation of AD may support the hypothesis of cognitive reserve capacity. In the hypothesis, cognitive reserve capacity refers to the ability to compensate for reduced cognitive function by neurodegeneration; education and lifestyle may actually provide the increase threshold for the emergence of the clinical features of AD would be increased despite advancing brain damage in the pathology. However, metabolic impairment measured by FDG-PET at initial diagnosis can reveal the advanced pathologic changes and would predict the outcome of the progression of the disease.

Meanwhile, the ability of FDG-PET showing early demonstration of metabolic impairment is particularly important to predict the disease outcome in MCI, of which about 10%–30% are progressed and newly diagnosed as AD in a year. In MCI patients, it has been demonstrated that similar patterns of FDG-PET hypometabolism in posterior cingulated, precuneus, parieto-temporal association cortex are exhibited in several studies, although the magnitude and spatial extent of hypometabolism was lesser than those in AD patients. And the hypometabolism in the medial temporal lobe is not significant, which is similar in very early AD. Furthermore, this characteristic finding of FDG-PET can accurately predict the conversion of AD in MCI.[87,94–96] The first noting the predictive power of posterior cingulate metabolism in patients with severe memory deficits for predicting progression was performed by Minoshima *et al.* in 1997.[87] A recent large cohort study also demonstrated the powerful prediction ability of FDG-PET (91% sensitivity and 80% specificity), in which more extensive hypometabolism was demonstrated in MCI subjects who converted to AD by 1 year than in MCI subjects who continued to be classified on clinical grounds as MCI, with correlation between the extent of abnormal hypometabolism and timing of conversion to AD.[97] Furthermore, this study demonstrated the excellent prediction power of FDG-PET regardless of the presence of the common neuropsychological comorbidities in elderly (e.g., depression, thyroid). FDG-PET seems to be superior to ApoE ε4 testing[98] in prediction of conversion to AD in MCI. Normal FDG PET in MCI indicates a low chance of progression within one year,

135

even if there is a severe memory deficit on neuropsychological testing.[99] In a meta-analysis, positive prediction power of FDG-PET with typical metabolic patterns of AD is approximately 89% in progression of MCI to AD, whereas the negative predictive value is 84.9%.[100] Confirmation of such results is likely to lead to greater clinical use of FDG-PET in evaluation of MCI patients.

4.3.2. *FDG-PET in differential diagnosis of dementia*

Several studies provided evidence for distinctive patterns of metabolic abnormalities to distinguish AD from other dementias. The first published series of dementia patients who underwent both PET and autopsy of the brain comprised 22 cases.[101] FDG-PET scans were visually graded for the presence of bilateral parieto-temporal hypometabolism. PET evaluations correctly identified AD in 79% of the cases and non-AD in 88% of the cases.[101]

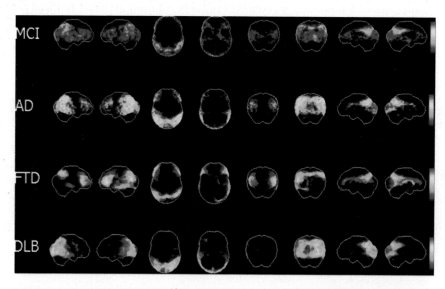

Fig. 4.14. Representative cortical [^{18}F] FDG-PET patterns in NL, AD, DLB, and FTD. Three-dimensional SSP maps and corresponding Z scores showing CMRglc reductions in clinical groups as compared with the NL database are displayed on a color-coded scale ranging from 0 (black) to 10. From left to right: 3D-SSP maps are shown on the right and left lateral, superior and inferior, anterior and posterior, and right and left middle views of a standardized brain image.[110]

DLB, the second most common cause of degenerative dementia in the elderly, is clinically characterized by the progressive cognitive decline with fluctuations in cognition and alertness, recurrent visual hallucinations, and Parkinsonism. The disorder shares clinical and pathological features with both AD and PD and is frequently misdiagnosed as AD. The metabolic patterns of DLB similarly display widespread cerebral hypometabolism with marked decreases in association cortices and relative sparing of subcortical structures and primary somatomotor cortex. But unlike AD, hypometabolism also affects the primary visual cortex and occipital association cortex (Brodmann Areas 17,18).[102–106] With this characteristic finding of FDG-PET, the overall sensitivity and specificity in differential diagnosis between DLB and AD are reported as about 90% and 80%, respectively.

In DLB, presence of visual hallucination is associated with metabolic impairment of visual association cortex rather than the primary visual cortex. Moreover, relative metabolic reductions in hallucinating patients with DLB as compared with non-hallucinating patients were found at the visual right temporo-occipital junction,[108] and the right middle frontal gyrus in some reports.[107] These brain regions are known to participate in the processing of visual stimuli, and they have been linked to visual hallucination in other neurodegenerative conditions such as Parkinson's disease.

Meanwhile, frontotemporal dementia (FTD) is a group of related conditions resulting from the progressive degeneration of the temporal and frontal lobes of the brain. It has a relatively earlier disease onset, therefore it has been the second most common type of dementia presented in patients

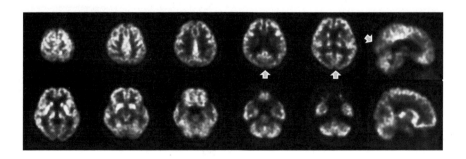

Fig. 4.15. A representative FDG-PET image in a patient with DLB.

137

younger than 65 years. In clinical practice, the diagnosis of FTD relies on observations from the patient's relatives and on identifying typical signs and symptoms. FTD is usually presented as progressive decline in behavior or language-associated degeneration of the frontal and anterior temporal lobes. Sometimes FTD patients may also have difficulty in walking, rigidity, tremor, or muscle weakness. Due to the symptoms, FTD can be mistaken for Alzheimer's disease, Parkinson's disease, or a primarily psychiatric disorder such as depression, manic depression, obsessive-compulsive disease, or schizophrenia. In cases of FTD, cognitive impairment is not prominent in early stage, however, it has rapid progression in compared with other neurodegenerative dementia, and moreover the treatment of anti-cholinesterase is less effective with FTD in contrast to AD. In particular, it tends to have a strong hereditary so that up to 40% of FTD patients have a history that is suggestive of familial transmission, with roughly 10% of patients showing an autosomal dominant inheritance pattern.

On structural MRI, cortical atrophy in the frontal and temporal lobes is often examined.[108,109] PET and SPECT studies have consistently shown anterior distribution of functional impairment in FTD. Reductions in glucose metabolism and blood flow in the frontal and anterior temporal cortices with frequent asymmetric patterns are observed.[109] Occasionally, metabolic or flow reduction in the striatum and thalamus has been observed.[110] Although the metabolic impairment is accentuated in the frontal lobes and anterior temporal lobes, the involvement of the parietal region is also noted by FDG-PET, and parietal pathological involvement has been recognized in post-mortem studies of patients with advanced FTD. FDG PET could

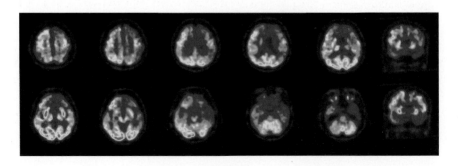

Fig. 4.16.   FDG-PET in a patient with FTD.

improve the diagnostic accuracy of subjects with dementia. Characteristic FTD pattern of hypometabolism on FDG-PET can differentiate AD and frontotemporal dementia, showing specificity of more than 97%.[112] However, frontal hypometabolism can be observed in other neurodegenerative disease such as progressive supranuclear palsy (PSP), spinocerebellar ataxia, or dementia induced by drug addiction. The FTD pattern of hypometabolism can be observed in some cases of AD, so that about 10% of clinically diagnosed AD patients clearly have an FTD pattern of hypometabolism in the frontal cortex.

4.3.3. *Amyloid plaque imaging in AD*

Confirmation of the clinical diagnosis of AD is based on the detection of amyloidplaques and neurofibrillary tangles in the brain. However, such measures, until recently, could only be done post-mortem. However, recent developments in radiotracers may now allow for the measurement of amyloid plaques and neurofibrillary tangles in the brain *in vivo*. The first *in vivo* imaging of AD pathology in living patients with AD was successfully conducted with [^{18}F] FDDNP (2-(I-{6-[2-[^{18}F]fluoroethyl]-(methyl)-amino}-2-napthyl)ethylene)malononitrile), which binds to the plaque and tangles. To date, [^{11}C]-labeled 6-OH-BTA (N-methyl-]2-(4'-methylaminophenyl)-6-hydroxybenzothiazole (6-OH-BTA), also known as Pittsburgh Compound B or PIB, has been most widely used in research studies with encouraging results. However, short half-life of [^{11}C] may limit the use of amyloid imaging in community-based diagnosis. Recently, several amyloid imaging agents labeled with [^{18}F] such as Flobetapir ([^{18}F]AV-45) and [^{18}F] Flutemetamol have been successfully tested in clinical trials, and begin to emerge.[113–117]

In Alzheimer's disease patients, cortical PIB retention is notably detected in the posterior cingulate/precuneus, medial inferior frontal cortex, and lateral temporal cortex, with sparing of sensorimotor areas and occipital cortex (Fig. 4.17). The neocortical PIB retention is also increased in the stage of early AD, supporting the fact that amyloid retention in the brain is an earlier pathologic process preceding metabolic changes. Interestingly, PIB retention is relatively spared in the hippocampus, amygdala, and parahippocampus compared with cortical association areas in AD, and the finding

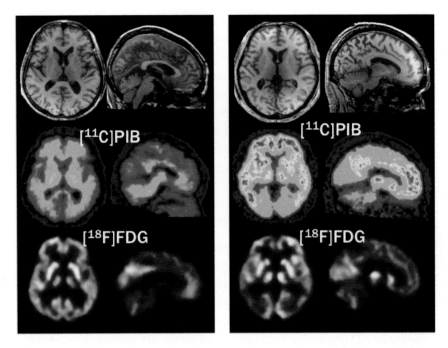

Fig. 4.17. Cortical PIB retention in posterior cingulated, medial inferior frontal cortex, and lateral temporal cortex in Alzheimer's disease.

is consistent that the hippocampus is spared from amyloid pathology at early stage of AD [45]. But, [^{18}F]FDDNP-PET has a high specific uptake in these structures,[118,119] which may result from the different binding affinity to neurofibrillary tangle, which is more abundant pathology in hippocampus in AD.

In quantitative analysis of [^{11}C] PIB-PET, cortical to cerebellar ratio for distribution volume (DVR; distribution volume ratio), or standard uptake value (SUVr: SUV ratio) are frequently used as quantitative parameters since cerebellum shows little PIB retention in AD as well as healthy controls.[120,121] Generally, a PIB-positive result is considered when the region to cerebellar ratio exceeds 1.4–1.5. A PIB-positive result can be detected in 89%–95% of patients with clinically diagnosed AD, while PIB-negative result can be observed in 10%–20% of patients with clinically diagnosed AD. This PIB-negative result in AD may be caused by not only failure of PIB in detection of amyloid deposits, but also a possibility of inaccurate clinical diagnosis, considering typical accuracy of clinical diagnosis is around 85%–90% compared with post-mortem histopathological diagnosis.[122,123]

Meanwhile, amyloid retention may be observed in cognitive healthy elderly. The frequency of a PIB-positive result in healthy elderly from most literature studies using PIB PET is 20% to 30%.[124,125] When significant PIB is present in healthy elderly, the distribution was similar to AD although PIB retention is generally less intense and less involved in the posterior cingulate/precuneus. The positivity of PIB seems to be similar with the prevalence of amyloid plaque as detected at postmortem in cognitively unimpaired subjects.[126–128] The prevalence of amyloid positivity in healthy elderly is affected by age. PIB retention steadily increases with age in healthy elderly, showing 18% of positivity in healthy elderly aged 60–69 years, to 37% in those of aged 70–79 years, and to 65% in those older than 80 years.[129] In recent large cohort studies from ADNI and AIBL[97,129] somewhat higher PIB positivity in healthy controls, showing up to 43%–47%, was reported. However, the data may not be generalized since high prevalence of ApoE4 carriers in those cohorts (twice than in general population) could increase the PIB positivity in healthy controls. ApoE4 allele, the major known genetic risk factor for AD, is considered with greater amyloid burden. *In vivo* imaging studies also demonstrated that carriers with at least one ApoE4 allele have higher PIB retention than non-carriers in healthy elderly or patients with MCI, but there are no differences in AD.[129–132]

In cases of MCI, variable PIB retention is expected from very PIB-negative to very PIB-positive.[131] About 55%–70% of MCI patients have a significant PIB retention, and more positive findings may be found in amnestic or multiple-domain MCI.[97] The distribution is the greatest in the frontal, anterior cingulate, precuneus, and lateral temporoparietal cortex like those in AD (Fig. 4.18). PIB positivity in MCI is considered as a prognostic marker for conversion to AD. In a follow-up study with PIB-PET, half of patients with PIB positivity converted to AD within one year of baseline, and these faster converters have higher PIB uptake than slower converters in the frontal cortex and anterior cingulated.[133]

Generally, the overall PIB retention is correlated with the metabolic impairment on FDG-PET typically in the parietal cortex.[134] In particular, PIB retention in healthy elderly and patients with MCI has a good correlation

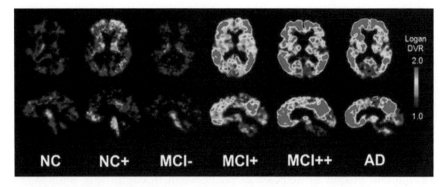

Fig. 4.18. Variable PIB retention in MCI with the greatest in frontal cortex, anterior cingulated, and lateral temporoparietal cortex like those in AD.

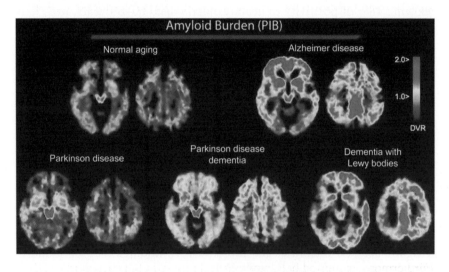

Fig. 4.19. PIB-PET images in healthy eldery, AD, PD, PDD and DLB.[139]

with cognitive impairments as well as metabolic changes, and the changes of PIB retention over the time may vary according to the initial status of the dementia (Fig. 4.19). However, no appreciable change in PIB retention over 1–2 year follow-up have been demonstrated in AD patients despite progressive deterioration in cerebral glucose metabolism as well as a clear decrease in cognitive function in some cases.[134,135] This relatively stable PIB retention might reflect a dynamic process in amyloid deposition reaching an equilibrium at the time of presentation of AD. The neuronal damage caused by amyloid deposition rather than amyloid deposition itself is thought to lead to the progression of cognitive impairment in clinically apparent AD, and this would be reflected as progressive metabolic decline on FDG-PET.

Amyloid PET imaging may provide helpful information to differentiate the dementic illness and underlying pathology in other dementic illness, although the data of amyloid PET imaging in dementia other than AD are not sufficient to make an agreement, yet.

In cases of DLB, about 80% patients are PIB positive, and the distribution of PIB retention has a similar pattern with that in AD. In particular, higher amyloid deposit in DLB is correlated with a lower MMSE score,[64] which is a consistent finding with post-mortem analysis of DLB patients.[136] There seems to be a correlation between cortical PIB uptake and the time interval between first sign of cognitive impairment recalled by the caregiver and development of diagnostic clinical features of DLB, and related with rapid progression of dementia.[131,138] Meanwhile, Parkinson's disease dementia (PDD) is another common dementia associated with movement disorders, which will be eventually developed in about 40% (up to 78%) of PD patients after an average of a decade of motor symptoms. Unlike Alzheimer's disease (AD), PD is known to have pathology of synucleinopathy instead of amyloidopathy; however, the presence of beta-amyloid has occasionally been reported in idiopathic PD, and this is more commonly a feature in patients with PD who have developed later dementia (PDD). In the studies with PIB-PET, the positivity of PIB can be observed in a minority of PDD cases.[136] And the pattern of distribution of amyloid deposition, when present in PDD, appears similar to that in DLB, targeting association cortical areas with a frontal and cingulate cortex.[139,140] Furthermore, increased beta-amyloid pathololgy in the striatum of PDD is detected in the recent work,[141] and mild increase in striatal PIB uptake in the absence of cortical amyloid in some PD subjects without dementia can be observed.

Amyloid plaque imaging will be of use not only in diagnosis of AD but also in the investigation of the temporal relationship between amyloid deposition, neuronal loss, and cognitive decline and assessment of the effects of drugs in disease progression. Also, this imaging technique may provide treatment for AD patients early in their disease when response to treatment is usually better.

References

1. Hattori N, *et al*. (1996) One-day protocol for cerebral perfusion reserve with acetazolamide. *J Nucl Med* **37**(12): 2057–2061.
2. Martin AJ, *et al*. (1991) Decreases in regional cerebral blood flow with normal aging. *J Cereb Blood Flow Metab* **11**(4): 684–689.
3. Ogawa A, *et al*. (1989) Regional cerebral blood flow with age: Changes in rCBF in childhood. *Neurol Res* **11**(3): 173–176.
4. Takahashi T, *et al*. (1999) Developmental changes of cerebral blood flow and oxygen metabolism in children. *AJNR Am J Neuroradiol* **20**(5): 917–922.
5. Catafau AM, *et al*. (1996) Regional cerebral blood flow pattern in normal young and aged volunteers: A 99mTc-HMPAO SPET study. *Eur J Nucl Med* **23**(10): 1329–1337.
6. Melamed E, *et al*. (1980) Reduction in regional cerebral blood flow during normal aging in man. *Stroke* **11**(1): 31–35.
7. Pantano P, *et al*. (1984) Regional cerebral blood flow and oxygen consumption in human aging. *Stroke* **15**(4): 635–641.
8. Yamaguchi T, *et al*. (1986) Reduction in regional cerebral metabolic rate of oxygen during human aging. *Stroke* **17**(6): 1220–1228.
9. Baird AE, *et al*. (1997) Sensitivity and specificity of 99mTc-HMPAO SPECT cerebral perfusion measurements during the first 48 hours for the localization of cerebral infarction. *Stroke* **28**(5): 976–980.
10. Brass LM, *et al*. (1994) The role of single photon emission computed tomography brain imaging with 99mTc-bicisate in the localization and definition of mechanism of ischemic stroke. *J Cereb Blood Flow Metab* **14**(Suppl 1): S91–S18.
11. Ezura M, Takahashi A, Yoshimoto T. (1996) Evaluation of regional cerebral blood flow using single photon emission tomography for the selection of patients for local fibrinolytic therapy of acute cerebral embolism. *Neurosurg Rev* **19**(4): 231–236.
12. Giubilei F, *et al*. (1990) Predictive value of brain perfusion single-photon emission computed tomography in acute ischemic stroke. *Stroke* **21**(6): 895–900.
13. Alexandrov AV, *et al*. (1996) Agreement on disease-specific criteria for do-not-resuscitate orders in acute stroke. Members of the Canadian and Western New York Stroke Consortiums. *Stroke* **27**(2): 232–237.
14. Bogousslavsky J, *et al*. (1990) Prolonged hypoperfusion and early stroke after transient ischemic attack. *Stroke* **21**(1): 40–46.
15. Hwang TL, *et al*. (1996) Brain SPECT with dipyridamole stress to evaluate cerebral blood flow reserve in carotid artery disease. *J Nucl Med* **37**(10): 1595–1599.
16. Yamada I, *et al*. (1996) SPECT and MRI evaluations of the posterior circulation in moyamoya disease. *J Nucl Med* **37**(10): 1613–1617.
17. Jeffree RL, Stoodley MA. (2009) STA-MCA bypass for symptomatic carotid occlusion and haemodynamic impairment. *J Clin Neurosci* **16**(2): 226–235.
18. So Y, *et al*. (2005) Prediction of the clinical outcome of pediatric moyamoya disease with postoperative basal/acetazolamide stress brain perfusion SPECT after revascularization surgery. *Stroke* **36**(7): 1485–1489.

19. Eo JS, Oh CW, Kim YK, Park EK, Lee WW, Kim SE. (2006) Hemodynamic outcome of successful bypass surgery in patients with atherosclerotic cerebrovascular disease: A study with acetazolamide and 99mTc-ECD SPECT. *Nucl Med Mol Imaging* **40**(6).

20. Kim JE, *et al.* (2008) Transient hyperperfusion after superficial temporal artery/middle cerebral artery bypass surgery as a possible cause of postoperative transient neurological deterioration. *Cerebrovasc Dis* **25**(6): 580–586.

21. Ozgur HT, *et al.* (2001) Correlation of cerebrovascular reserve as measured by acetazolamide-challenged SPECT with angiographic flow patterns and intra- or extracranial arterial stenosis. *AJNR Am J Neuroradiol* **22**(5): 928–936.

22. Kim SK, *et al.* (2002) Combined encephaloduroarteriosynangiosis and bifrontal encephalogaleo(periosteal)synangiosis in pediatric moyamoya disease. *Neurosurgery* **50**(1): 88–96.

23.

24. Lee SK, *et al.* (2000) The clinical usefulness of ictal SPECT in temporal lobe epilepsy: The lateralization of seizure focus and correlation with EEG. *Epilepsia* **41**(8): 955–962.

25. Shin WC, *et al.* (2002) Ictal hyperperfusion patterns according to the progression of temporal lobe seizures. *Neurology* **58**(3): 373–380.

26. Kim SK, *et al.* (2001) Diagnostic performance of [18F]FDG-PET and ictal [99mTc]-HMPAO SPECT in occipital lobe epilepsy. *Epilepsia* **42**(12): 1531–1540.

27. Lee SA, Spencer DD, Spencer SS. (2000) Intracranial EEG seizure-onset patterns in neocortical epilepsy. *Epilepsia* **41**(3): 297–307.

28. Lee DS, *et al.* (2000) Late postictal residual perfusion abnormality in epileptogenic zone found on 6-hour postictal SPECT. *Neurology* **55**(6): 835–841.

29. Devous MD, Sr., *et al.* (1998) SPECT brain imaging in epilepsy: A meta-analysis. *J Nucl Med* **39**(2): 285–293.

30. Chang DJ, *et al.* (2002) Comparison of statistical parametric mapping and SPECT difference imaging in patients with temporal lobe epilepsy. *Epilepsia* **43**(1): 68–74.

31. McNally KA, *et al.* (2005) Localizing value of ictal-interictal SPECT analyzed by SPM (ISAS). *Epilepsia* **46**(9): 1450–1464.

32. O'Brien TJ, *et al.* (1998) Subtraction ictal SPECT co-registered to MRI improves clinical usefulness of SPECT in localizing the surgical seizure focus. *Neurology* **50**(2): 445–454.

33. Brinkmann BH, *et al.* (2000) Voxel significance mapping using local image variances in subtraction ictal SPET. *Nucl Med Commun* **21**(6): 545–551.

34. Kazemi NJ, *et al.* Ictal SPECT statistical parametric mapping in temporal lobe epilepsy surgery. *Neurology* **74**(1): 70–76.

35. Lee JD, *et al.* (2000) Evaluation of ictal brain SPET using statistical parametric mapping in temporal lobe epilepsy. *Eur J Nucl Med* **27**(11): 1658–1665.

36. Ryvlin P, *et al.* (1992) Functional neuroimaging strategy in temporal lobe epilepsy: A comparative study of 18FDG-PET and 99mTc-HMPAO-SPECT. *Ann Neurol* **31**(6): 650–656.

37. Gaillard WD, *et al.* (1995) FDG-PET and volumetric MRI in the evaluation of patients with partial epilepsy. *Neurology* **45**(1): 123–126.

38. Knowlton RC, *et al.* (1997) Magnetoencephalography in partial epilepsy: Clinical yield and localization accuracy. *Ann Neurol* **42**(4): 622–631.

39. Ryvlin P, *et al.* (1998) Clinical utility of flumazenil-PET versus [18F]fluorodeoxyglucose-PET and MRI in refractory partial epilepsy. A prospective study in 100 patients. *Brain* **121**(Pt 11): 2067–2081.

40. Kim YK, *et al.* (2003) Differential features of metabolic abnormalities between medial and lateral temporal lobe epilepsy: Quantitative analysis of (18)F-FDG PET using SPM. *J Nucl Med* **44**(7): 1006–1012.

41. Carne RP, *et al.* (2004) MRI-negative PET-positive temporal lobe epilepsy: A distinct surgically remediable syndrome. *Brain* **127**(Pt 10): 2276–2285.

42. Theodore WH, *et al.* (1992) Temporal lobectomy for uncontrolled seizures: The role of positron emission tomography. *Ann Neurol* **32**(6): 789–794.

43. O'Brien DF. (2008) Epilepsy surgery: A proven neurosurgical treatment and a multidisciplinary team practice. *Ir Med J* **101**(9): 266–267.

44. Wong CH, *et al.* The topography and significance of extratemporal hypometabolism in refractory mesial temporal lobe epilepsy examined by FDG-PET. *Epilepsia.*

45. O'Brien TJ, *et al.* (2008) The cost-effective use of 18F-FDG PET in the presurgical evaluation of medically refractory focal epilepsy. *J Nucl Med* **49**(6): 931–937.

46. Theodore WH, *et al.* (1986) Neuroimaging in refractory partial seizures: Comparison of PET, CT, and MRI. *Neurology* **36**(6): 750–759.

47. Sperling MR, *et al.* (1990) Subcortical metabolic alterations in partial epilepsy. *Epilepsia* **31**(2): 145–155.

48. Akman CI, *et al.* Epilepsy duration impacts on brain glucose metabolism in temporal lobe epilepsy: Results of voxel-based mapping. *Epilepsy Behav* **17**(3): 373–380.

49. Van Paesschen W, *et al.* (2003) SPECT perfusion changes during complex partial seizures in patients with hippocampal sclerosis. *Brain* **126**(Pt 5): 1103–1111.

50. Takaya S, *et al.* (2006) Prefrontal hypofunction in patients with intractable mesial temporal lobe epilepsy. *Neurology* **67**(9): 1674–1676.

51. Theodore WH, *et al.* (1997) FDG-positron emission tomography and invasive EEG: Seizure focus detection and surgical outcome. *Epilepsia* **38**(1): 81–86.

52. Juhasz C, *et al.* (2000) Electroclinical correlates of flumazenil and fluorodeoxyglucose PET abnormalities in lesional epilepsy. *Neurology* **55**(6): 825–835.

53. Jokeit H, *et al.* (1997) Prefrontal asymmetric interictal glucose hypometabolism and cognitive impairment in patients with temporal lobe epilepsy. *Brain* **120**(Pt 12): 2283–2294.

54. Choi JY, *et al.* (2003) Extratemporal hypometabolism on FDG PET in temporal lobe epilepsy as a predictor of seizure outcome after temporal lobectomy. *Eur J Nucl Med Mol Imaging* **30**(4): 581–587.

55. Wong CH, *et al.* The topography and significance of extratemporal hypometabolism in refractory mesial temporal lobe epilepsy examined by FDG-PET. *Epilepsia* **51**(8): 1365–1373.

56. Newberg AB, *et al.* (2000) Ipsilateral and contralateral thalamic hypometabolism as a predictor of outcome after temporal lobectomy for seizures. *J Nucl Med* **41**(12): 1964–1968.

57. Lee SK, *et al.* (2002) FDG-PET images quantified by probabilistic atlas of brain and surgical prognosis of temporal lobe epilepsy. *Epilepsia* **43**(9): 1032–1038.

58. Kim MA, *et al.* (2006) Relationship between bilateral temporal hypometabolism and EEG findings for mesial temporal lobe epilepsy: Analysis of 18F-FDG PET using SPM. *Seizure* **15**(1): 56–63.

59. Hashiguchi K, *et al.* (2007) Thalamic hypometabolism on 18FDG-positron emission tomography in medial temporal lobe epilepsy. *Neurol Res* **29**(2): 215–222.

60. Takaya S, *et al.* (2009) Improved cerebral function in mesial temporal lobe epilepsy after subtemporal amygdalohippocampectomy. *Brain* **132**(Pt 1): 185–194.

61. Lee TM, Yip JT, Jones-Gotman M. (2002) Memory deficits after resection from left or right anterior temporal lobe in humans: A meta-analytic review. *Epilepsia* **43**(3): 283–291.

62. Joo EY, *et al.* (2005) Postoperative alteration of cerebral glucose metabolism in mesial temporal lobe epilepsy. *Brain* **128**(Pt 8): 1802–1810.

63. Kim SK, *et al.* (2000) Focal cortical dysplasia: Comparison of MRI and FDG-PET. *J Comput Assist Tomogr* **24**(2): 296–302.

64. Swartz BE, *et al.* (2002) The use of 2-deoxy-2-[18F]fluoro-D-glucose (FDG-PET) positron emission tomography in the routine diagnosis of epilepsy. *Mol Imaging Biol* **4**(3): 245–252.

65. da Silva EA, *et al.* (1997) Identification of frontal lobe epileptic foci in children using positron emission tomography. *Epilepsia* **38**(11): 1198–1208.

66. Lee JJ, *et al.* (2008) Frontal lobe epilepsy: Clinical characteristics, surgical outcomes and diagnostic modalities. *Seizure* **17**(6): 514–523.

67. Van Bogaert P, *et al.* (2000) Statistical parametric mapping of regional glucose metabolism in mesial temporal lobe epilepsy. *Neuroimage* **12**(2): 129–138.

68. Lee JJ, *et al.* (2005) Diagnostic performance of 18F-FDG PET and ictal 99mTc-HMPAO SPET in pediatric temporal lobe epilepsy: Quantitative analysis by statistical parametric mapping, statistical probabilistic anatomical map, and subtraction ictal SPET. *Seizure* **14**(3): 213–220.

69. Lin TW, *et al.* (2007) Predicting seizure-free status for temporal lobe epilepsy patients undergoing surgery: Prognostic value of quantifying maximal metabolic asymmetry extending over a specified proportion of the temporal lobe. *J Nucl Med* **48**(5): 776–782.

70. Nelissen N, *et al.* (2006) Correlations of interictal FDG-PET metabolism and ictal SPECT perfusion changes in human temporal lobe epilepsy with hippocampal sclerosis. *Neuroimage* **32**(2): 684–695.

71. Kim YK, *et al.* (2002) (18)F-FDG PET in localization of frontal lobe epilepsy: Comparison of visual and SPM analysis. *J Nucl Med* **43**(9): 1167–1174.

72. Plotkin M, *et al.* (2003) Use of statistical parametric mapping of (18) F-FDG-PET in frontal lobe epilepsy. *Nuklearmedizin* **42**(5): 190–196.

73. Kennedy AM, Newman SK, Frackowiak RS, *et al.* (1995) Chromosome 14 linked familial Alzheimer's disease. A clinico-pathological study of a single pedigree. *Brain* **118**(Pt 1): 185–205.

74. Kennedy AM, Frackowiak RS, Newman SK, *et al.* (1995) Deficits in cerebral glucose metabolism demonstrated by positron emission tomography in individuals at risk of familial Alzheimer's disease. *Neurosci Lett* **186**(1): 17–20.

75. Alexander GE, Chen K, Pietrini P, Rapoport SI, Reiman EM. (2002) Longitudinal PET evaluation of cerebral metabolic decline in dementia: A potential outcome measure in Alzheimer's disease treatment studies. *Am J Psychiatry* **159**(5): 738–745.

76. Reiman EM, Chen K, Alexander GE, *et al.* (2004) Functional brain abnormalities in young adults at genetic risk for late-onset Alzheimer's dementia. *Proc Natl Acad Sci U S A* **101**(1): 284–289.

77. Reiman EM, Chen K, Alexander GE, *et al.* (2005) Correlations between apolipoprotein E epsilon4 gene dose and brain-imaging measurements of regional hypometabolism. *Proc Natl Acad Sci U S A* **102**(23): 8299–8302.

78. Mosconi L. (2005) Brain glucose metabolism in the early and specific diagnosis of Alzheimer's disease. FDG-PET studies in MCI and AD. *Eur J Nucl Med Mol Imaging* **32**(4): 486–510.

79. Mosconi L, Sorbi S, de Leon MJ, *et al.* (2006) Hypometabolism exceeds atrophy in presymptomatic early-onset familial Alzheimer's disease. *J Nucl Med* **47**(11): 1778–1786.

80. Chetelat G, Desgranges B, Landeau B, *et al.* (2008) Direct voxel-based comparison between grey matter hypometabolism and atrophy in Alzheimer's disease. *Brain* **131**(Pt 1): 60–71.

81. Jhoo JH, Lee DY, Choo IH, *et al.* Discrimination of normal aging, MCI and AD with multimodal imaging measures on the medial temporal lobe. *Psychiatry Res* **183**(3): 237–243.

82. Caroli A, Geroldi C, Nobili F, *et al.* Functional compensation in incipient Alzheimer's disease. *Neurobiol Aging* **31**(3): 387–397.

83. Johnson JK, Head E, Kim R, Starr A, Cotman CW. (1999) Clinical and pathological evidence for a frontal variant of Alzheimer disease. *Arch Neurol* **56**(10): 1233–1239.

84. Smith GS, de Leon MJ, George AE, *et al.* (1992) Topography of cross-sectional and longitudinal glucose metabolic deficits in Alzheimer's disease. Pathophysiologic implications. *Arch Neurol* **49**(11): 1142–1150.

85. Ishii K, Sasaki M, Kitagaki H, *et al.* (1997) Reduction of cerebellar glucose metabolism in advanced Alzheimer's disease. *J Nucl Med* **38**(6): 925–928.

86. Chen K, Langbaum JB, Fleisher AS, *et al.* Twelve-month metabolic declines in probable Alzheimer's disease and amnestic mild cognitive impairment assessed using an empirically pre-defined statistical region-of-interest: Findings from the Alzheimer's Disease Neuroimaging Initiative. *Neuroimage* **51**(2): 654–664.

87. Minoshima S, Giordani B, Berent S, Frey KA, Foster NL, Kuhl DE. (1997) Metabolic reduction in the posterior cingulate cortex in very early Alzheimer's disease. *Ann Neurol* **42**(1): 85–94.

88. Salmon E, Collette F, Degueldre C, Lemaire C, Franck G. (2000) Voxel-based analysis of confounding effects of age and dementia severity on cerebral metabolism in Alzheimer's disease. *Hum Brain Mapp* **10**(1): 39–48.

89. Choo IH, Lee DY, Youn JC, *et al.* (2007) Topographic patterns of brain functional impairment progression according to clinical severity staging in 116 Alzheimer disease patients: FDG-PET study. *Alzheimer Dis Assoc Disord* **21**(2): 77–84.

90. Small GW, Ercoli LM, Silverman DH, *et al.* (2000) Cerebral metabolic and cognitive decline in persons at genetic risk for Alzheimer's disease. *Proc Natl Acad Sci U S A* **97**(11): 6037–6042.

91. Reiman EM, Caselli RJ, Chen K, Alexander GE, Bandy D, Frost J. (2001) Declining brain activity in cognitively normal apolipoprotein E epsilon 4 heterozygotes: A foundation for using positron emission tomography to efficiently test treatments to prevent Alzheimer's disease. *Proc Natl Acad Sci U S A* **98**(6): 3334–3339.

92. Mosconi L, Nacmias B, Sorbi S, *et al.* (2004) Brain metabolic decreases related to the dose of the ApoE e4 allele in Alzheimer's disease. *J Neurol Neurosurg Psychiatr* **75**(3): 370–376.

93. Kim EJ, Cho SS, Jeong Y, *et al.* (2005) Glucose metabolism in early onset versus late onset Alzheimer's disease: An SPM analysis of 120 patients. *Brain* **128**(Pt 8): 1790–1801.

94. Berent S, Giordani B, Foster N, *et al.* (1999) Neuropsychological function and cerebral glucose utilization in isolated memory impairment and Alzheimer's disease. *J Psychiatr Res* **33**(1): 7–16.

95. Arnaiz E, Jelic V, Almkvist O, *et al.* (2001) Impaired cerebral glucose metabolism and cognitive functioning predict deterioration in mild cognitive impairment. *Neuroreport* **12**(4): 851–855.

96. Chetelat G, Desgranges B, de la Sayette V, Viader F, Eustache F, Baron JC. (2003) Mild cognitive impairment: Can FDG-PET predict who is to rapidly convert to Alzheimer's disease? *Neurology* **60**(8): 1374–1347.

97. Jagust WJ, Bandy D, Chen K, *et al.* The Alzheimer's Disease Neuroimaging Initiative positron emission tomography core. Alzheimers Dement; **6**(3): 221–229.

98. Drzezga A, Grimmer T, Riemenschneider M, *et al.* (2005) Prediction of individual clinical outcome in MCI by means of genetic assessment and (18)F-FDG PET. *J Nucl Med* **46**(10): 1625–1632.

99. Anchisi D, Borroni B, Franceschi M, *et al.* (2005) Heterogeneity of brain glucose metabolism in mild cognitive impairment and clinical progression to Alzheimer disease. *Arch Neurol* **62**(11): 1728–1733.

100. Yuan Y, Gu ZX, Wei WS. (2009) Fluorodeoxyglucose-positron-emission tomography, single-photon emission tomography, and structural MR imaging for prediction of rapid conversion to Alzheimer disease in patients with mild cognitive impairment: A meta-analysis. *AJNR Am J Neuroradiol* **30**(2): 404–410.

101. Hoffman JM, Welsh-Bohmer KA, Hanson M, *et al.* (2000) FDG PET imaging in patients with pathologically verified dementia. *J Nucl Med* **41**(11): 1920–1928.

102. Albin RL, Minoshima S, D'Amato CJ, Frey KA, Kuhl DA, Sima AA. (1996) Fluorodeoxyglucose positron emission tomography in diffuse Lewy body disease. *Neurology* **47**(2): 462–466.

103. Ishii K, Imamura T, Sasaki M, *et al.* (1998) Regional cerebral glucose metabolism in dementia with Lewy bodies and Alzheimer's disease. *Neurology* **51**(1): 125–130.

104. Imamura T, Ishii K, Hirono N, *et al.* (1999) Visual hallucinations and regional cerebral metabolism in dementia with Lewy bodies (DLB). *Neuroreport* **10**(9): 1903–1937.

105. Minoshima S, Foster NL, Sima AA, Frey KA, Albin RL, Kuhl DE. (2001) Alzheimer's disease versus dementia with Lewy bodies: Cerebral metabolic distinction with autopsy confirmation. *Ann Neurol* **50**(3): 358–365.

106. Small GW. (2004) Neuroimaging as a diagnostic tool in dementia with Lewy bodies. *Dement Geriatr Cogn Disord* **17**(Suppl 1): 25–31.

107. Perneczky R, Drzezga A, Boecker H, Forstl H, Kurz A, Haussermann P. (2008) Cerebral metabolic dysfunction in patients with dementia with Lewy bodies and visual hallucinations. *Dement Geriatr Cogn Disord* **25**(6): 531–538.

108. Whitwell JL, Josephs KA, Rossor MN, *et al.* (2005) Magnetic resonance imaging signatures of tissue pathology in frontotemporal dementia. *Arch Neurol* **62**(9): 1402–1408.

109. Grossman M, McMillan C, Moore P, *et al.* (2004) What's in a name: Voxel-based morphometric analyses of MRI and naming difficulty in Alzheimer's disease, frontotemporal dementia and corticobasal degeneration. *Brain* **127**(Pt 3): 628–649.

110. Mosconi L, Tsui WH, Herholz K, *et al.* (2008) Multicenter standardized 18F-FDG PET diagnosis of mild cognitive impairment, Alzheimer's disease, and other dementias. *J Nucl Med* **49**(3): 390–398.

111. Jeong Y, Cho SS, Park JM, *et al.* (2005) 18F-FDG PET findings in frontotemporal dementia: An SPM analysis of 29 patients. *J Nucl Med* **46**(2): 233–239.

112. Foster NL, Heidebrink JL, Clark CM, *et al.* (2007) FDG-PET improves accuracy in distinguishing frontotemporal dementia and Alzheimer's disease. *Brain* **130**(Pt 10): 2616–2635.

113. Lin KJ, Hsu WC, Hsiao IT, *et al.* Whole-body biodistribution and brain PET imaging with [18F]AV-45, a novel amyloid imaging agent — a pilot study. *Nucl Med Biol* **37**(4): 497–508.

114. Wong DF, Rosenberg PB, Zhou Y, *et al.* In vivo imaging of amyloid deposition in Alzheimer disease using the radioligand 18F-AV-45 (florbetapir [corrected] F 18). *J Nucl Med* **51**(6): 913–920.

115. Koole M, Lewis DM, Buckley C, *et al.* (2009) Whole-body biodistribution and radiation dosimetry of 18F-GE067: A radioligand for in vivo brain amyloid imaging. *J Nucl Med* **50**(5): 818–822.

116. Vandenberghe R, Van Laere K, Ivanoiu A, *et al.* (18)F-flutemetamol amyloid imaging in Alzheimer disease and mild cognitive impairment: A phase 2 trial. *Ann Neurol.*

117. Braak H, Braak E. (1991) Demonstration of amyloid deposits and neurofibrillary changes in whole brain sections. *Brain Pathol* **1**(3): 213–216.

118. Shin J, Lee SY, Kim SH, Kim YB, Cho SJ. (2008) Multitracer PET imaging of amyloid plaques and neurofibrillary tangles in Alzheimer's disease. *Neuroimage* **43**(2): 236–244.

119. Tolboom N, Yaqub M, van der Flier WM, *et al.* (2009) Detection of Alzheimer pathology *in vivo* using both 11C-PIB and 18F-FDDNP PET. *J Nucl Med* **50**(2): 191–197.

120. Lopresti BJ, Klunk WE, Mathis CA, *et al.* (2005) Simplified quantification of Pittsburgh Compound B amyloid imaging PET studies: A comparative analysis. *J Nucl Med* **46**(12): 1959–1972.

121. Ikonomovic MD, Klunk WE, Abrahamson EE, *et al.* (2008) Post-mortem correlates of *in vivo* PiB-PET amyloid imaging in a typical case of Alzheimer's disease. *Brain* **131**(Pt 6): 1630–1645.

122. Gearing M, Mirra SS, Hedreen JC, Sumi SM, Hansen LA, Heyman A. (1995) The Consortium to Establish a Registry for Alzheimer's Disease (CERAD). Part X. Neuropathology confirmation of the clinical diagnosis of Alzheimer's disease. *Neurology* **45**(3 Pt 1): 461–466.

123. Lim A, Tsuang D, Kukull W, *et al.* (1999) Clinico-neuropathological correlation of Alzheimer's disease in a community-based case series. *J Am Geriatr Soc* **47**(5): 564–569.

124. Johnson KA, Gregas M, Becker JA, *et al.* (2007) Imaging of amyloid burden and distribution in cerebral amyloid angiopathy. *Ann Neurol* **62**(3): 229–234.

125. Pike KE, Savage G, Villemagne VL, *et al.* (2007) Beta-amyloid imaging and memory in non-demented individuals: Evidence for preclinical Alzheimer's disease. *Brain* **130**(Pt 11): 2837–2844.

126. Davies L, Wolska B, Hilbich C, *et al.* (1988) A4 amyloid protein deposition and the diagnosis of Alzheimer's disease: Prevalence in aged brains determined by immunocytochemistry compared with conventional neuropathologic techniques. *Neurology* **38**(11): 1688–1693.

127. Braak H, Braak E. (1997) Diagnostic criteria for neuropathologic assessment of Alzheimer's disease. *Neurobiol Aging* **18**(4 Suppl): S85–S88.

128. Sugihara S, Ogawa A, Nakazato Y, Yamaguchi H. (1995) Cerebral beta amyloid deposition in patients with malignant neoplasms: Its prevalence with aging and effects of radiation therapy on vascular amyloid. *Acta Neuropathol* **90**(2): 135–141.

129. Rowe CC, Ellis KA, Rimajova M, *et al.* Amyloid imaging results from the Australian Imaging, Biomarkers and Lifestyle (AIBL) study of aging. *Neurobiol Aging* **31**(8): 1275–1283.

130. Kemppainen NM, Aalto S, Wilson IA, *et al.* (2007) PET amyloid ligand [11C]PIB uptake is increased in mild cognitive impairment. *Neurology* **68**(19): 1603–1606.

131. Rowe CC, Ng S, Ackermann U, *et al.* (2007) Imaging beta-amyloid burden in aging and dementia. *Neurology* **68**(20): 1718–1725.

132. Reiman EM, Chen K, Liu X, *et al.* (2009) Fibrillar amyloid-beta burden in cognitively normal people at 3 levels of genetic risk for Alzheimer's disease. *Proc Natl Acad Sci U S A* **106**(16): 6820–6825.

133. Okello A, Koivunen J, Edison P, *et al.* (2009) Conversion of amyloid positive and negative MCI to AD over 3 years: An 11C-PIB PET study. *Neurology* **73**(10): 754–760.

134. Engler H, Forsberg A, Almkvist O, *et al.* (2006) Two-year follow-up of amyloid deposition in patients with Alzheimer's disease. *Brain* **129**(Pt 11): 2856–2866.

135. Jack CR, Jr., Lowe VJ, Weigand SD, *et al.* (2009) Serial PIB and MRI in normal, mild cognitive impairment and Alzheimer's disease: Implications for sequence of pathological events in Alzheimer's disease. *Brain* **132**(Pt 5): 1355–1365.

136. Maetzler W, Liepelt I, Reimold M, *et al.* (2009) Cortical PIB binding in Lewy body disease is associated with Alzheimer-like characteristics. *Neurobiol Dis* **34**(1): 107–112.

137. Braak H, Rub U, Jansen Steur EN, Del Tredici K, de Vos RA. (2005) Cognitive status correlates with neuropathologic stage in Parkinson disease. *Neurology* **64**(8): 1404–1410.

138. Foster ER, Campbell MC, Burack MA, *et al.* Amyloid imaging of Lewy body-associated disorders. *Mov Disord* **25**(15): 2516–2523.

139. Gomperts SN, Rentz DM, Moran E, *et al.* (2008) Imaging amyloid deposition in Lewy body diseases. *Neurology* **71**(12): 903–910.

140. Brooks DJ. (2009) Imaging amyloid in Parkinson's disease dementia and dementia with Lewy bodies with positron emission tomography. *Mov Disord* **24**(Suppl 2): S742–S747.

141. Kalaitzakis ME, Graeber MB, Gentleman SM, Pearce RK. (2008) Striatal beta-amyloid deposition in Parkinson disease with dementia. *J Neuropathol Exp Neurol* **67**(2): 155–161.

Chapter 5

Scintigraphic Imaging of Cerebral Spinal Fluid Flow, Blockage, and Leakage

Franklin C. Wong and E. Edmund Kim

5.1. Introduction

Human cerebrospinal fluid (CSF) flows in the subarachnoid space. It is produced mostly by the choroid plexus in the roof at the lateral ventricles at about 750 ml/day but occupies about 150 ml of volume. The major functions of HSF are to insulate the brain and spinal cord from direct contact with bone structures and to eliminate toxic metabolic and biologic byproducts of the central nervous system. The path of human CSF is via the third ventricle, fourth ventricle, basal cistern and then partly upward to the Sylvian and Rolandic cisterns and cerebral convexity and downward to the posterior compartment of spinal canal before returning to the basal cistern via the anterior compartment of the spinal canal. From the close compartment of subarachnoid space, CSF returns to the general circulation via multiple pathways, predominantly under hydraulic or bulk flow, at obviously rapid pace of about five times turnover daily. About 80% of CSF leaves to return to the general circulation via the cristae villa in the parasagittal veins, while the rest returns via transependymal flow or through sleeves of the spinal root. Any structural, metabolic, or functional anomalies in the brain and spinal cord may manifest in CSF compositions or alternation of CSF flow dynamics.

Early manifestation of brain diseases may present in the CSF as abnormal biomarkers, elevated protein levels, depressed glucose levels, increased leukocyte numbers, or hemorrhage. When the production or absorption of

CSF is affected, the CSF dynamics will be altered and detected. Altered dynamics may result in non-specific symptoms of headache. Increased intracranial pressure occurs mostly because of decreased CSF return from either regional structural blockade or inflammation of meninges. Decreased intracranial pressure may result from iatrogenic or spontaneous CSF leakage, resulting in loss of the insulation function to protect CNS. Scintigraphic imaging is the most sensitive non-invasive method to detect altered CSF dynamics, especially in the evaluation of normal pressure hydrocephalus (NPH), spinal fluid blockade, spinal fluid leakage, and patency of ventriculo-peritoneal shunts. In addition to the FDA-approved agent of ^{111}In-DTPA, ^{131}I-radioiodide human serum albumin (RISA), ^{99m}Tc DTPA, [131]I NaI, and ^{111}In octreotide have been reported in intrathecal studies. This chapter reviews scintigraphic imaging of human CSF in different diseases.

Conventional cisternograms involve serial sets of planar images of the lumbar spine, thoracic spine, head, and neck two to three days after lumbar injection of tracers. The procedures are lengthy and interpretation difficult because of non-uniformity between images. Quantification is also difficult. Nevertheless, CSF obstruction manifests as prolonged retention of tracer, as often observed in hydrocephalus. Spinal fluid leakage may be identified as visualization of tracer outside of the cranium or spine. Ventriculo-peritoneal shunts are studied over shorter period of 1–2 h to confirm tracer arrival to the abdomen.

Whole-body imaging has supplemented conventional methods by providing fast uniform sets of images at 2, 4, 24 and 48 h after the administration of the radionuclide that allow semi-quantification.[1,2] Uneven body depth is accounted for using geometric means of regions of interest (Fig. 5.1). Using whole-body imaging method, whole-body serial imaging over 48 h reported normal range of effective half-life (Te) of [111]In- DTPA in the CSF pathways to be 10–20 h. Symptoms of increased intracranial pressure indicating CSF obstruction was found to be >20 h[3] while CSF leak was correlated with Te <10 h[4] in preliminary reports.

With more advances in hybrid imaging, SPECT-CT may also be applied to provide anatomic correlation to localize and quantify normal and abnormal CSF tracers.

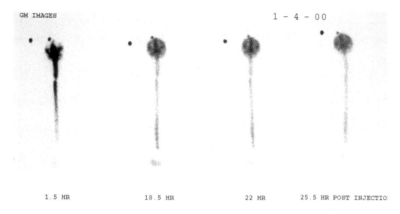

Fig. 5.1. A cancer patient with leptomeningeal metastasis received 0.5 mCi ^{111}In-DTPA via an Ommaya reservoir over the right frontal scalp. There is prompt flow of tracer down to the spine and back over to the convexity. A small area of decreased tracer activity is seen in all 4 serial images over 26 h. Te is in the normal range. Thoracic spine MRI revealed narrowing of the CSF space at T4, with no blockade.

5.2. CSF Blockade

The CSF flow may be blocked at any level from the lateral ventricle, third ventricle, fourth ventricle, difference cisterns, spinal cord, or cerebral convexity. The etiology may be trauma, inflammation, or infection. In addition, local loculation of radiopharmaceuticals may occur as epidural injection during lumbar puncture or as interstitial injection in the brain from malpositioning of intraventricular catheter.

Because of the high turnover of CSF, acute blockade of CSF within the ventricular system may lead to elevated pressure proximal to the block. Blockade of CSF at any level may be identified as retention of tracer proximal to the CSF path and decrease or absence of tracer distal to the block. It is easier to identify on scintigrams with blockade at the spinal cord level (Fig. 5.2[A] and [B]). When the block occurs within the ventricular system, it is often associated with hydrocephalus, especially in acute settings, because the buildup of pressure from continuous production of CSF easily overcomes compensatory mechanisms in increased transependymal flow. Anatomic imaging modalities CT and MRI are the initial procedures of choice to evaluate suspected hydrocephalus because of resolution of

155

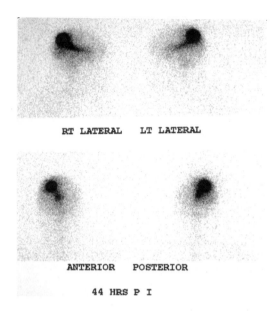

RT LATERAL   LT LATERAL

ANTERIOR   POSTERIOR

44 HRS P I

Fig. 5.2. A patient with leptomeningeal metastasis from breast cancer underwent surgical placement of an Ommaya reservoir for intrathecal chemotherapy. She became obtunded after the first intrathecal chemotherapy. Upon injection of 0.5 mCi ^{111}In-DTPA, serial static images of the head revealed loculation of injectate at the tip of the catheter indicating interstitial placement. Following advice based on scintigraphy, surgical revision of the catheter normalized the subsequent imaging findings and the patient had no adverse effect from more intrathecal infusion.

exquisite details and brief procedures to allow prompt interpretation to direct clinical management. Nevertheless, cisternogram is useful to confirm sub-acute and chronic disease such as NPH, which is associated with dementia, incontinence, and ataxia. The etiology is decreased absorption of CSF to the general circulation at the cerebral convexity. Cisternogram is performed after exclusion of structural pathologies such as tumor, stroke, multi-infarct, and multiple sclerosis. It starts with lumbar puncture followed by intrathecal injection of 0.5 mCi of [111]In- DTPA. Abnormal and prolonged visualization of tracer in the ventricle and cerebral convexity is often observed up to four days.

Blockade of CSF in the brain and spinal cord levels have been reported in patients with leptomeningeal metastases from different cancers.[5] It occurs because of inflammation of meninges from tumor invasion and from intrathecal chemotherapeutic agents. Meningitis leads to loss of compliance of one-way valves in the cristae villi in the venous sinus in which the CSF returns to systemic circulation. These CSF blocks are associated with poor prognosis. Furthermore, patients who had normalized block by radiotherapy had better outcome.[6]

5.3. CSF Leakage

Leakage of CSF can result from trauma, disease process such as spontaneous intracranial hypotension, or surgical procedures traversing the subarachnoid space. Spontaneous intracranial hypertension occurs with headache similar to those after lumbar puncture and is associated with small meningeal tear in the nerve roots, typically at the thoracic level. It takes meticulous attention to the scintigram, especially the earlier images, to detect the leakage at the sleeves of the nerve root paramedian locations.[7,8] Leakage of CSF may also occur with metastases or surgical procedures that erode into the thecal sac[9] as seen in Fig. 5.3.

After head trauma or transsphenoidal resection of pituitary adenoma, patients often have rhinorrhea, which may be related to irritation of mucosal membranes or leakage of CSF. Cisternography is a good method to distinguish the two entities. Typically, after intrathecal injection of 0.5 mCi of [111]In- DTPA via lumbar puncture, serial static images are acquired starting at 4 h and 24 h. Visualization of extrathecal tracer activities in the skull or even in the GI tract is indicative of CSF leakage. However, the sensitivity of detecting CSF leak is low using scintigram alone.

The detection rate of CSF leak in the nasopharyngeal region can be augmented by placement of multiple marked nasal pledgetts into the nostrils at different locations before injection of tracer. They are removed at 4 h, usually after the scintigrams are acquired along with blood draw of 3–5 ml of blood. The radioactivity counts for each pledgett is compared with 0.5 ml of serum to get the pledgett/serum ratio. Ratios greater than 2 is considered suspicious with CSF leak.[10] Often, this ratio has to be relaxed to maintain higher specificity because of the arbitrary nature of nasal mucus production and variable leakage rates. The ratios between the different plegetts are also important indicators of whether CSF leak is present.

Even when CSF leak is confirmed, such as by visualization of GI track, the exact localization of a leak to a particular tissue is difficult. Recent

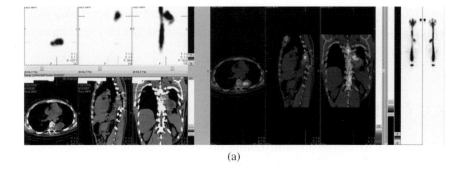

(a)

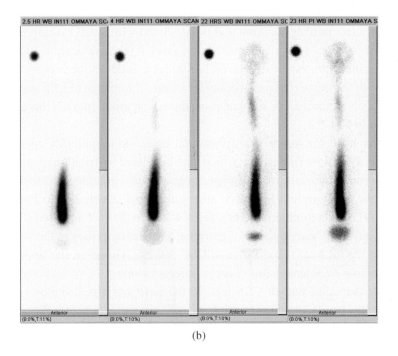

(b)

Fig. 5.3. (A) A patient with melanoma invading the thoracic vertebra underwent cisternogram (right-most images) followed by SPECT-CT of the thorax. Abnormal tracer is localized to left T6–T7 paravertebral space consistent with CSF leak. (B) Upon surgical resection of tumor and repair of the dura, there is narrowing of the CSF space at T7–T8 and slow ascent of tracer from the lumbar spine, indicating CSF block which is confirmed by MRI of spine. However, an earlier finding of CSF leak has resolved.

advances in hybrid imaging have enabled fused SPECT-CT to localize minute amount of radioactivity such as in Fig. 5.3(A). It is a promising tool to detect and localize CSF leaks.

5.4. VP Shunts

Increased intracranial pressure (ICP) occurs often after a chronic course of intracranial hemorrhage, meningeal metastasis, meningitis, tumor, or obstruction of ventricle. A VP shunt can relieve the chronically elevated ICP by diverting the bulk flow of CSF to the peritoneal cavity, which would rapidly absorb the fluid. It may have an on–off valve to allow external control. Some of the valves have internal setting to open to high-, medium-, or low- pressure gradients. Malfunctioning of VP shunt may occur when protein deposits obstruct the catheter, resulting in no CSF flow down the shunt and resurgence of increase ICP and headache.

Patency of the VP shunt can be studied by injection of 0.5 mCi of ^{111}In-DTPA into the reservoir (often it is an Ommaya type) and perform dynamic imaging of the head, thorax, and abdomen [Fig. 5.4]. For those VP shunts

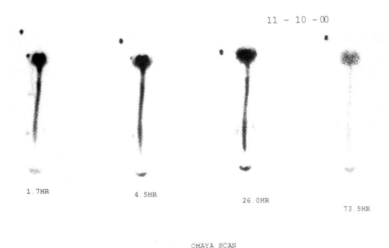

Fig. 5.4. A patient had a VP shunt placed because of increase intracranial pressure and a shunt study was performed to evaluate patency. Prompt transit of tracer down to the abdomen in the first hour indicates patency. However, persistent tracer activity in the CSF space is noted with clearance at 74 h. The determination of total tracer exposure may be able to guide intrathecal chemotherapy.

with a valve, one can evaluate tracer distribution in the CSF before and after the valve is turned on (open position). Often, there is substantial amount of tracer visualized inside the ventricle and spine, indicating significant remaining CSF in spite of the requirement of the shunt. Since the amounts of ^{111}In-DTPA are directly proportional to chemotherapeutic agents inside the CSF,[11] having a VP shunt does not always preclude patients from receiving intrathecal chemotherapy. Instead, the ability to visualize tracer distribution in the CSF and to obtain the temporal profile of CSF kinetics may allow the quantitative determination of the area-under-curve of the tracer as a surrogate to make adjustment of intrathecal chemotherapy dosage.

5.5. Discussion

Advances in scintigraphic imaging have allowed optimal use of imaging modalities to manage CNS and CSF anomalies. While traditional cisternograms have given way to CT and MRI to evaluate structural anomalies such as hydrocephalus, newer techniques of whole-body scanning and serial imaging enable quantitative assessment of CSF tracer distribution and kinetics. These kinetics studies in turn provide better understanding and more accurate assessment of CSF blockade and leakage and also allow evaluation of the degree of blockade such as in patient requiring VP shunt. Hybrid imaging of SPECT-CT is another newer tool that may prove effective in improving ability of scintigram to localize CSF leak. While traditional imaging of CSF only use the bulk flow agent [111]In- DTPA, CSF imaging may further benefit from better understanding and utilization of radiopharmaceutical with unique molecular properties.

References

1. Wong FC, Podoloff DA. (2001) Evaluation of ventricular shunts and pumps via radionuclide technique. In: *Nuclear Oncology: Diagnosis and Therapy*, Khalkhali I, Maublant J, Goldsmith S, eds., Lippincott, Williams & Wilkins, Philadelphia, 183–186.
2. Moriyama E *et al.* (2004) Quantitative analysis of radioisotope cisternography in the diagnosis of intracranial hypotension. *J Neurosurg* **101**(3): 421–426.
3. Wong FC, Kim E, Groves M, Conrad C, McCutcheon I, Podoloff D. (2002) The clearance rates of In-111 DTPA from CSF vary with different sites of CSF blockade. *Eur J Nucl Med* **29**(8): S286.

4. Wong FC, McCutcheon IE, Groves M, Kim EE. (2010) Evaluation of CSF flow by whole-body scintigraphy. *J Nucl Med* **51**(Suppl 2): 378P.
5. Chamberlain MC. (1995) Spinal 111Indium-DTPA CSF flow studies in leptomeningeal metastasis. *J Neurooncol* **25**(2): 135–141.
6. Chamberlain MC. (1998) Radioisotope CSF flow studies in leptomeningeal metastases. *J Neurooncol* **38**(2–3): 135–140.
7. Thomas DL, Menda Y, Graham MM. (2009) Radionuclide cisternography in detecting cerebrospinal fluid leak in spontaneous intracranial hypotension: A series of four case reports. *Clin Nucl Med* **34**(7): 410–416.
8. Hyun SH *et al.* (2008) Potential value of radionuclide cisternography in diagnosis and management planning of spontaneous intracranial hypotension. *Clin Neurol Neurosurg* **110**(7): 657–661.
9. Hentschel SJ, Rhines LD, Wong FC, Gokaslan ZL, McCutcheon IE. (2004) Subarachnoid-pleural fistula after resection of thoracic tumors. *J Neurosurg* **100**(4 Suppl): 332–336.
10. Frick M, Rosler H, Escher F. (1977) [Isotopic cisternography in detection of CSF Rhinorrhea] (author's translation). *HNO* **25**(2): 67–71.
11. Mason WP, Yeh SD, DeAngelis LM. (1998) 111Indium-diethylenetriamine pentaacetic acid cerebrospinal fluid flow studies predict distribution of intrathecally administered chemotherapy and outcome in patients with leptomeningeal metastases. *Neurology* **50**(2): 438–444.

Chapter 6
Nuclear Endocrinology

Ho-Young Lee, June-Key Chung and E. Edmund Kim

6.1. Thyroid Gland

6.1.1. *Anatomy, physiology and metabolism*

The thyroid is located below the thyroid cartilage and in the front of the trachea. It is composed of two lobes that are connected by the isthmus. The average length of the thyroid is about 4 cm and the thickness is $\sim$2–2.5 cm and it weighs $\sim$15–20 g.

6.1.1.1. *Iodide metabolism and the physiology of thyroid*

(1) Iodide metabolism in the other organs

Orally administered iodide is almost completely taken up in the proximal part of small bowel. In the blood, iodide is metabolized as chloride. About 80% of iodide in the serum is excreted through the urinary system. The thyroid clearance is normally about $\sim$5–40 mL/min; during iodide deficiency, it increases to 100 mL/min. However, in iodide excess state, it decreases to $\sim$2–5 mL/min.

(2) Synthesis and secretion of thyroid hormone

The synthesis and secretion of thyroid hormone is composed of iodide trapping, oxidation and organization, linking, and secretion (Fig. 6.1).

(3) Delivery and metabolism of thyroid hormone

After release into blood, most of the triiodothyronine (T3) and thyroxine (T4) are bound to thyroxine-binding globulin, transthyretin, and albumin. Only a small fraction of the circulating hormone is unbound. The free form of the hormone had biological activity in the peripheral sites. In blood, the

163

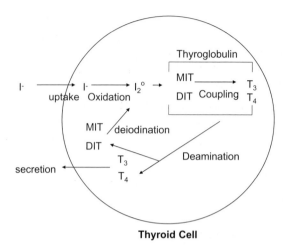

Thyroid Cell

Fig. 6.1. Process of thyroid hormones synthesis. (a) iodine uptake; (b) oxidation and organization of iodine; (c) coupling; (d) deamination and secretion; (e) deiodination.

Table 6.1. Biological activity and property of thyroid hormone in normal population.

Hormone	Serum Concentration (μg/dl)	Metabolic Rage (L/day)	Synthetic Rate (μg/day)	T1/2 in Serum (day)	Biological Activity
T_4	8	1	80	7	1
T_3	0.12	25	30	1	3–4
rT_3	0.04	100	40	0.2	0

T_4: Thyroxine, T_3: triiodothyronine, rT_3: reverse triiodothyronine

fraction of free thyroxine is 0.03% of the total thyroxine, the portion of free T3 is 0.3% of total T3. In the serum, the half-life of T4 is 7 days, whereas that of T3 is 1 day. However, the biological activity of T3 is higher than T4 (Table 6.1). Thyroid hormone is metabolized by four pathways: (1) it is catalyzed by deiodination; (2) it is metabolized through transamination, deamination, and decarboxylation process; (3) it is catalyzed by conjugation and iodine conjugated protein formation; (4) it is metabolized through catalyzation of ether conjugated site. Deiodination is the major route of thyroid hormone metabolism and it is catalyzed by 5′-monodeiodinase in the thyroid and pituitary glands, liver, muscle, and kidney. About 80% of T4 is deiodinized, and about 80%–85% of total T3 results from the deiodination of T4 and only 15% of total T3 is synthesized in thyroid.

(4) The regulation of thyroid function

Thyrotropin-releasing hormone (TRH) secreted from hypothalamus stimulates the secretion and synthesis of thyroid-stimulating hormone (TSH) of pituitary gland. TSH stimulates thyroid and increases the level of T3 and T4 in blood. In contrary, T3 and T4 in blood control the hypothalamus to inhibit the secretion of TSH from pituitary gland. This feedback system maintains the constant level of T3 and T4 in blood.

6.1.1.2. *Thyroid function test*

(1) Radioisotope

There are several kinds of radioisotopes that could be used for thyroid function test (Table 6.2). ^{131}I is used for thyroid scan and radioactive iodine uptake test. ^{123}I could be used for radioimmunoassay. ^{99m}Tc is appropriate for thyroid scan due to lower radiation exposure and energy level.

(2) *In vivo* test

A. Radioactive iodine uptake

The uptake in thyroid within regular interval after administration of radioactive iodine reflects the metabolic activity of thyroid. Radioactive iodine uptake (RAIU) could evaluate the general function of thyroid.

Table 6.2. Radioisotope used for thyroid function test.

	^{123}I	^{125}I	^{131}I	^{99m}Tc
Half life	13 hours	60.2 day	8.06 day	6 hours
Main energy (keV)	159	35	364	140
Dose for uptake test (uCi)	20	☐	5–10	☐
Dose for soan (mCi)	0.15–0.4	☐	0.05–0.1	2–5
Radiation exposure (rads/mCi)				
whole body	0.027	0.29	0.47	0.014
thyroid	24.–13.0	140–790	260–1300	0.13

The indications of RAIU are:

(1) To decide the therapeutic dose of radioactive iodine for patient with hyperthyroidism
(2) To diagnosis subacute thyroiditis or painless thyroiditis
(3) Perchlorate discharge test
(4) T3-inhibitory test
(5) To evaluate the general function of thyroid

RAIU generally uses the uptake rate at 24 h after administration of radioactive iodine. However, in patients with hyperthyroidism, the uptake of radioactive iodine could increase earlier and decrease at 24 h. In that cases, the monitoring the uptake at 2, 4, and 6 h is necessary.

A) ^{131}I thyroid uptake test

After oral administration of 5~20 uCi of ^{131}I, the 24-h delay uptake of thyroid is measured.

$$Uptake\ (\%) = (count/min\ of\ neck - count/min\ of\ thigh)/$$
$$(count/min\ of\ standard\ source)$$

The normal range of uptake at 24 h is ~10%–40%.

B) ^{123}I thyroid uptake test

The test method is same as ^{131}I thyroid uptake test. ^{131}I is replaced by 400 uCi of ^{123}I.

C) ^{99m}Tc thyroid uptake test

The thyroid uptake is measured as ^{131}I thyroid uptake test, 20 min after the intravenous injection of 500 uCi of Tc99mO4. The normal range of uptake is 1.7%~4%.

B. Perchlorate discharge test

This test evaluates the impairment of iodine organization in thyroid hormone synthesis. In fasting state, 20 uCi of ^{131}I is orally administered and after 2 h the uptake in thyroid is measured. After the measurement, 1 g of $KClO_4^-$ is orally administered and the thyroid uptake is remeasured. If the uptake decreases more than 15%, it is interpreted as positive (Fig. 6.2). Patients with Hashimoto's thyroiditis or congenital goiter due to thyroid peroxidase deficiency or anti-thyroid drug could show positive results.

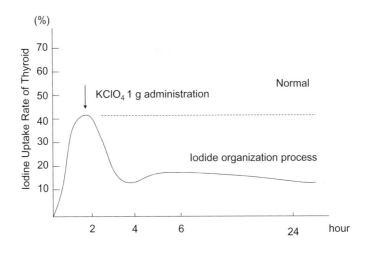

Fig. 6.2. Perchlorate discharge test.

(3) *In vitro* test

A. Measurement of total T4 and T3 in serum.

A) Method

Total T3 and T4 could be measured by radioimmunoassay method. In general, the normal range of total T4 in serum is 5∼13 *ug*/dL, and T3 is 80∼200 *ug*/dL.

B) Clinical significance of measurement of total T4 and T3 in serum

Total T4 and T3 in serum include not only the protein-bound form but also the free form of T4 and T3, which are biologically active. Accordingly, the total amount of T4 and T3 could be affected by the amount of binding protein and the binding condition between binding protein and thyroid hormone.

The increment of total T4 results from hyperthyroidism or excess of binding protein. The decrement of total T4 could induced by factors such as hypothyroidism, deficiency of binding protein, drugs inhibiting the binding between protein and hormone, non-thyroid disease, and T3 administration. Most of the T3 results from the deiodination of T4. Factors that inhibit the deiodination of T4 could affect the total T3 level.

B. Measurement of free thyroxine

There are two methods of radioimmunoassay to measure free thyroxine (T4). The two-step method is widely used due to its accuracy. However, the method using ^{125}I-conjugated T4 analogue is simple but it could be affected by the albumin, serum protein, and anti-T4 antibody.

C. Measurement of TSH

Serum THS could be measured by radioimmunoassay or immunoradiometric assay (IRMA). The normal range of TSH is $\sim$0.4–4 uU/mL.

D. TRH stimulation test

TRH is a tripeptide secreted from hypothalamus and stimulates pituitary gland to secrete TSH. Therefore, the measurement of TSH after TRH administration could evaluate the functional axis of hypothalamus-pituitary gland-thyroid. After intravenous injection of $\sim$200–500 ug synthesized TRH, TSH is measured at 0, 30, 60 90, 120, 180 min.

TRH stimulation test is used to evaluate the reason of hypothyroidism (Table 6.3). The IRMA method for TRH measure is widely used. The measurement of basal TRH level is enough to evaluate the functional axis of pituitary gland-thyroid. TRH stimulating test is replaced by TRH measurement.

6.1.1.3. *Thyroid scan*

(1) Radioisotope

For thyroid scan, ^{131}I, ^{123}I, and ^{99m}Tc are used. According to physiology, radioactive iodine is appropriate, but considering the physical characteristics, ^{99m}TcO$_4^-$ is widely used for thyroid scan.

Table 6.3.   Differentiation diagnosis of hypothyroidism.

Test	Primary Hypothyroidism	Pituitary Hypothyroidism	Hypothalamus Hypothyroidism
Total T$_4$	Decrease	Decrease	Decrease
TSH	Increase	Decrease, normal	Decrease, normal
TRH test	Over response	No response	Normal or delayed response

(2) Image acquisition

Image is acquired ∼10–20 min after intravenous injection of ∼185–370 MBq of $^{99m}TcO_4^-$ Generally, the pinhole collimator is used to change the size of thyroid on image by changing the distance between thyroid and collimator. Therefore, size marker is used together.

(3) Normal finding of thyroid scan

A normal thyroid scan shows a clear margin of thyroid with definite and even uptake of the radioisotope. The lateral margin of thyroid is linear or slightly convex. In case of concave lateral margin, the extrathyroid lesion should be considered.

(4) Abnormal finding of thyroid scan

A. Non-visualized thyroid

(1) Increase of iodine pool in serum (excess administration of iodine)
(2) Acute phase of subacute thyroiditis, painless thyroiditis.
(3) Chronic thyroiditis or primary myxedema
(4) Anti-thyroid treatment
(5) Thyroidectomy state or after ablation of residual thyroid
(6) Congenital thyroid abnormality
(7) Ectopic thyroid

B. Thyroid nodule

By the functionality or the number of thyroid nodules, the treatment of choice could be different. Therefore, the finding on thyroid scan is important.

A) Cold nodule

Cold nodule refers to the nodule with a lower uptake of radioisotope rather than the normal thyroid (Fig. 6.3). Cold nodule could be found in case of cyst, malignant tumor, benign tumor, thyroiditis, fibrosis, calcification, etc.

B) Warm nodule and hot nodule

Hot nodule refers to the nodule with higher uptake of radioisotope rather than normal thyroid (Fig. 6.4). Warm nodule shows similar uptake as normal thyroid. Some hot nodules have autonomy. Most of the toxic autonomously functioning nodules are benign tumors. Some patients with

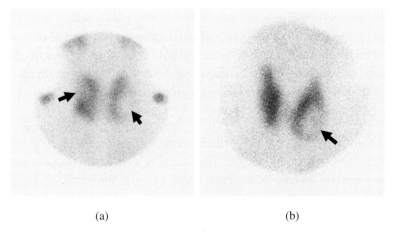

(a)   (b)

Fig. 6.3. Cold nodule. (a) multiple cold nodules in both thyroid lobes; (b) Solitary cold nodule in left thyroid lobe.

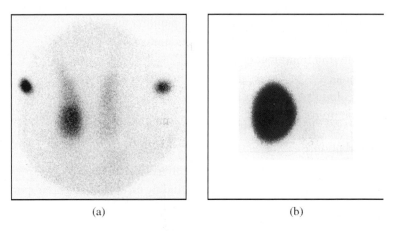

(a)   (b)

Fig. 6.4. Hot nodule. (a) Hot nodule with mild uptake in normal thyroid tissue; (b) Hot nodule without uptake of other tissue.

toxic autonomously functioning nodules could have hyperthyroidism due to excess secretion thyroid hormone from nodule.

When hot nodules with normal thyroid uptake are detected on thyroid scan, the toxic autonomously functioning nodule shows no change of uptake with decrease uptake of normal thyroid after administration of T3

(75~100 ug/day) for ~7–10 days. If the uptake of hot nodule and normal thyroid decreases after administration of T3, nodule results from compensating hypertrophy. When hot nodule shows only uptake in nodule without uptake in normal thyroid, thyroid scan after intramuscular injection of recombinant human TSH (rhTSH ~5–10 U/day, 3 days) could differentiate toxic autonomously functioning nodule.

C. Thyroiditis

Thyroiditis could be categorized as acute, sub-acute, and chronic phases. Acute thyroiditis is caused by viral or bacterial infection, and is sometimes accompanied with abscess. Sub-acute thyroiditis is usually acquired after upper respiratory infection and is accompanied with pain in early phase. The finding on thyroid scan is different depending on the phase of disease. In the early phase, thyroid is not visualized and RAIU is severely decreased. In the recovery phase, thyroid uptake is recovered or increased on the scan, and RAIU is recovered or increased. In some cases, sub-acute thyroiditis involves the other lobe after few days of unilateral lobe involvement. In those cases, it could be confused with cold nodule. After 3 to 6 months, RAIU and thyroid scan show normal finding (Fig. 6.5).

Painless thyroiditis shows similar finding of thyroid scan and RAIU as subacute thyroiditis.

Chronic thyroiditis is clinically common and most of them are Hashimoto's thyroiditis. It typically shows enlarged thyroid with uneven

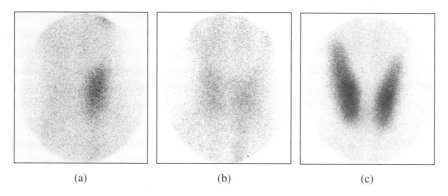

| (a) | (b) | (c) |

Fig. 6.5. Creeping-type Subacute Thyroiditis. (a) Initially subacute thyroiditis involves right lobe; (b) two weeks later, left lobe was also involved; (c) After then, recovered from thyroiditis.

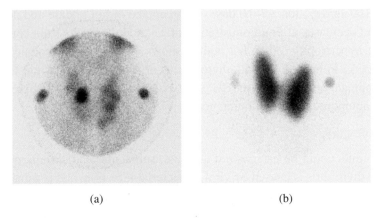

(a)   (b)

Fig. 6.6. Chronic Thyroiditis and Graves' disease. (a) Thyroid scan of Hashimoto's thyroiditis; (b) thyroid scan of Graves' disease.

uptake on thyroid scan (Fig. 6.6[A]). In some cases, it shows small cold nodules. Due to atrophy of thyroid, it shows like thyroid aplasia. Thyroid function test is normal or decreased.

D. Graves disease

In diagnosis or Graves disease, thyroid scan is not mandatory. However, thyroid scan is performed accompanying thyroid nodule or adenoma. Graves' disease shows evenly increased uptake in thyroid scan (Fig. 6.6[B]).

E. Metastasis of thyroid cancer

[131]I whole-body scan (WBS) is performed to evaluate metastasis of well-differentiated thyroid cancer such as papillary cancer and follicular cancer. Four to six weeks after radical total thyroidectomy, restriction of thyroid hormone and TSH more than 30 uU/mL is pre-requisite for ^{131}I WBS scan. To shorten thyroid hormone restriction period, T3 agent could administered for 2 weeks until ~2–3 weeks prior to ^{131}I WBS. Two weeks prior to ^{131}I WBS, it is necessary for the patient to follow an iodine-free diet. Without thyroid hormone restriction, rhTSH could be used by daily intramuscural injection two days prior to ^{131}I WBS.

[131]I WBS performed 24~72 h after 0.5~5 mCi oral administration of [131]I. WBS with higher dose of ^{131}I is more sensitive to detect metastasis. However, it could induce stunning effect in case of radioactive iodine

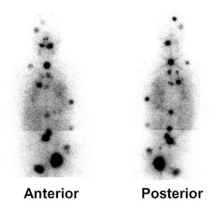

Anterior   **Posterior**

Fig. 6.7. ^{131}I whole-body scan of thyroid cancer patient with multiple metastasis. On ^{131}I whole-body scan, functioning metastasis was detected in skull, spines, pelvic bones, mediastinum, and lungs.

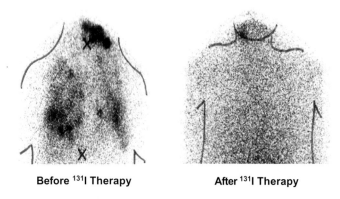

Before ^{131}I Therapy   **After ^{131}I Therapy**

Fig. 6.8. ^{131}I whole-body scan of thyroid cancer patient with pulmonary metastasis. (a) ^{131}I whole-body scan of thyroid cancer patient with pulmonary metastasis. ^{131}I uptake was detected in both lung fields; (b) After radioactive treatment, patient achieved complete remission of pulmonary metastasis.

therapy. Commonly, metastasis of thyroid cancer is detected in neck nodes, lung, and bone (Fig. 6.7). Normal uptake of radioactive iodine is found in salivary gland, stomach, colon, breast, and bladder. ^{131}I-WBS is also useful to follow-up after radioactive iodine therapy (Fig. 6.8).

F. Ectopic thyroid

Ectopic thyroid is commonly located in lingual area, mediastinum, and ovary. Thyroid develops from basal portion of tongue in embryonic stage

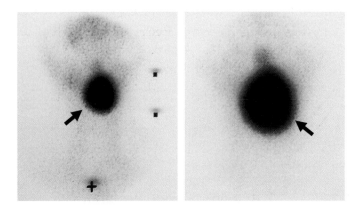

Fig. 6.9. Lingual thyroid. Front and expanded view of patient with lingual thyroid.

and moves down below thyroid cartilage. Lingual thyroid is thyroid left in the base of tongue. In thyroid scan, it is detected in the base of tongue (Fig. 6.9).

In case of mediastinal thyroid, ^{131}I scan is more appropriate than the other isotopes due to chest wall attenuation.

6.1.1.4. *FDG-PET in thyroid disease*

In the detection of recurrent thyroid cancer, serum thyroglobulin is very sensitive. However, radioactive iodine WBS shows only ∼30%–50% of sensitivity. The low sensitivity of WBS is due to (1) small tumor; (2) recurrent tumor, which could produce thyroglobulin without iodine uptake; (3) patient with increased serum iodine level; (4) patient with insufficient increase of TSH; and (5) patient with residual thyroid tissue.

In some cases, differentiated thyroid cancer has dedifferentiation and loses the ability to uptake iodine with increase of glucose metabolism (flip-flop phenomenon). Therefore, FDG-PET is meaningful in patients with increased thyroglobulin and negative in ^{131}I WBS.

6.1.2. *Radioactive iodine therapy*

1) Hyperthyroidism

The first ^{131}I therapy was performed to patient with hyperthyroidism in 1941. After then it was applied to therapy to differentiated thyroid cancer.

Its efficacy and safety is already well known. Iodine is a part of tyrosine and it is uptake by follicular cell in thyroid. Retention in follicular cells depends on the metabolic rate of the cell. Iodine could be detected in the cell even one month after radioactive iodine therapy. ^{131}I is specifically taken up by thyroid (effective half-life ~3–5 days). ß-ray from ^{131}I destroy thyroid and inhibit function of follicular cell. Long-term follow up is necessary even in patients with normalized thyroid function after treatment, due to delayed iatrogenic hypothyroidism.

1) Hyperthyroidism

(1) Indications

Hyperthyroidism results from Graves disease and toxic autonomous functioning nodules. Sub-acute thyroiditis, Jod–Basedow disease, and drug-induced hyperthyroidism also cause hyperthyroidism but those are not indication for radioactive iodine therapy. In general, radioactive iodine therapy is appropriate for middle-aged patients. Indications of radioactive iodine therapy are (1) hyperthyroidism; (2) removal of thyroid in thyrotoxicosis patient with heart failure; (3) toxic autonomous functioning nodule (5) size reduction of normal function goiter. The best indications are cases of severe state of hyperthyroidism, resistant to anti-thyroid treatment, recurrent hyperthyroidism, hyperthyroidism accompanying with other diseases such as cardiac disease, diabetes, pulmonary disease, patient with inoperable state, hypersensitivity to anti-thyroid agents, and patient's refusal to operation.

^{131}I therapy had no correlation with genetic disorder, leukemia, and thyroid cancer. In case of necessity, radioactive iodine therapy could be applied to patients younger than 20 years. It is recommended to get pregnant six months after radioactive iodine therapy. During pregnancy, PTU is recommended and nursing women should not perform radioactive iodine therapy as iodine is secreted through milk.

In general, patients with such condition: (1) no experience of therapy, (2) without exophthalmos and with mild symptom, (3) small thyroid adenoma, (4) high uptake of ^{131}I, (5) with long half time of ^{131}I, are expected to have a good response.

(2) Administration method and dose determination

A. Administration protocol

Prior to radioactive iodine therapy, thyroid scan using Tc-99m sodium pertechnetate or ^{123}I sodium iodide is necessary. Within two weeks of administration of radioactive iodine, iodine diet and contrast agents should be prohibited. Prior to radioactive iodine therapy, normalizing thyroid function by medication is helpful to avoid the aggravation of thyrotoxicosis after radioactive iodine treatment. If patient have severe thyrotoxicosis or cardiac disease, using ß-blocker or digoxin, anti-thyroid agents could inhibit acute aggravation of symptoms due to excess secretion of thyroid hormone. Lithium could improve the therapeutic effect of radioactive iodine by elongating the retention time of iodine in thyroid.

B. Dose determination

A) Fixed-dose method

This method uses regular dose of ^{131}I at each time ($\sim$2–15 mCi). In some case, hypothyroidism is induced by removal of thyroid and thyroid function is controlled with thyroid agents.

B) Mircrocurie per gram method

Expected ^{131}I uptake of 1g thyroid is considered as $\sim$50–110 uCi and the dose will be calculated with the size of thyroid and RAIU (Table 6.4).

Larger the size of thyroid is more resistant to ^{131}I therapy. Therefore, patient with a large thyroid needs higher dose than calculated dose.

C) Delivered rads method

The dose is calculated using measured the sized and RAIU of thyroid to reach absorbed dose about $\sim$40–100 Gy. This method is theoretically most accurate but there is debate about the formula.

D) Other methods

Symptoms after radioactive iodine therapy should be controlled with medication. In first year after therapy, $\sim$7%–25% of patients reach hypothyroidism and 15 years after $\sim$35%–70% of patients will have hypothyroidism. Regardless of the administered dose, careful follow-up is necessary throughout the patient's life.

Table 6.4. Therapeutic dose for hyperthyroidsim by size.

Thyroid Size (g)	24 Hours Accumulation Demand in Thyroid (uCi/g)	Averaged Accumulation Demand (rad)
10–20	40	3,310
21–30	45	3,720
31–40	50	4,135
41–50	60	4,960
51–60	70	5,790
61–70	75	6,200
71–80	80	6,620
81–90	85	7,030
91–100	90	7,440
100$\leq$	100	8,270

(3) Side effects

A. Radiation thyroiditis

Radiation thyroiditis will develop ∼1–3 days after therapy. It accompanies tenderness but will disappear in a few days.

B. Aggravation of thyroxicosis and thyroid crisis

By ^{131}I administration, thyroid tissue is destructed and thyroid hormone in follicular cell will abruptly be secreted. Within ∼4–10 days after therapy, symptom of thyrotoxicosis could be aggravated. Two to three days after ^{131}I administration, the patient should restart anti-thyroid agent to inhibit synthesis of thyroid hormone and peripheral conversion of T4. Propranolol could improve the symptoms of peripheral organs.

(4) Clinical course after therapy

Within 5 to 6 weeks, subjective symptoms, including goiter, will be improved. The maximal effect comes three to four months after therapy. Within six months, most of patients could be determined whether they are resolved of the disease. If patients do not reach remission, repeated radioactive iodine therapy should be determined with careful follow-up for more than six months.

(5) Hypothyroidism after ^{131}I therapy

After therapy, some patients do not realize the symptoms of hypothyroidism. TSH level should be carefully monitored for early detection of hypothyroidism. Patients with hypothyroidism should take thyroid hormone agents. It is easy to perform and had lesser side effects than anti-thyroid hormone for hyperthyroidism.

2) Thyroid cancer

(1) Introduction

Primary therapy for thyroid cancer is surgical resection. Depending on the stage of thyroid cancer, neck dissection could be added. However, there are many cases with metastasis, which could not be resolved by surgery. In case of metastasis, well-differentiated thyroid cancer such as follicular carcinoma and papillary carcinoma could be treated by radioactive iodine therapy. Radioactive iodine could be used for purpose of diagnosis, ablation of residual thyroid, treatment. Papillary thyroid cancer (85%) and follicular thyroid cancer had good prognosis. Therefore, surgical resection should be primarily performed. Lobectomy is enough in case of cancer with tumor less than 1.5 cm diameter. Total thyroidectomy should be done in cases of large-size cancer or invasion to extrathyroid tissue.

(2) Diagnosis

A. Thyroglobulin

Patient with thyroid cancer shows high level of thyroglobulin (Tg). There is close correlation between serum thyroglobulin level and thyroglobulin of tumor. However, synthesis of thyroglobulin and radioactive iodine uptake are independent in well-differentiated thyroid cancer. Serum thyroglobulin has correlation with the number of cells synthesizing thyroglobulin and with the differentiation of cancer.

B. Techniques such as scan, ultrasonography, and fine needle aspiration

Tc-99m scan is most widely used; ^{131}I and ^{123}I are also used for scanning. While scanning with ^{131}I or ^{123}I represents organization process, Tc-99m scan only represents a trapping function.

Most hot nodules are benign nodule but cold nodule needs fine needle aspiration to confirm. By the advancement of ultrasonography technique,

1- to 2-mm sized nodule could be detected, and small nodules need regular observation. Fine needle aspiration is a simple and safe technique for diagnosis. Its false negative is about $\sim$2%–37% in nodules less than 1 cm.

(3) Radioactive iodine therapy after surgical resection

The ablation of residual thyroid had several advantages; (1) increased sensitivity of radioactive iodine whole body scan, (2) increased sensitivity of serum thyroglobulin to detect recurrence, (3) increase efficacy of ^{131}I treatment. Residual thyroid uptakes iodine and secretes thyroglobulin. Patients with tumor larger than 1.5 cm, invasion to extrathyroid tissue, lymph node metastasis, or distant metastasis needs radioactive iodine therapy (Fig. 6.10 [A] and [B]).

(4) Administration method and dosage

Patients should stop the administration of thyroid hormone for four weeks prior to ^{131}I therapy and raise serum TSH level by more than 30 uU/mL. Two weeks prior to ^{131}I therapy, patients should restrict their dietary iodine uptake. Before oral administration of ^{131}I, blood sample was acquired to measure serum thyroglobulin (Tg) and TSH. Within five to seven days after the oral administration of radioactive iodine, post-therapy scan or diagnostic scan should be performed to evaluate the effect of ^{131}I therapy. For the ablation of residual thyroid, $\sim$1.15–5.55 GBq of ^{131}I is used.

[131]I is in form of capsule or solution and orally administered. In general, ^{131}I should be administered in fasting state with water more than 200 mL. To enhance absorbance from stomach and small bowel, the patient is recommended to walk around.

More than 200 Gy should be delivered to lesion for treatment. In first trial, the maximal dose which patient could tolerate is recommended. In general, $\sim$3.7–5.55 GBq is used in patients with cancer limited in thyroid, 7.4 GBq for distant metastasis. In case using more than 7.4 GBq, careful consideration of side effects is necessary.

A. Fixed dose method

The conventional method is the administration of a fixed empirical dose regardless of tumor ^{131}I uptake.

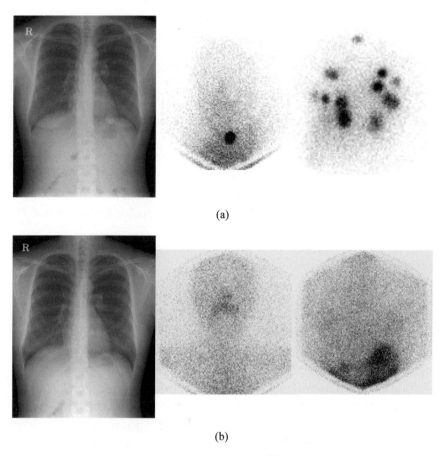

(a)

(b)

Fig. 6.10. Patient with multiple pulmonary metastases. (a). ^{131}I whole-body scan of thyroid cancer patient with pulmonary metastasis. ^{131}I uptake was detected in both lung fields; (b) after radioactive treatment, patient achieved complete remission of pulmonary metastasis.

B. Maximal safety dose method

Maximal safety dose method is the administration of a maximum safe dose (MSD) calculated to deliver a maximum of 2 Gy (200 rad) to blood

C. Retionic acid method

To treat the lesion without iodine uptake, Retinoid acid administration for several weeks induce redifferentiation of lesion and the lesion recovers the ability to uptake iodine (Fig. 6.11).

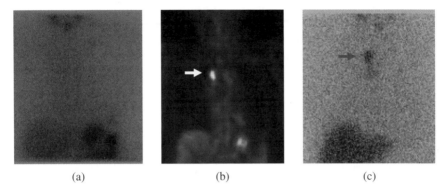

(a)   (b)   (c)

Fig. 6.11. A case with mediastinal lymph node metastasis with retinoic acid combined therapy. The metastatic lesion without ^{131}I accumulation (a) was detected in FDG-PET (b). After six weeks of retinoic acid administration, the lesion restored the accumulation (c).

(5) Side effects

A. Short-term side effects

A) Transient sialoadenitis

Transient sialoadenitis happens in patient underwent ^{131}I therapy ($\sim$3.7–7.4 GBq), due to iodine retention salivary glands. Within three days of therapy, pain, swelling, and edema could occur, especially in dehydrated patients. Within 24 h of therapy, hydration and stimulating salivary gland could reduce possibility to sialoadenitis.

B) Radiation gastritis

By drinking water, this condition could be prevented. About 5% of patients with 5.55~7.4 GBq have symptoms of vomiting.

C) Acute radiation disease

Symptoms such as fatigue, headache, and nausea could occur within 24 h after high-dose therapy. Sometimes, vomiting could occur but it is rare in patients with $\sim$5.55–7.4 GBq.

D) Marrow suppression

Marrow suppression could happen within one month after high-dose therapy and most of them are transient.

E) Others

By radiation-induced inflammation, tenderness, hemorrhage, edema could happen in metastatic lesions. In case of brain metastasis, cerebral hemorrhage or edema could happen.

B. Long-term side effects

A) Myeloid leukemia and other cancers

Myeloid leukemia or other malignancy could happen in less than 0.1% of patients. About 85% of the malignancies is acute leukemia and mostly occurs in female patients older than 50 years. Chronic leukemia is another malignancy that occurs in patients.

B) Azoospermia

There are debates about the presence of azoospermia after radioactive iodine therapy. However, azoospermia after 12.95 GBq of ^{131}I therapy was reported.

C) Pulmonary fibrosis

Patients with pulmonary metastasis has risk or pulmonary fibrosis after ^{131}I therapy. After cumulative dose of more than 37 GBq, pulmonary function test should be performed regularly. In some cases, steroid could be used to treat pulmonary fibrosis.

(6) Evaluation of therapeutic effect and patient care

Using simple X-ray or palpation, recurrent cancer could be detected. However, WBS after ^{131}I therapy is more sensitive. The lesions that are not detected in diagnostic scan (1~10 mCi) could be detected in WBS after ^{131}I therapy. Pulmonary metastasis, which could not be detected in chest X-ray, could show ^{131}I uptake in WBS.

Six month to one year after ^{131}I therapy WBS and measurement of Tg should be done and ^{131}I therapy should be planned by the results of WBS and Tg level. Repeated ^{131}I therapy could induce dedifferentiation of cancer cell and results in decrease of iodine uptake. Retinoic administration for several weeks could induce redifferentiation of cancer cell and recovery of iodine uptake.

Serum Tg should be measured three to six months after ^{131}I therapy. Follicular thyroid cancer shows highest level of Tg. As Tg from metastatic lesion is affected by TSH level, low Tg level during thyroxine administration could increase after discontinuing thyroxine. About 10%~15% of patients with high Tg level are negative in WBS. In those cases, FDG-PET could be useful to detect lesions (sensitivity: 85%~94%, specificity: 90%~95%).

(7) Combination therapy

To treat bone metastasis, ^{131}I therapy alone is not enough. It should be treated by ^{131}I therapy combined with surgical resection, and radiation therapy.

(8) Isolation and excrement treatment

To prevent environmental pollution and radiation exposure, the patient should be isolated for two days after administration of ^{131}I over 1.11 GBq. Urine and stool should be collected in a special septic tank until the activity decreases under permitted activity.

(9) Conclusion

After ^{131}I therapy, recurrent rate is 32%. Recurrent rate of patient who underwent surgical resection without ^{131}I therapy is 11%. In contrast, recurrent rate is only 2.7% in patients who performed ^{131}I therapy after surgical resection. In special cases, the recurrent rate of pulmonary metastasis is much lower in patients underwent ^{131}I therapy. Survival period is 16~19 years in patients who undergo ^{131}I therapy after surgical resection, which is three times longer than the survival period of other cancer patients who undergo chemotherapy. In general, thyroid cancer patients performed radial thyroidectomy and ^{131}I therapy.

6.2. Parathyroid Glands

There are four parathyroid glands located posterior to the lateral lobes of the thyroid, and each measures 5 mm in length and weighs about 35 mg. In approximately 10%–15%, there are a variable numbers of supernumerary glands, most commonly a fifth gland in a thymic area. The superior parathyroids originate from the fourth branchial pouch and migrate to posterior portions of thyroid lobes (type A behind the superior pole of thyroid lobe; type B in upper thyroesophageal groove) (Figs. 6.12 and 6.13). Less than 10% of superior glands are ectopically located. Type D one is behind the middle of thyroid lobe where the recurrent laryngeal nerve is located.

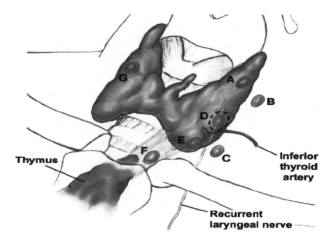

Fig. 6.12. Schematic diagram of various locations of parathyroid adenomas (A–G types).

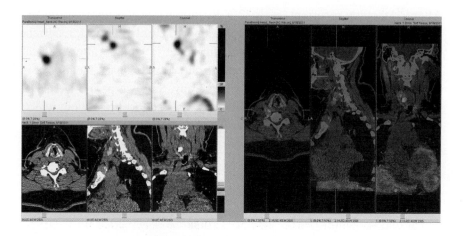

Fig. 6.13. Type A parathyroid adenoma on the right side.

The inferior parathyroids arise from the third branchial pouch and descend along with the thymus into mediastinum. Only 60% of them are found in the region of inferior poles of the thyroid (type E behind the inferior pole of thyroid lobe; type C in the lower thyroesophageal groove). Type F one is in the mediastinum (Fig. 6.14). Intrathyroidal parathyroid adenoma (type G) is found in 2%–5% of cases.

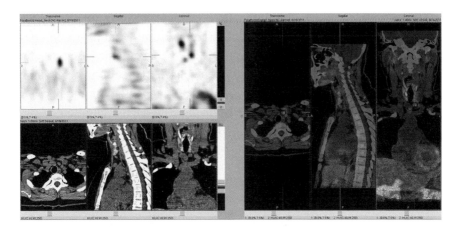

Fig. 6.14. Type F parathyroid adenoma on the left side.

Routine test for serum calcium has resulted in earlier detection of patients with hyperparathyroidism. More than 80% of them are asymptomatic or have non-specific symptoms, with renal stones present in less than 15%. Primary hyperparathyroidism results from a solitary adenoma in 80% of cases, and secondary hyperparathyroidism with chronic renal failure is also related to diffuse parathyroid hyperplasia and may require a surgical therapy due to progressive bone disease. Treatment by surgery has a success rate of 90%–95%, and recurrent or persistent hyperparathyroidism is related to aberrant or ectopic parathyroid glands. Preoperative non-invasive localization improves the cure rate of second surgery from 50%–60% up to 90%.

Tc-99m sestamibi (MIBI) has been found to accumulate in a variety of tumors including parathyroid adenomas. It is distributed in proportion to blood flow and is sequestered intracellularly within the mitochondria. The large number of mitochondria in the cells of parathyroid adenomas, especially oxyphil cells, may be responsible for the avid uptake and slow release of Tc-99m sestamibi in parathyroid adenomas compared to surrounding thyroid tissue. Typically parathyroid scintigraphy is performed as a double-phase study using Tc-99m sestamibi. Following the injection of 20–25 mCi of Tc-99m sestamibi, two sets of planar static images of the neck and chest are obtained using a low-energy collimator. The initial images at

185

15–30 min after radionuclide injection corresponds to the thyroid phase and a second set at 1.5-3 h post-injection to the parathyroid phase. Single-photon emission computed tomography (SPECT) or computed tomography (CT) of neck and chest at 1.5–2 h has been helpful to precisely localize the parathyroid adenoma (Figs. 6.12–6.14). A focus of activity in the neck or mediastinum that either progressively increases over the duration of the study or persists on delayed imaging is interpreted as differential washout consistent with parathyroid adenoma, particularly corresponding to nodular density on CT.

Using high-frequency transducer, ultrasonography can reliably detect enlarged parathyroid adenoma. CT often shows artifacts from metallic clips or anatomic distortion related to post-surgical scarring. Without the use of contrast agent it is not easy to differentiate adenoma from lymph node. MRI has shown approximately 82%–88% sensitivity in contrast to 79%–85% sensitivity by Tc-99m sestamibi for the localization of parathyroid pathology in patients with recurrent or persistent hyperparathyroidism.

6.3. Adrenal Glands

The adrenal disorders have been simply evaluated by sensitive and specific biochemical tests and high-resolution CT or MRI. Each adrenal gland lies in the retroperitoneal perinephric space, weighing about 4 g and <10-mm thickness. The right gland is triangular and lies above the superior pole of the right kidney, posterior to inferior vena cava. The left gland is crescent shaped and lies medial to the left kidney above the left renal vein. The adrenal medulla secretion of catecholamine and epinephrine (adrenaline) is under central sympathetic nervous control. The adrenal cortical steroid hormones are synthesized from cholesterol and secreted from the three cortical zones. Aldosterone secretion from the outmost zona glomerulosa is modulated by the rennin-angiotensin-aldosterone system while cortisol secretion from the zona fasciculate and androgen secretion from the innermost zona reticularis are under control of the hypothalamic-pituitary-adrenal axis.

[131]I 6-beta-iodomethyl-19-norcholesterol (known as NP-59) has been used for adrenal cortical imaging. Although radiotracer uptake reaches its maximum by 48 h, imaging is usually delayed to day 4 or 5 to allow clearance

of the background activity. The right adrenal activity frequently appears more intense than the left one due to its more posterior location. Bilateral symmetrical uptake is seen in ACTH-dependent Cushing's syndrome related to pituitary hypersecretion (Cushing disease) or ectopic ACTH secretion. Aldosteronomas are typically less than 2 cm in diameter and cannot be differentiated from non-functioning adenomas by CT or MRI. Dexamethasone suppression, 4 mg for 7 days before and continued for 5–7 days post-injection, results in scans in which the normal cortex is not visualized before fifth day following iodocholesterol injection. Unilateral adrenal visualization before fifth day post-injection is consistent with adenoma.

Pheochromocytomas are catecholamine-secreting tumors arising from chromatin cells, and approximately 10% are malignant, 10% are bilateral, 10% occur in children, and 10%–20% are extra-adrenal (paraganglioma), usually in the abdomen or pelvis but occasionally in mediastinum or neck. Bilateral extra-adrenal sites are more common in children. The diagnosis of pheochromocytoma is made by the elevated levels of catecholamine in the plasma and/or urine. Although the sensitivity of CT for the detection of metastatic and extra-adrenal pheochromocytoma is high, CT specificity is relatively poor in the post-surgical case. Adrenal medullary scintigraphy plays a pivotal role in the management of pheochromocytoma or paraganglioma. Metaiodobenzylguanidine (MIBG) is similar to norepinephrine that is taken up by adrenergic tissue via plasma norepinephrine transporters and intracellular monoamine transporters. Uptake may be inhibited by sympathomimetics, antidepressants, and some antihypertensives. Serial whole body images at 4 and 24 h after injection of 10 mCi of ^{123}I MIBG are routinely obtained. SPECT/CT is very helpful to localize precisely focal increased activity and characterized the abnormality based on CT findings (Fig. 6.15). Due to a release of free iodine, the administration of stable iodine is needed to block thyroid uptake. Malignant pheochromocytoma may dedifferentiate and thus no longer accumulate MIBG. In these cases, In-111 octreotide SPECT/CT or F-18 FDG PET/CT may better demonstrate the extent of metastatic disease (Fig. 6.16). Octreotide scan has been reported to be highly sensitive for the detection of head and neck paraganglioma but has a low sensitivity for the detection of adrenal pheochromocytoma. Dopamine is a better substrate for the norepinephrine transporter than other amines, and the use of F-18 fluorodopamine PET is promising for the determination

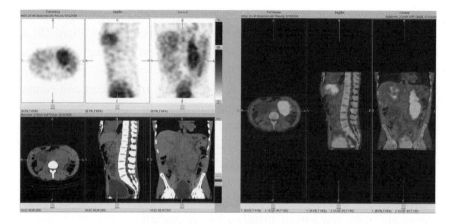

Fig. 6.15. ^{123}I MIBG uptake in a large pheochromocytoma in the left adrenal gland.

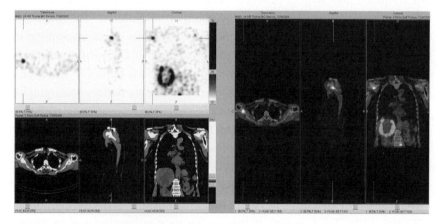

Fig. 6.16. ^{111}In octreotide uptake in the periphery of the metastatic lesion of pheochromocytoma in the liver with central necrosis. Also noted is an octreotide uptake in the metastasis in the glenoid portion of right scapula.

of metastatic disease extent, especially in patients whose tumor is not MIBG-avid.

Bibliography

Benua RS, Cicale NR, Sonenberg M, *et al.* (1962) The relation of radioiodine dosimetry to results and complications in the treatment of metastatic thyroid cancer. *Am J Roentgenol Radium Ther Nucl Med* **87**: 171–182.

Bernier MO, Leenhardt L, Hoang C, *et al.* (2001) Survival and therapeutic modalities in patients with bone metastases of differentiated thyroid carcinomas. *J Clin Endocrinol Metab* **86**: 1568–1573.

Burrow GN, Oppenheimer JH, Volpe R. (1989) *Thyroid Function and Disease*. WB Saunders Co, Philadelphia.

Choi CW, Moon DH, Lee MC, *et al.* (1986) Clinical study on thyroid cancer. *Korean J Nucl Med* **20**: 59–65.

Choi JY, Lee KS, Kim HJ, Shim YM, Kwon OJ, Park K, Baek CH, Chung JH, Lee KH, Kim BT. (2006) Focal thyroid lesions incidentally indentified by integrated ^{18}F-FDG PET/CT: Clinical significance and improved characterization. *J Nucl Med* **47**: 609–615.

Chung JK. (2001) Treatment of patients with serum Tg positive and negative in radioactive iodine whole body scan. *Journal of Korean Endocrine Society* **16** (Suppl 1): 42–46.

DeGroot LJ. (1989) *Endocrinology*. 2nd edn, WB Saunders Co, Philadelphia.

Ell PJ, Gambhir SS. (eds.) (2004). *Nuclear medicine in Clinical Diagnosis and Treatment*. 3rd edn, Churchill Livingstone, New York.

Fernandes JK, Day TA, Richardson MS, *et al.* (2005) Overview of the management of differentiated thyroid cancer. *Curr Treat Options Oncol* **6**: 47–57.

Filetti S, Bidart JM, Arturi F, *et al.* (1999) Sodium/iodide symporter: A key transport system in thyroid cancer cell metabolism. *Eur J Endocrinol* **141**: 443–457.

Gotway MB, Reddy GP, Webb WR, *et al.* (2001) Comparison between MRI and Tc-99m MIBI scintigraphy in the evaluation of recurrent or persistent hyperparathyroidism. *Radiology* **218**: 783–790.

Grünwald F, Pakos E, Bender H, *et al.* (1998) Redifferentiation therapy with retinoic acid in follicular thyroid cancer. *J Nucl Med* **39**: 1555–1558.

Hamburger JI. (1990) *Diagnostic methods in Clinical Thyroidology*. Raven Press, New York.

Haq M, Harmer C. (2005) Differentiated thyroid carcinoma with distant metastases at presentation: Prognostic factors and outcome. *Clin Endocrinol* **63**: 87–93.

Ilias I, Yu J, Carrasquillo JA, *et al.* (2003) Superiority of 6-F-18-fluorodopamine PET versus I131 MIBG scintigraphy in the localization of metastatic pheochmocytoma. *J Clin Endocrinol Metab* **88**: 4083–4087.

Ingbar Sh, Braverman LE. (1986) *Werner's The Thyroid. A Fundamental and Clinical Text*. 5th edn, Philadelphia: JB Lippincott Co.

Kim JM, Ryu JS, Kim TY, Kim WB, Kwon GY, Gong G, Moon DH, Kim SC, Hong SJ, Shong YK. (2007) ^{18}F-FDG PET does not predict malignancy in thyroid nodules cytologically diagnosed as follicular neoplasm. *J Clin Endocrinol Metab* **92**: 1630–1634.

Kim TY, Kim WB, Ryu JS, Gong G, Hong SJ, Shong YK. (2005) ^{18}F-fluorodeoxyglucose uptake in thyroid from positron emission tomogram for evaluation in cancer patients: High prevalence of malignancy in thyroid PET incidentaloma. *Laryngoscope* **115**: 1074–1078.

Kim YK, Chung J-K, Lee DS, *et al.* (1997) Ablation of remnant thyroid tissue with I-131 in well differentiated thyroid cancer after surgery. *Korean J Nucl Med* **31**: 339–345.

Kurebayashi J, Tanaka K, Otsuki T, *et al.* (2000) All-trans-retinoic acid modulates expression levels of thyroglobuine and cytokines in a new human poorly differentiated papillary thyroid carcinoma cell line, KTC-1. *J Clin Endocrinol Metab* **85**: 2889–2896.

Lee JJ, Chung JK, Kim SE, *et al.* (2008) Maximal safe dose of I-131 after failure of standard fixed dose therapy in patients with differentiated thyroid carcinoma. *Ann Nucl Med* **22**: 727–734.

Lee YJ, Chung JK, Shin JH, *et al.* (2004) *In vitro* and *in vivo* properties of a human anaplastic thgyroid carcinoma cell line transfected with the sodium iodide symporter gene. *Thyroid* **14**: 889–895.

Machens A, Holzhausen HJ, Dralle H. (2005) The prognostic value of primary tumor size in papillary and follicular thyroid carcinoma. *Cancer* **203**: 2269–2273.

Maxon HR, Thomas SR, Hertzberg VS, *et al.* (1983) Relation between effective radiation dose and outcome of radioiodine therapy for thyroid cancer. *N Engl J Med* **309**: 937–941.

Mazzaferri El, Jhiang SM. (1994) Long-term impact of initial surgical and medical therapy on papillary and follicular thyroid cancer. *Am J Med* **97**: 418–428.

Schmutzler C, Winxer R, Meissner-Weigl J, *et al.* (1997) Retinoic acid increases sodium/iodide symporter mRNA levels in human thyroid cancer cell lines and suppresses expression of functional symporter in nontransformed FRTL-5 rat thyroid cells. *Biochem Biophys Res Commun* **240**: 832–838.

Simon D, Koehrle J, Reiners C, *et al.* (1998) Redifferentiation therapy with retinoids: Therapeutic option for advanced follicular and papillary thyroid carcinoma. *World J Surg* **22**: 569–574.

Simon D, Körber C, Krausch M, *et al.* (2002) Clinical impact of retinoids in redifferentiation therapy of advanced thyroid cancer — final results of a pilot study. *Eur J Nucl Med Mol Imaging* **29**: 775–782.

Shoup M, Stojadinovic A, Nissan A, *et al.* (2003) Prognostic indicators of outcomes in patients with distant metastases from differentiated thyroid carcinoma. *J Am Coll Surg* **197**: 191–197.

Stojadinovic A, Shoup M, Ghossein RA, *et al.* (2002) The role of operations for distant metastatic well-differentiated thyroid carcinoma. *Surgery* **131**: 636–643.

Van Nostrand D, Atkins F, Yeganeh F, *et al.* (2002) Dosimetrically determined doses of radioiodine for the treatment of metastatic thyroid carcinoma. *Thyroid* **12**: 121–134.

Venkataraman GM, Yatin M, Marcinek R, *et al.* (1999) Restoration of iodide uptake in dedifferentiated thyroid carcinoma: Relationship to human Na+/I- symporter gene methylation status. *J Clin Endocrinol Metab* **84**: 2449–2257.

Wagner HN, Szabo Z, Buchanan JM, (eds.) (1995) *Principles of Nuclear Medicine.* 2nd edn, Saunders, New York.

Zeiger MA, Dackiw PB. (2005) Follicular thyroid lesions, element that affect both diagnosis and prognosis. *J Surg Oncol* **89**: 108–113.

Chapter 7
Nuclear Cardiac Imaging

Jin-Chul Paeng and Dong-Soo Kim

7.1. Myocardial Perfusion Imaging

Heart disease, including coronary artery disease (CAD), is the most common cause of death in the United States, and second most common cause of death in the world. Although anatomical coronary imaging of coronary angiography (CAG) or computed tomography (CT) CAG may show atherosclerotic narrowing of coronary arteries, nuclear imaging for myocardial perfusion is still the most practical and most accurate study for evaluation of myocardial perfusion.

7.1.1. Radiopharmaceuticals

For an ideal radiopharmaceutical for myocardial perfusion imaging, high first-pass extraction rate is crucial. Currently used radiopharmaceuticals have first-pass extraction rate of more than 50% (Table 7.1). With decrease of first-pass extraction rate, myocardial perfusion is underestimated in high-perfusion area,[1] and thus, sensitivity of lesion detection is decreased.

For single-photon emission computed tomography (SPECT), ^{201}Tl, ^{99m}Tc-sestamibi, and ^{99m}Tc-tetrofosmin are used in most institutes. ^{201}Tl is produced in cyclotron and has physical half-life of 74 h. It emits several γ- and X-rays, among which X-rays of 69~83 keV are used for imaging. The Usual administered dose is 111 MBq (3 mCi). ^{201}Tl is similar to potassium *in vivo* and is taken up by a cell via Na/K channel. Therefore, it reflects potassium pool of a body at delayed phase, while it reflects perfusion status immediately after injection. Delayed uptake of ^{201}Tl by redistribution is

Table 7.1.   Radiopharmaceuticals for myocardial perfusion imaging.

Radiopharmaceuticals	First-pass Extraction Rate	Half-life	Radiation Dose (Injection Dose)	Mechanism of Uptake
^{15}O-water	100%	2 min	2.1 mSv (2,220 MBq)	Diffusion
^{13}N-ammonia	80%~100%	10 min	1.6 mSv (740 MBq)	Diffusion and Metabolism
^{201}Tl	85%~87%	74 h	10.0 mSv (74 MBq)	Na/K Channel
^{99m}Tc-sestamibi	64%~70%	6 h	12.0 mSv (1,480 MBq)	Diffusion and electrostatic binding
^{82}Rb	50%~60%	1.25 min	4.2 mSv (1,110 MBq)	
^{99m}Tc-tetrofosmin	50%~58%	6 h	9.6 mSv (1,480 MBq)	Diffusion and electrostatic binding

used as a marker for viability because intact cell maintains Na/K channel in the cell membrane.

^{99m}Tc-sestamibi is better for imaging than ^{201}Tl due to its 140-keV γ-ray and shorter half-life of 6 h. ^{99m}Tc-sestamibi is lipophilic and can diffuse into a cell. In a cell, it is bound to mitochondrial membrane by electrostatic power because ^{99m}Tc-sestamibi has 1+ positive charge. There is an ignorable amount of redistribution for ^{99m}Tc-sestamibi in comparison with ^{201}Tl. ^{99m}Tc-tetrofosmin is similar to ^{99m}Tc-sestamibi in its uptake mechanism and biodistribution. Although first-pass extraction rate is lower, excretion via hepatic and biliary system is somewhat faster than that of ^{99m}Tc-sestamibi. Usual dose of administration is 925~1110 MBq (20~30 mCi) for both the ^{99m}Tc radiopharmaceuticals.

For myocardial perfusion PET, ^{82}Rb, and ^{13}N-ammonia are commonly used in practice. Although ^{15}O-water has best physiological characteristics such as first-pass extraction rate of 100% with free diffusion, it cannot be used easily due to very short half-life of 2 min. ^{13}N-ammonia has half-life of 10 min and is produced in a cyclotron. ^{13}N-ammonia passes through capillary and cell membrane through passive diffusion and retained in a cell in the form of ^{13}N-glutamine. The usual dose is 740 MBq with 340 MBq for each of stress and rest image. [82]Rb is converted to a cation in the body like potassium and transported into a cell via Na/K channel, like [201]Tl. However, first-pass extraction rate of [82]Rb is lower than that of ^{201}Tl, as 50%~60%. [82]Rb can be extracted from an [82]Sr/[82]Rb generator, which can be used for about a month as half-life of [82]Sr is 25.3 days. The half-life of [82]Rb is very short (1.25 min), so a relatively high dose of 1,110 MBq (30 mCi) can be administered with better radiation safety.[2]

7.1.2. Stress study

In the progression of CAD, deterioration of coronary flow reserve (CFR) occurs earlier than that of basal perfusion.[3] Therefore, stress study to assess coronary flow reserve is essential in early diagnosis of CAD. Stress studies used in nuclear cardiology are classified into three types, that is, physical exercise, inotropic drugs, and vasodilator drugs.

Exercise stress using treadmill or bicycle is a conventional method. Although it is most physiological, demand ischemia may occur, resulting in fatal complications as it increases myocardial oxygen consumption. CFR recruited in exercise stress is about two to three folds of rest perfusion. Various exercise protocols such as Bruce, modified Bruce, and Naughton are adopted for exercise stress. Radiopharmaceuticals are injected after 6~12 min of exercise, which is sustained at least for 2 min after injection. Drugs such as beta blockers, calcium channel blockers, and nitrate derivatives should be withdrawn before exercise stress.

While exercise stress study is physiological, it is often unavailable in patients who cannot exercise enough. In such cases, pharmacological stress can be used as a robust and well-standardized method. In inotropic pharmacologic stress, dobutamine is used for a stress agent, which induces increase in contractility. Therefore, myocardial oxygen demand is also increased during dobutamine stress, such as exercise stress. Recruitment of CFR is similar to that of exercise stress as two to three folds. Dobutamine is started at the dose of 10 μg/kg/min, which is increased up to 40 μg/kg/min by

10 μg/kg/min every 3 min. Dobutamine injection is maintained until 2 min after injection of radiopharmaceuticals. If dobutamine-related symptoms persist after cessation of dobutamine, 0.5 mg/kg of esmolol may be injected over 1 min.

However, the most commonly adopted stress method in nuclear cardiology is pharmacologic stress using adenosine. Adenosine is a kind of vasodilator working on coronary artery via A2a receptor. Theoretically, it does not induce increase in oxygen consumption of the myocardium. Fatal complications for adenosine include bronchospasm, arrhythmia of A-V block, and very rarely, myocardial infarction. CFR recruitment with adenosine is about three to five fold of rest perfusion. Recently an A2a receptor-specific agonist was introduced and reported to be free of complications caused by activation of other receptor subtypes. With this specific agonist, complications such as bronchospasm related to A3 receptor and A-V block related with A1 receptor may be decreased. Furthermore, time for stress is also markedly shortened. Adenosine is injected at the dose of 0.14 mg/kg/min for 6 min, during which radiopharmaceuticals are injected at 3 min. In case of A2a specific agonist, radiopharmaceuticals are injected 10~20 sec after bolus injection of stress agent.

7.1.3. *Imaging and analysis*

Imaging protocol for myocardial perfusion imaging depends on the adopted radiopharmaceuticals and condition of each institute. Most commonly used protocols are summarized in Fig. 7.1. SPECT imaging is usually performed with a step-and-shoot method, and the usual acquisition time is 15~25 min, which is varied according to the characteristics of each instrument. However, more rapid acquisition is available with recently developed heart-dedicated SPECT cameras, in which rotation of detector is not needed.

Images are usually reconstructed by filtered back projection. Commonly used filters are Ramp, Butterworth, Hamming, and Hanning filters. At present, iterative algorithms are also applied for image reconstruction. Reconstructed images are displayed in the orientation of short-axis, vertical and horizontal long-axis views. Anatomical orientations of each image are displayed in Fig. 7.2. In addition to visual qualitative analysis by experts, quantitative analysis using automatic software is now available

A. ²⁰¹Tl

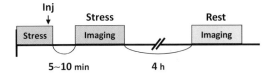

B. ⁹⁹ᵐTc Agents

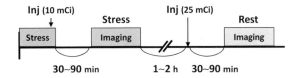

C. Dual Isotopes

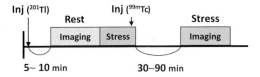

D. ¹³N-ammonia PET

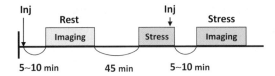

E. ⁸²Rb PET

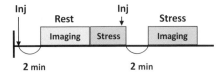

Fig. 7.1. Commonly used imaging protocols for various myocardial perfusion imaging agents.

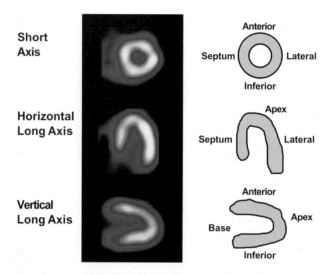

Fig. 7.2. Normal myocardial perfusion imaging using ^{99m}Tc-sestamibi and orientation of each view image.

with many commercialized software packages. An example of automatic analysis software is shown in Fig. 7.3. Regional myocardial perfusion and function can be quantified in addition to global function like ejection fraction.

In the analysis of images, there are many chances of artifacts.[4] These artifacts can be roughly categorized into three groups; patient factor, equipment factor, and technologist factor (Fig. 7.4). Among these artifacts, attenuation artifact is most significant and inevitable even if whole the imaging process is cautiously controlled. Commonly observed attenuation artifacts are breast attenuation of female patients in the anterior wall and diaphragmatic attenuation of male patients in the inferior wall. Currently, new fusion devices such as PET/CT and SPECT/CT can be solutions for this kind of artifacts.

7.1.4. *Application in CAD*

CAD is presented as reversible or even persistent perfusion defect in the affected coronary territories (Fig. 7.5). The diagnostic sensitivity and specificity of myocardial perfusion SPECT are about 89% and 76%, respectively, with CAG as a gold standard. Diagnostic accuracy for

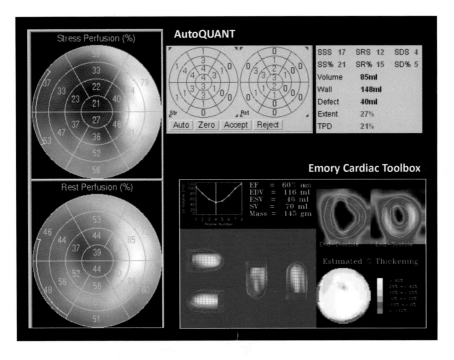

Fig. 7.3. Commonly used software for quantitative analysis of myocardial perfusion image.

one-vessel, two-vessel, three-vessel diseases are 73%~83%, 87%~93%, and 95%~97%, respectively.[5] However, the difference between physiology and anatomy should be considered in the interpretation of these data. There may be no physiological ischemia even if anatomically "significant" stenosis is present, and vice versa.[6] CT angiography, which is expanding recently, is another imaging method for coronary anatomy. The physiological significance of anatomically detected lesions often needs to be determined, and myocardial perfusion imaging can be an answer to this question.

In acute coronary syndrome, myocardial perfusion imaging is effective in the early diagnosis of myocardial infarct without elevation in level of cardiac enzyme. In addition, myocardial perfusion imaging is very valuable in the prediction of cardiac events in cases of equivocal acute coronary syndrome. In emergency rooms, myocardial perfusion imaging can be used for determination of discharge, with proven cost-effectiveness. Stress imaging is also one of the recommended options in acute coronary syndrome.[7]

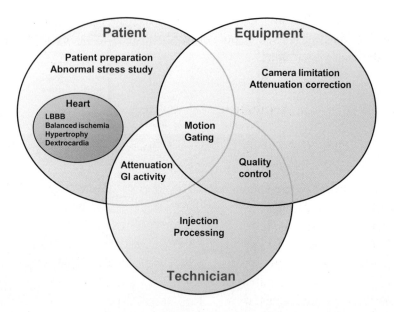

Fig. 7.4. Common causes for artifacts in myocardial perfusion imaging.

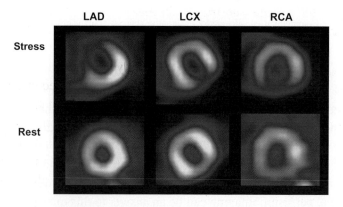

Fig. 7.5. Typical dual isotope (^{99m}Tc-sestamibi stress and ^{201}Tl rest) images of reversible perfusion defect that is matched with each coronary arterial territory of left anterior descending (LAD), left circumflex (LCX), and right coronary artery (RCA).

In addition to diagnosis of CADs, myocardial perfusion imaging is known to be a significant prognostic marker. The extent and severity of perfusion defect on myocardial perfusion imaging can predict coronary events such as myocardial infarct or sudden cardiac death, in general population and various specific conditions.[8] Preoperative myocardial perfusion imaging is used to predict perioperative cardiac events in non-vascular major operations.[9]

7.2. Myocardial Metabolism and Viability

7.2.1. *Energy metabolism of myocardium and radiopharmaceuticals*

Myocardium can utilize various substrates for energy production, including glucose, fatty acids, lactate, ketone, amino acid, pyruvate, and acetate. In normal myocardium with sufficient oxygen, long-chain fatty acids such as palmitate are basic sources of energy. Fatty acids provide 60%~85% of total energy requirement in normal resting myocardium. The selection of energy source depends on various factors including concentration of each substrate, hormonal status, workload of myocardium. For example, insulin induces more utilization of glucose as energy source. Hypoxic condition also induces anaerobic glycolysis and increases glucose utilization.

Among the various substrates, glucose is the most important one in hypoxic condition. Glucose is transported into a cell via glucose transporter (GLUT) on the cell membrane. In myocardium GLUT-4 is the main subtype of GLUT, like other muscle cells. Through glycolysis, glucose is metabolized to pyruvate, which goes through Kreb's cycle or stored in the form of lactate (Fig. 7.5). Glucose metabolism of myocardium can be assessed by ^{18}F-fluorodeoxyglucose (FDG). FDG is an analogue of glucose, which is transported into a cell and retained in the form of FDG-6-phosphate after phosphorylation by hexokinase. Therefore, uptake of FDG is determined by GLUT and hexokinase activity. ^{18}F-FDG is labeled with ^{18}F that has half-life of 110 min.

Fatty acid is transported into mitochondria after taken up by a cell. Afterward, Acetyl-CoA is continuously produced by β-oxidation of fatty acid and goes through Kreb's cycle (Fig. 7.6). In hypoxic condition, both β-oxidation and Kreb's cycle are inhibited and unmetabolized fatty acid is stored in triglyceride pool of a cell. Radiopharmaceuticals to assess fatty acid metabolism are classified into two groups, one of which is straight-chain fatty acids and the other is modified fatty acids. Straight-chain fatty

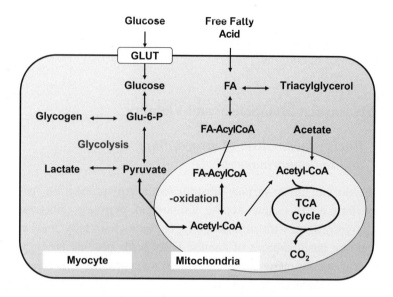

Fig. 7.6. Energy metabolism of myocardium.

acid is metabolized finally to CO_2 and eliminated from a cell. Therefore, elimination rate rather than uptake is the main focus of imaging. Iodine-labeled IHDA or *p*-IPPA for SPECT and ^{11}C-plamitate for PET are representative straight-chain fatty acids. Modified fatty acids are free from β-oxidation and trapped in a cell. Therefore, the uptake of modified fatty acid can reflect metabolism status of fatty acid. Iodine-labeled BMIPP is most widely used modified fatty acid.

7.2.2. *Imaging protocol*

The protocol of ^{18}F-FDG PET for myocardial imaging is different from that of oncologic imaging. In oncologic imaging, uptake of ^{18}F-FDG in normal tissue, including myocardium, should be suppressed. In case of myocardial imaging, however, myocardial uptake should be induced to assess metabolic potential of myocardium for which methods such as insulin clamp or glucose loading are used. In a glucose-loading method, patient is kept fasting for more than 12 h, and 75 g of glucose is administered by oral intake. ^{18}F-FDG is injected 45~60 min after oral intake of glucose and image acquisition is started in another 40~60 min. In case of a patient with diabetes, the protocol is modified with use of insulin, and insulin clamp may also used for more strict control of serum insulin and glucose level. Injection dose of ^{18}F-FDG is 172~444 MBq (6~12 mCi). Glucose metabolism of myocardium is usually assessed visually. However, absolute quantification of metabolic rate of FDG is available by dynamic image acquisition and tracer kinetic analysis using three-compartmental model.

[11]C-palmitate PET is performed by dynamic image acquisition after fasting more than 6 h. Usual injection dose is 740~925 MBq (20~25 mCi). Elimination rate calculated by monoexponential curve fitting correlates well with myocardial oxygen consumption. ^{123}I-BMIPP SPECT is also performed in fasting state. Image is acquired 30 min after injection of 111 MBq (3 mCi). BMIPP imaging is used as "ischemic memory imaging," because deterioration of fatty acid metabolism is sustained until several days after recovery from acute ischemic insult.

7.2.3. *Myocardial viability assessment*

Heart failure due to ischemic cardiomyopathy is the main cause of death in CAD. Within the ischemic dysfunctional myocardium, considerable portion is viable myocardium, which shows functional recovery after successful revascularization. Diagnosis of viable myocardium is important because aggressive revascularization is required for it to heal. Pathophysiologically, ischemic viable myocardium is coined as stunned or hibernating myocardium. Stunning refers to the condition of dysfunction just after transient ischemic insult, and hibernation refers to the dysfunction related with chronic hypoperfusion. According to the theoretical definition, a hibernating myocardium will show a varied range of perfusion decrease. Although basal perfusion itself measured on SPECT may be used for viability assessment, diagnostic performance, especially sensitivity, is not very high.

Several enhanced methods for viability assessment have been developed based on the pathophysiological differences between viable and infarct myocardium. First, muscle cells are intact in viable myocardium while fibrous tissue replaces them in infarct. This intactness of cell may be assessed on ^{201}Tl-delayed redistribution SPECT. Delayed uptake of ^{201}Tl is observed in viable myocardium with intact cells while initial uptake is in proportion to perfusion status. Usually, 24-h delayed imaging is performed for this

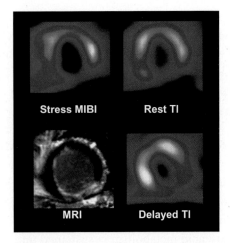

Fig. 7.7. Delayed ^{201}Tl imaging for viability assessment and delayed enhancement presented on cardiac MRI. The inferolateral wall shows no uptake on ^{201}Tl-delayed scan and whole transmural delayed enhancement on MRI. The inferior wall shows partial improvement on ^{201}Tl-delayed scan and about 50% transmural delayed enhancement on MRI.

purpose (Fig. 7.7). Reinjection of 37 MBq (1 mCi) ^{201}Tl is performed in some institutes to enhance sensitivity.

In spite of the usefulness of ^{201}Tl SPECT, the most effective method for viability assessment in nuclear medicine is ^{18}F-FDG PET.[10] In ischemic viable myocardium, glucose metabolism is increased, or at least, maintained due to hypoxic condition. While the metabolic rates of glucose in normal myocardium are about 0.15 μmol/min/g in fasting condition and about 0.6 μmol/min/g after meal, it is about 0.4 μmol/min/g in ischemic myocardium regardless of fasting. In visual analysis of ^{18}F-FDG-PET, myocardium that shows ^{18}F-FDG uptake more than 50% of that of normal myocardium is considered viable (Fig. 7.8).

Contractile reserve is another point that can differentiate infarct from viable myocardium. Ischemic dysfunctional but viable myocardium maintains contractile reserve and will show biphasic response to dobutamine challenge. During low-dose dobutamine challenge, viable myocardium shows improved function with recruitment of contractile reserve. However, with high-dose dobutamine challenge, it lapses back to dysfunction. This functional response to dobutamine challenge is assessed usually on

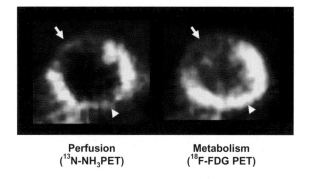

Perfusion
(^{13}N-NH$_3$PET)   **Metabolism**
(^{18}F-FDG PET)

Fig. 7.8. Match (arrow) and mismatch (arrowhead) between perfusion (^{13}N-NH$_3$) and metabolism (^{18}F-FDG) defect. Matched defect suggests myocardial infarct and mismatched defect suggests viable myocardium.

echocardiography, and cardiac magnetic resonance (CMR) imaging also may be used.

More recent developments in radiological viability assessment is delayed enhanced (DE) CMR, which is based on the difference of extracellular space between infarct and viable myocardium. As fibrous tissue in infarct area has larger extracellular space than viable myocardium, delayed enhancement is prominent in infarct tissue.[11] DE-CMR is an imaging technique that shows what is non-viable, while delayed ^{201}Tl SPECT or ^{18}F-FDG PET shows what is viable.

7.3. Other Cardiovascular Imaging

7.3.1. *Functional imaging*

First-pass radionuclide angiography (FP-RNA) is used for the assessment of left ventricular ejection fraction (LVEF) or cardiac shunt. Although it is seldom used at present for the assessment of LVEF because there are many other easy methods, it is still useful for the assessment of left-to-right (L–R) cardiac shunt.

For FP-RNA, any radiopharmaceuticals can be used if they can pass through pulmonary circulation. Among them, ^{99m}Tc-pertechnetate and ^{99m}Tc-DTPA are commonly used because they are readily available or impose low radiation dose due to fast excretion. Radiopharmaceuticals should be prepared in a small volume less than 1 mL because bolus injection is crucial in the quality of the study. Images are acquired at the rate of 2~4 frames/sec for shunt study or 20~25 frames/sec for LVEF study. Region of interest (ROI) is set on the lung and time-activity curve is acquired. In case L–R shunt exists, there are several peaks in the time-activity curve. For each peak, area under the curve is calculated using gamma-variate fitting, and shunt fraction is calculated from these areas. Shunt fraction calculated from this method is very accurate, if bolus injection is reliable. The reliable range of shunt fraction measured on FP-RNA is 1.2~3.0.

Gated blood pool (GBP) scan, also called as multi-gated radionuclide angiography (MUGA), is used for accurate measurement of LVEF. Although there are many methods for assessment of LVEF, including echocardiography, gated SPECT, gated CMR, and gated cardiac CT, GBP scan is still the most accurate method for the assessment of LVEF unless gating is inappropriate due to arrhythmia. GBP is based on the radioactivity of blood pool, while all other methods are based on the LV volume delineated on images. ^{99m}Tc-labeled red blood cells or other radiopharmaceuticals that remain in intravascular space can be used for GBP scan. After injection of radiopharmaceuticals, anterior, left anterior oblique, and lateral view images are acquired. LVEF is calculated from the end-systolic and end-diastolic radioactivity of LV.

7.3.2. *Molecular imaging*

In nuclear molecular imaging for cardiovascular system, the most intriguing field at present is vulnerable plaque imaging. Because all atherosclerotic plaques do not rupture and result in fatal complications such as myocardial or cerebral infarct, the detection and differentiation of rupture-prone vulnerable plaque is promising for the prevention of fatal complications and monitoring of therapeutic efficacy. Many radiopharmaceuticals have been reported or are under development. Imaging targets of vulnerable plaque include inflammation, apoptosis, angiogenesis, aggregation of platelet, proteolytic enzymes, and activated cytokines. Among them, the most feasible method at present is ^{18}F-FDG PET. As is well known, ^{18}F-FDG is accumulated in active inflammatory lesions, because activated leukocytes, especially, macrophages shows much enhanced glucose metabolism. Likewise, ^{18}F-FDG is accumulated in vulnerable plaques due to active inflammatory process in them. ^{18}F-FDG can be used for detection of vulnerable plaques, grading of inflammatory activity, and efficacy monitoring of antiatherosclerotic treatment. Furthermore, recent studies suggest that ^{18}F-FDG PET can be a prognostic factor in the prediction of cardiovascular events.[12] For this, uptakes of ^{18}F-FDG in major arteries or specific putative arteries are measured.

A more conventional molecular imaging in cardiovascular system is infarct imaging. Infarct imaging may be used in acute coronary syndrome or myocardial viability assessment. ^{99m}Tc-pyrophosphate is one of the early developed radiopharmaceuticals for infarct imaging. It is taken up in calcium-depositing lesions like infarct tissue. ^{111}In-labeled anti-myosin antibody is targeting for myosin heavy chain, which is insoluble and remains *in situ* after infarct. ^{99m}Tc-annexin V is binding to a cell membrane component of phosphatidyl serine that is exposed in case of apoptosis. Although there is some controversy on the role of apoptosis in infarct, ^{99m}Tc-annexin V has been reported as an imaging agent for infarct.

Hypoxia imaging is under development for ischemic myocardium imaging. Derivatives of nitroimidazole and dithiosemicarbazone such as ^{18}F-FMISO and ^{64}Cu-ATSM have been reported. Imaging for sympathetic nervous system is also useful in cardiac imaging. Sympathetic innervation status of heart is regarded to be related with prognosis in ischemic heart disease, heart failure, arrhythmia, and heart transplantation. ^{123}I-MIBG and ^{11}C-hydroxyephedrine have been developed for imaging of sympathetic nervous system.

References

1. Heller GV, Hendel RC. (2003) *Nuclear Cardiology. Practical Applications.* McGraw-Hill.
2. Stabin MG. (2008) Radiopharmaceuticals for nuclear cardiology: Radiation dosimetry, uncertainties, and risk. *J Nucl Med* **49**: 1555–1563.
3. Camici PG, Rimoldi OE. (2009) The clinical value of myocardial blood flow measurement. *J Nucl Med* **50**: 1076–1087.
4. Burrell S, MacDonald A. (2006) Artifacts and pitfalls in myocardial perfusion imaging. *J Nucl Med Technol* **34**: 193–211.

5. Zaret BL, Beller GA. (2004) *Clinical Nuclear Cardiology, State of the Art and Future Directions.* 3rd ed. Elsevier-Mosby.

6. Van Werkhoven JM, Schuijf JD, Gaemperli O, *et al.* (2009) Prognostic value of multislice computed tomography and gated single-photon emission computed tomography in patients with suspected coronary artery disease. *J Am Coll Cardiol* **56**: 623–632.

7. Klocke FJ, Baird MG, Lorell BH, *et al.* (2003) ACC/AHA/ASNC guidelines for the clinical use of cardiac radionuclide imaging–executive summary: A report of the American College of Cardiology/American Heart Association Task Force on Practice Guidelines (ACC/AHA/ASNC Committee to Revise the 1995 Guidelines for the Clinical Use of Cardiac Radionuclide Imaging). *Circulation* **108**: 1404–1418.

8. Shaw LJ, Berman DS, Maron DJ, *et al.* (2008) Optimal medical therapy with or without percutaneous coronary intervention to reduce ischemic burden: Results from the Clinical Outcomes Utilizing Revascularization and Aggressive Drug Evaluation (COURAGE) trial nuclear substudy. *Circulation* **117**: 1283–1291.

9. Brown KA, Rowen M. (1993) Extent of jeopardized viable myocardium determined by myocardial perfusion imaging best predicts perioperative cardiac events in patients undergoing noncardiac surgery. *J Am Coll Cardiol* **21**: 325–330.

10. Di Carli MF, Davidson M, Little R, *et al.* (1994) Value of metabolic imaging with positron emission tomography for evaluating prognosis in patients with coronary artery disease and left ventricular dysfunction. *Am J Cardiol* **73**: 527–533.

11. Kim RJ, Wu E, Rafael A, *et al.* (2000) The use of contrast-enhanced magnetic resonance imaging to identify reversible myocardial dysfunction. *N Engl J Med* **343**: 1445–1453.

12. Rudd JHF, Myers KS, Bansilal S, *et al.* (2009) Relationships among regional arterial inflammation, calcification, risk factors, and biomarkers. A prospective fluorodeoxyglucose positron-emission tomography/computed tomography imaging study. *Circ Cardiovasc Imaging* **2**: 107–115.

Chapter 8
Pulmonary Nuclear Medicine

E. Edmund Kim and Franklin Wong

8.1. Introduction

Studies in pulmonary imaging predominantly depict the distribution of pulmonary perfusion or the ventilation–perfusion balance for the detection of pulmonary embolism (PE), obstructive airway disease, and lung carcinoma. Much work has been done using ^{133}Xe to study both regional ventilation and blood flow. This work has led to a greater understanding of regional blood flow and ventilation, lung anatomy and morphometry, mechanical factors that influence lung function, and biochemical and other non-respiratory functions of the lung.

The physical parameters measured in radionuclide emission studies are the temporal and spatial relations in the distribution of tracer in the lungs. Tracers that are diffusible will wash into and out of the lungs at a rate proportional not only to flow but also to membrane permeability. If the radionuclide label is attached to microspheres or macro-aggregates, the amount lodging in any portion of the lung can be related to relative flow in the lung.

The problems encountered in assessing the value of ventilation–perfusion scans for the diagnosis of PE are concern with improving specificity, but also with better estimation of the prior probability of PE in the patient being evaluated. Well-defined diagnostic criteria and uniform diagnostic algorithms are the key elements for reducing the variability in ventilation–perfusion image interpretation. It is also possible that PE will be detected with better sensitivity and specificity by use of emission tomography, but at present time, SPECT and PET have not been evaluated sufficiently to demonstrate this definitively.

8.2. Anatomy and Physiology

The tracheobronchial airways divide about 16 times, in an irregular dichotomous fashion, between the trachea and the terminal bronchioles. Beyond this level, the respiratory bronchioles divide two to seven times to reach alveolar ducts, alveolar sacs, and alveoli. The cross-sectional area of the bronchial tree begins to increase very rapidly at the level of the terminal bronchioles, so that beyond this point, the airflow rates, pressure differences, and airway resistance are very low during normal breathing. The alveoli are packed together and surrounded by a network of collagen and elastic fiber. This structural arrangement ensures considerable stability because changes in one alveolus will be mitigated by opposite changes in surrounding alveoli. The communications between alveoli (pores of Kohn) become more numerous in older subjects and allow collateral ventilation.

The pulmonary arterial branches follow the divisions of the bronchial tree. The pulmonary arterioles that accompany the terminal bronchioles are about $100\,\mu$m in diameter, whereas the precapillary vessels are about $35\,\mu$m in diameter and number 250 to 300 million, each vessel serving one alveolus, which is surrounded by about 1000 capillaries. Anastomoses between the pulmonary capillaries and bronchial capillaries may be found along the respiratory bronchioles. The capillaries are between 7 and $10\,\mu$m in diameter. The pulmonary veins drain blood from the alveolar capillaries as well as from the peripheral parts of the airways and the pleura. The bronchial arteries usually arise from the aorta and accompany the airways, nourishing them as well as the pulmonary arteries and veins. The pleura is richly supplied with lymphatic vessels, but lymphatics are not found around alveoli. There are approximately 300 million alveoli in each lung.

The lungs are remarkable because the full cardiac output passes through at such low pressure (11 mmHg mean pulmonary artery pressure). Vascular resistance (the ratio of pressure to flow) is much lower in the lungs than in the systemic circulation. Even when there is high cardiac output, the pulmonary arterial pressure rises very little. Gravity, acceleration, and posture play important parts in the distribution of blood flow.

Once pulmonary arterial pressure exceeds alveolar pressure, blood flow increases and the flow rate then depends on the difference between these two pressures. Pulmonary venous pressure exceeds alveolar pressure farther down in the lung, and at this point the driving force for blood flow is the difference between pulmonary arterial pressure and pulmonary venous pressure.

In the upright position with breathing at functional residual capacity, ventilation per unit volume increases 1.5 to 2 fold between the upper zones and the lower zones, whereas blood flow increases three to five fold. However, the overall performance of the lungs leads to a fall of only 4 mmHg in the PO_2 gradient between arterial PO_2 and alveolar PO_2, giving a convenient measure of how closely ventilation (V) and perfusion (Q) are matched. The worse the match, the greater the PO_2 difference, indicating the presence of disease.

Determination of the ratio of physiologic dead space to tidal volume (V_D/V_T) provides a useful indication of the inefficiency of ventilation by showing what portion of each breath is wasted. The distribution of pulmonary blood flow is altered by changes in cardiac output, and also by changes in resistance in the pulmonary arteries or veins. It should be remembered that alveolar hypoxia is a powerful vasoconstrictor of the pulmonary arterioles. Resistance in airways may be increased by mucous plugs, bronchoconstriction, bronchial-wall thickening, or grossly distorted airways. Compliance increases in emphysema but diminishes in other parenchymal processes. In pneumonic consolidation and atelectasis, blood flow is reduced and acts as a right-to-left shunt. A number of disease processes directly affect the pulmonary arterial tree, the most common problem being PE. Compression or invasion of the pulmonary arteries may also cause changes in blood flow. Increases in left atrial pressure in mitral stenosis or in left ventricular failure cause a redistribution of blood flow from the base towards the apex.

Measurements of regional ventilation and blood flow are generally of little clinical value in restrictive lung disease. They are considerably more useful in obstructive airway disease, partly because early disease is quite readily recognized.

8.3. Radiopharmaceuticals

8.3.1. *Gases*

Xc-133 is the most widely used gas for the study of regional ventilation although its low energy and solubility in blood and fat are disadvantages. Xenon-127 has higher gamma energy peaks.

8.3.2. *Aerosols*

Aerosol scans have been used as an indication of regional ventilation. Aerosol deposition depends on a number of factors, including the size, shape, and density, and the electrostatic charge on the particle as well as lung geometry and the pattern of ventilation. Satisfactory scans can be obtained by use of 20 to 50 mCi of Tc-99m labeled pentetic acid (diethylene triamine pentaaceticacid, DTPA) or Tc-99m sulfur colloid in a volume of 3 to 4 mL. Only about 10% of this activity reaches the lung. In general, particles larger than 10 to 15 pm are removed by the nose or deposited in the larger airways, and the smaller particles (less than 2 to 4 pm) reach the alveoli.

8.3.3. *Particles*

Regional perfusion is most commonly studied following by the intravenous injection of labeled microspheres or macroaggregates of human serum albumin (MAA). The number of particles necessary for the scan in normal individuals is >60,000 but injecting more than 200,000 particles will not improve the scan quality. If 200,000 particles are given to a normal subject, fewer than 0.1% of the total number of arterioles are blocked, giving a safety margin of about 1000:1. The dose of MAA should be reduced by 50% in pregnant women and children by a factor that relates to body weight. Prior to the withdrawal of a patient's dose into a syringe, the vial containing the MAA should be shaken to disaggregate the particles, and the MAA is then injected slowly with the subject breathing normally.

8.4. Venous Thromboembolism

A deep vein thrombosis (DVT) often originates in the veins of the calf muscles or the venous valves of the iliofemoral veins in the thigh. DVT and pulmonary emboli (PE) are related aspects of the same dynamic process. They not only share risk factors and treatment but also require a coordinated approach to diagnosis. It is thought that there are at least 200,000 cases of venous thromboembolism (TE) in the USA each year comprising 105,000 DVT and 95,000 PE of whom 25% die within 7 days. Survival after the first episode of DVT was found to be 96% but after PE it decreased to 76%. Patients with DVT by duplex ultrasound have a high clinical pre-test probability of PE. The first screening test for VTE is often rapid quantitative ELISA (Vidas) D-dimer measurement for fibrin derivatives. A negative D-dimer test below 500 ng/ml can accurately exclude VTE with the specificity of 95%. It is acceptable to withhold anticoagulant therapy in patients suspected DVT but with negative ultrasound. However, it is unacceptable to withhold the therapy in suspected PE with negative ultrasound result. ^{111}In-labeled platelet or peptide for platelet receptor is useful to detect a new blood clot.

8.5. Lung Imaging Techniques

8.5.1. *Ventilation imaging*

Ventilation (V) imaging studies using Xe-133 gas are most commonly performed in three phases. The first phase begins with the patient inhaling 10 to 20 mCi of Xe-133 gas to vital capacity, followed by breath holding for 15 to 20 sec. During this time, an image of this single-breath distribution is obtained. The patient then begins the second (tidal breathing) phase, at which time Xe-133 gas is rebreathed through a closed-loop ventilation system. This equilibrium phase should last for at least 3-min duration to allow the gas to enter poorly ventilated areas. If there is a shorter rebreathing phase, the abnormal areas may not accumulate or retain the gas during the third (washout) phase which is composed of 60-sec images acquired for at least 5 consecutive min after the beginning of Xe-133 clearance. The second phase is the least sensitive for revealing the presence of obstructive pulmonary disease. By definition, Xe-133 distribution at equilibrium represents the distribution of accelerated lung volume, not the distribution of tidal ventilation. The Xe-133 single-breath inhalation image is more likely to reveal inhomogeneities in ventilation than is the equilibrium phase

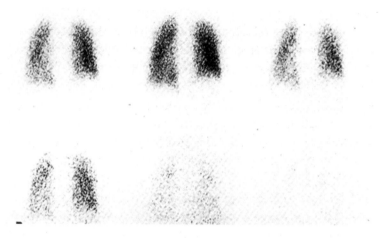

Fig. 8.1. Normal ventilation study with Xe-133 gas. Note good wash-in and -out of radioxenon gas.

image. Abnormalities of regional ventilation are revealed as defects in the single-breath distribution. Because Xe-133 has a low-energy photon, sub-stantial scatter occurs in the body, and it is hard to resolve small ventilation abnormalities. The single-breath maneuver is effort-dependent, and 10% to 20% of studies are technically unsatisfactory. Xenon-133 washout images are more likely to show regional obstructive airway disese. Uniform Xe-133 retention during the first two minutes of clearance can be seen in normal patients (Fig. 8.l), but uneven distribution at any time or Xe-133 retention at 3 min or later is abnormal, regardless of whether it is diffuse or regional. Knowledge of the minute-ventilation rate (respiratory rate × tidal volume) is needed to exclude hypoventilation as the cause of transient diffuse Xe-133 retention.

Hepatic uptake of Xe-133 gas is most commonly seen in alcoholic fatty infiltration, diabetes mellitus, and obesity. The extent of Xe-133 uptake is closely correlated with the degree of steatosis seen histologically. Other agents for the ventilation study in Xe-127 and Kr-81m gases as well as aerosols. Because Xe-127 allows ventilation imaging after perfusion scan, it can be a useful agent. However, similar sensitivity and specificity have been reported in a series of patients who had angiography with either Xe-133 or Xe-127, and the Xe-127 is not readily available commercially.

Krypton-81m gas has a 13-sec half-life and is eluted from an Rb-81 generator that has a 4.5-h half-life. Because of its short half-life, Kr-81m provides steady-state images in which activity is proportional to regional tidal ventilation, with less than 100 mrad to the lungs for typically six to eight views. Its disadvantage is in its inability to obtain the washout phase of standard ventilation imaging. Radioaerosols allow evaluation of regional ventilation as they are deposited in the lungs by impaction into bronchial walls, by sedimentation out of the air stream, or by random collisions with alveolar walls during diffusion in distal air spaces (Fig. 8.2). When a settling bag is placed between the patient and the nebulizer, patients inhale a more uniform and small-sized aerosol. Large particles tend to impact on central airway walls. After the perfusion scan is performed with 1 or 2 mCi Tc-99m labeled particles, the patient breathes the Tc-99m–labeled DTPA aerosols until the lung count rate is three to four times that obtained with the perfusion agent alone, and multiple views are obtained. When regional ventilation is normal, good peripheral deposition of the activity occurs even if pulmonary emboli are present. The overall results of aerosol-perfusion imaging agreed with those of Xe-133 ventilation-Tc-99m perfusion imaging in 90% of patients in one series. An alternative approach employs a low-dose (1 mCi) Tc-99m aerosol imaging prior to a conventional (4 mCi) Tc-99m MAA perfusion scan (Fig. 8.3).

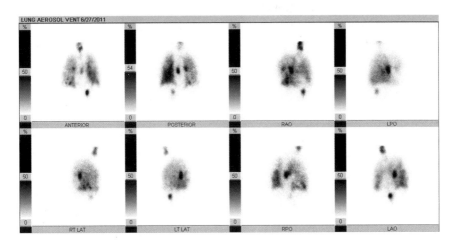

Fig. 8.2. Ventilation study with Tc-99m DTPA aerosols. Note focal activities retained in the bilateral main bronchi due to inadequate inhalation.

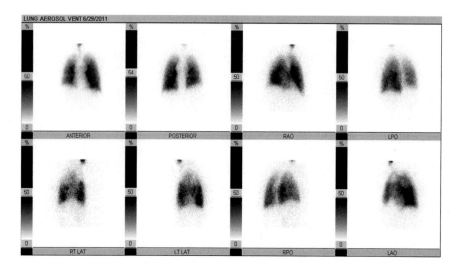

Fig. 8.3. Normal ventilation with Tc-99m DTPA aerosols.

8.5.2. *Perfusion imaging*

Regional pulmonary perfusion is most conveniently studied following the intravenous injection of 2 to 5 mCi Tc-99m–labeled microspheres or macro-aggregates of human serum albumin. Their distribution is proportional to pulmonary arterial blood flow. Absolute blood flow to any region can be determined only if cardiac output is measured at the same time. When Xe-133 in saline solution is used, images obtained during breath-holding show the relative capillary blood flow to reach the region. Routine imaging in anterior, posterior, and lateral views (Fig. 8.4) shows smooth outline of the lungs with relatively less activity in the apexes, and it may fail to visualize small defects on account of "shinethrough" from normally perfused areas in front of or behind the defect. Bilateral posterior oblique views reduce the frequency of equivocal interpretation from 30% to 15% because they give improved delineation of small defects and also identify many perihilar defects. About 25% to 30% of the counts detected in a lateral view come from the opposite side of the chest. In obese patients, the costophrenic angles are usually blunted. Patients injected in the supine position are usually asked to take two or three deep breaths during the injection to promote an even distribution of the particles. When the injection is given in a sitting position,

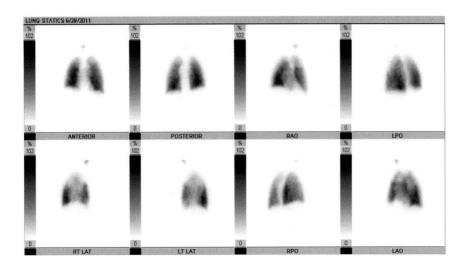

Fig. 8.4. Normal perfusion with Tc-99m MAA particles.

a gravity effect on pulmonary blood flow is apparent. The particles should be shaken well prior to injection. If a few large particles are given or if small clots form in the syringe, several large hot spots are seen on the subsequent scan. Most particles are believed to break up as a result of phagocytosis and pulmonary flow and to eventually pass through the lungs. With the use of doses having between 60,000 and 150,000 particles, fewer than 1 in 1000 pulmonary terminal arterioles are obstructed. However, the presence of pulmonary hypertension and right-to-left shunts should be careful due to possible development of acute right heart failure, pulmonary chemoreflex, or stroke. Intravenous Xe-133 in saline solution should pose no hazard in these circumstances.

8.5.3. *Pulmonary emboli*

Pulmonary embolism is the most common acute pulmonary disorder encountered in hospitalized patients. This disorder is a complication of a venous thrombosis originating elsewhere in the body. The clinical diagnosis of PE is notoriously difficult because of non-specific signs and symptoms. The most frequent presenting symptoms are dyspnea, pleuritic chest pain, apprehension, and cough. The most frequent sign is tachypnea (90%), and other signs include fever, tachycardia, and accentuation of the pulmonic component of the second heart sound. Physical findings of deep vein thrombosis in the lower extremities are noted in fewer than one third of patients. Arterial hypoxemia occurs frequently with pneumonia, congestive heart failure, and other disorders that may simulate PE clinically. Results of chest radiography may appear normal in 25% to 60% of patients, and other non-specific findings include diaphragmatic elevation, pulmonary consolidation, atelectasis, and pleural effusion. Pulmonary infarction is present in less than 10% of patients.

The development of CT technology has changed substantially the role of VQ scan. VQ scan with a normal chest X-ray can correctly exclude PE in patients with low or medium pre-test probability. VQ scan with normal chest X-ray also can pick up PE correctly with a high probability. Those with intermediate or indeterminate VQ scan then undergo further investigation with CT pulmonary angiography (PA). Currently, VQ scan is the screening test for suspected PE when D-dimer is abnormal, chest X-ray is normal, and when pre-test clinical probability is low or medium.

8.5.4. *VQ scan interpretation*

All perfusion defects are non-specific in truth, but perfusion defects that conform to segmental or lobar boundaries, particularly when multiple and bilateral with a normal accompanying ventilation, are highly correlated with acute or previous PE (Fig. 8.5). Most experienced reporters of VQ scans use probability terms based on modified prospective investigation of pulmonary embolism diagnosis (PIOPED) (Table 8.1).

A very low probability category scan is least likely to indicate acute PE while high probability category is most likely. Many patterns of abnormalities are indefinite, but abnormalities on the chest X-ray allow us to predict when VQ imaging will provide an indeterminate result and to move smartly to CTPA in the first instance if available. The first step for the consistent and accurate interpretation of VQ scan is the integration of the perfusion and ventilation studies with the chest X-ray. The second step is the assessment of the pre-test clinical probability of PE. The third step is the integration of the scan result with the pre-test clinical probability of PE to provide the final post-test diagnosis.

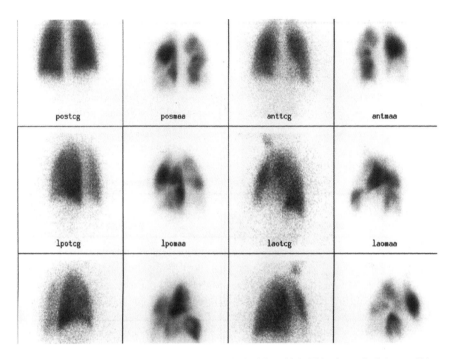

| postcg | posmaa | anttcg | antmaa |
| lpotcg | lpomaa | laotcg | laomaa |

Fig. 8.5. High probability of acute pulmonary emboli with multiple V/Q mismatched abnormalities in the bilateral lungs.

Several principles can be recognized for VQ scan service for clinical and radiological colleagues. The first one states that normal perfusion scan excludes PE for clinical purpose. The second one states that PE can present with any perfusion abnormality but the risk of acute PE will depend on the pattern of the abnormality in part. The larger the perfusion abnormality, the more segmental its appearance and the more normal ventilation, the greater the risk of PE becomes. The third principle states that a good quality erect and contemporaneous chest X-ray is essential for accurate VQ scan interpretation. The fourth principle states that the pre-test clinical probability of PE is itself an independent risk factor for PE. The fifth one states that VQ scan and chest X-ray should be interpreted and its category determined whenever possible. The last principle states that D-dimer level less than 500 units excludes VTE and need for VQ scan or CTPA.

Preservation of a peripheral parenchymal stripe of activity, a stripe sign, seems to suggest that the perfusion defect in the lung is non-

Table 8.1.   Criteria for VQ scan interpretation based on modified PIOPED.

Probability	Criteria
High probability	Two or more moderate/large mismatched perfusion defects. Prior heart and lung disease probably requires more abnormalities. Triple match in one lung with one or more mismatches in the other lung.
Intermediate probability	Single VQ mismatch or match without corresponding chest X-ray abnormality. Difficult to categorize or not described, including cases of chest X-ray abnormality.
Low probability	Large or moderate VQ matches involving no more than 50% of combined lung fields with no corresponding chest X-ray abnormalities. Small VQ mismatches with normal chest X-ray.
Very low probability	Small VQ matches with normal chest X-ray.

embolic in origin. Ventilation study may fail to detect airway disease associated with many small perfusion defects, and angiography also cannot detect the extremely small emboli that may have caused the perfusion defects.

There seems to be a low probability that angiographically detectable emboli are present when only very small perfusion defects are seen on perfusion images. The most frequently encountered non-embolic causes of ventilation–perfusion (V/Q) mismatches are previous PE, bronchogenic carcinoma, and previous radiation therapy. Vasculitis, intravenous drug abuse, lymphagitic carcinomatosis, and pulmonary venoocclusive disease are less common causes. Quantitative lung perfusion study is helpful to determine an operability of lung cancer (Fig. 8.6).

The simultaneous presence of airway disease and emboli makes the scintigraphic diagnosis of PE more difficult than usual. However, limited regions of airway disease do not interfere with the scintigraphic diagnosis of embolism. The sensitivity and specificity of ventilation–perfusion imaging for detection of PE are generally very high.

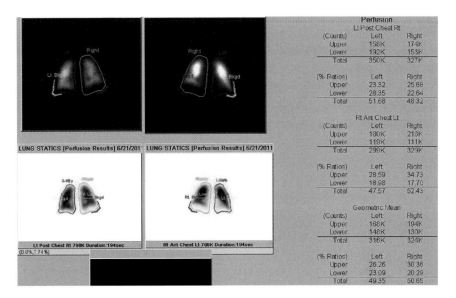

	Perfusion	
	Lt Post Chest Rt	
(Counts)	Left	Right
Upper	158K	174K
Lower	192K	153K
Total	350K	327K
(% Ratios)	Left	Right
Upper	23.32	25.68
Lower	28.35	22.64
Total	51.68	48.32
	Rt Ant Chest Lt	
(Counts)	Left	Right
Upper	180K	218K
Lower	119K	111K
Total	299K	329K
(% Ratios)	Left	Right
Upper	28.59	34.73
Lower	18.98	17.70
Total	47.57	52.43
	Geometric Mean	
(Counts)	Left	Right
Upper	168K	194K
Lower	148K	130K
Total	316K	324K
(% Ratios)	Left	Right
Upper	26.26	30.36
Lower	23.09	20.29
Total	49.35	50.65

Fig. 8.6. Quantitative lung perfusion study in a patient with small lung cancer in the right lower lobe. Right to left lung perfusion ratio is approximately 51 to 49, and thus at least 1.7 L/sec FEV1 is required for optimal right pneumonectomy.

8.5.5. *Post-test VQ investigation and follow-up of PE*

Final diagnosis of VQ scan has sufficient diagnostic power to permit immediate decision regarding treatment. Negative duplex ultrasound of legs would likely exclude the probability of PE to 5%–7%. It will be necessary to decide whether an abnormal chest X-ray, a 5%–10% clinical risk or 10% plus risk of PE following VQ scan should be a agreed trigger for CTPA. In PE patients treated with heparin alone, there is about 30%–40% improvement in perfusion in 5–7 days, 55% improvement in 2 weeks, and finally plateau value of 80% in one year.

Bibliography

American College of Emergency Physicians. Clinical Policy. (2003) Critical issues in the evaluation and management of adult patients presenting with suspected pulmonary embolism. *Ann Emerg Med* **41**: 257–270.

British Thoracic Society guidelines for the management of suspected acute pulmonary embolism. (2003) *Thorax* **58**: 470–483.

Gray HW. (2002) The natural history of venous thromboembolism: Impact on ventilation/perfusion scan reporting. *Semin Nucl Med* **32**: 159–172.

Perrier A. (2004) D-dimer for suspected pulmonary embolism: Whom should we test? *Chest* **125**: 807–809.

Schoepf UJ, Costello P. (2004) CT angiography for diagnosis of pulmonary embolism: State of the art. *Radiology* **230**: 329–337.

Wicki J, Perneger TV, Junod AF, *et al.* (2001) Assessing clinical probability of pulmonary embolism in the emergency ward: A simple score. *Arch Intern Med* **161**: 92–97.

Chapter 9
Gastrointestinal Nuclear Medicine

Gi-Jeong Cheon and E. Edmund Kim

9.1. Introduction

The recent development of functional and structural imaging techniques has resulted in redefining the role of scintigraphy in diagnosis of the various disorders of liver, gastrointestinal (GI) tract, and abdominal organs. Despite the ability to delineate structural changes, modern structural imaging fails to detect many pathologic states in the early stage of the disease. This is due to not only the lack of sensitivity of gross structural imaging techniques in detecting functional alterations and/or molecular activity of the physiologic and pathologic states but also to its poor specificity to differentiate between the active and inactive disease states.[1,2] Radionuclide scintigraphy remains a unique non-invasive modality with quantitative capability for the evaluation of functional disorders. Using various radiopharmaceuticals, nuclear medicine techniques can play complementary and supplementary roles to the anatomical imaging for the further categorization with molecular imaging information, particularly in difficult clinical settings that are frequently encountered in GI disorders.[1-3]

9.2. General Scintigraphy

9.2.1. *Gastric emptying scintigraphy*

Gastric emptying scintigraphy is a simple, well-established, physiologic procedure for the assessment of GI motility disorder. The conventional protocol measures the rate of transit of radiolabeled liquid (0.5–1.0 mCi

221

of Tc-99m DTPA) or solid food (commonly 0.5–1.0 mCi of Tc-99m sulfur colloid in scrambled eggs or oatmeal). Gastric emptying is performed after a 12-h overnight fast and discontinuation of any medication likely to interfere with gastric motility. Imaging is performed preferably with the patient sitting or standing. Using a modern dual-head gamma camera system, a series of 1-min dynamic images is obtained in the anterior and posterior views for at least 90 min. Depth attenuation must be corrected for by calculation of the geometric mean of gastric counts.[4]

The emptying pattern for solid food is biphasic, initiated by lag phase and followed by continuous emptying. The lag phase is the time required for the antrum to grind food (Fig. 9.1). Several quantitative data can be obtained from the time-activity curve: Lag phase (T_{lag}) in minutes, i.e., the first part of curve without emptying, the emptying rate in percentage of emptying per minute, and the half emptying time ($T_{1/2}$) in minutes. Half time of gastric emptying is slightly longer with egg than that with oatmeal. Gastric emptying curve findings of common clinical application are summarized in Table 9.1.

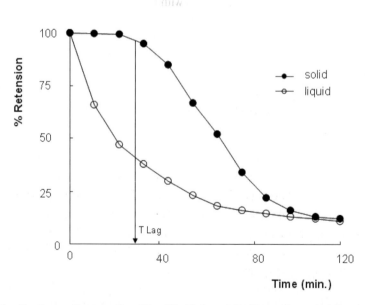

Fig. 9.1. Gastric emptying curve for solid and liquid phase. A liquid emptying curve follows a mono-exponential pattern. A solid emptying curve is biphasic pattern with an initial plateau (lag phase) followed by a linear emptying phase and a late slow portion.

Table 9.1. Typical findings of gastric emptying curve in clinical application.

	Findings of Gastric Emptying Curve
Healthy subjects (normal)	$T_{1/2}$ 60 ± 30 min for solid phase* and 30 ± 15 min for liquid phase Length of lag phase (T_{lag}) > 45 min considered abnormality* Percent of gastric emptying at 90 min < 35% considered abnormality*
Diabetes mellitus	Delay in solid gastric emptying is very common in symptomatic and asymptomatic long-standing diabetes (mainly due to prolonged lag phase) Rapid gastric emptying observed in early stage of diabetes autonomic neuropathy Liquid emptying is only abnormal when solid phase is severely impaired
Idiopathic dyspepsia	Prolonged lag phase and slow emptying rate
Gastric surgery	In patients with partial gastrectomy, no lag phase and slow empting rate (similar pattern in solid and liquid emptying)

*Variables depending on the content of the meal.

9.2.2. GI bleeding scintigraphy

GI bleeding scan is performed in order to evaluate the evidence or significance of GI bleeding and to localize the site of bleeding. Scintigraphy of the abdominal blood pool following intravenous (IV) administration of a patient's red blood cells (RBCs) labeled with Tc-99m pertechnate is tolerated and well-established procedure that is complementary to endoscopy and angiography for the detection and localization of GI bleeding. Both *in vivo* and *in vitro* red cell labeling methods are available.[5] The detection and localization of bleeding sites have been improved by the use of the improved *in vitro* labeling procedure (>98% labeling efficacy). The images provide a high sensitivity for the detection of a low bleeding rate and allow continuous monitoring for several hours. Bleeding rate detection varies from 0.05 to 0.1 ml/min, depending on the labeling efficacy and other technical factors.

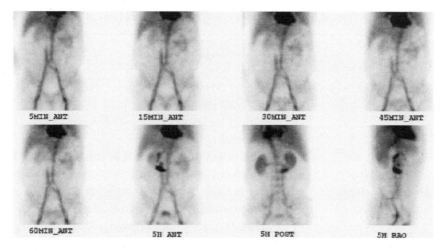

Fig. 9.2. Gastrointestinal bleeding scan. A 69-year-old man with a history of esophagojejunal stomy due to stomach cancer showed intermittent GI bleeding. GI bleeding scan shows an active bleeding focus in mid-abdomen at 5-h images. In this case, endoscopy which was performed just after the 5-h delay image demonstrated active jejunal bleeding.

Although contrast angiography provided exact anatomic detail, there must be bleeding at a rate of greater than 1 ml/min at the time of contrast injection. GI bleeding scan may be useful and complementary to angiography, especially in case of the intermittent nature of GI bleeding (Fig. 9.2). The cine display of continuous dynamic set of images helps the visualization and the precise localization of the bleeding sites. If the patient is bleeding profusely, a quick transfer is organized for the urgent management of bleeding control, either to interventional radiology or the operation room for surgery.

9.2.3. *Hepatobiliary scintigraphy*

Hepatobiliary scintigraphy is performed after IV administration of 5–10 mCi of a Tc-99m-labeled iminodiacetic acid (IDA) derivative such as disofenin (DISIDA) or mebrofenin (BrIDA). These compounds are first-pass agents and extracted by the hepatocyte via anion transport carrier as bilirubin.

Acute cholecystitis caused by the occlusion of cystic duct is the most common clinical indication for performing a hepatobiliary scintigraphy

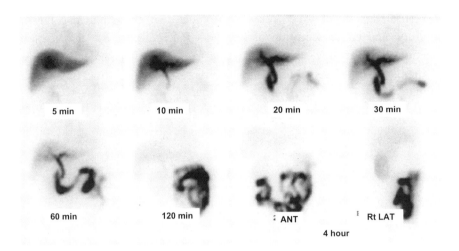

| 5 min | 10 min | 20 min | 30 min |

| 60 min | 120 min | ANT | Rt LAT |

4 hour

Fig. 9.3. Hepatobiliary scintigraphy of acute cholecystitis. Gallbladder activity is not visualized until the 4-h delayed images. Cystic duct obstruction causes non-visualization of gallbladder, whereas initial liver uptake and biliary excretion to CBD and intestinal loops show normal appearance.

(Fig. 9.3). Normal examination exhibits homogenous liver uptake (hepatocyte phase; 5–20 min) with uniform washout to biliary tracts (biliary tract phase; 10–60 min), resulting in visualization of the gallbladder and bowel (intestinal phase; 30–60 min). Patients need to be fasting for 2–5 h prior to the test to enable visualization of the gallbladder. If the gallbladder fails to visualize at 1 h after injection, delayed images are acquired until 4 h post injection or another 30 min acquisition after IV administration of 0.05 mg/kg of morphine sulfate if the cystic duct obstruction is suspected. Morphine augments the tone of the sphincter of Oddi and increases the luminal pressure of the common bile duct (CBD) by 10 times. If the cystic duct is patent, this increase of pressure is sufficient to enable bile flow into the gallbladder. Morphine-augmented cholescintigraphy increased the sensitivity in assessing cystic duct patency. A history of drug abuse, an allergy to the drug, pancreatitis, and significant obstruction of CBD are contraindications to the administration of morphine.[4]

As a non-invasive procedure, cholescintigraphy is used for the evaluation of functional hepatobiliary disorder. The gallbladder ejection fraction (GBEF) is determined by IV infusion of $0.02 \, \mu g/kg$ CCK (sincalide) over a period of 30 min or fatty meal administration. Cholecystagogues cause the gallbladder to contract, relax the sphincter of Oddi, enhance bowel motility, and cause secretion of bile and pancreatic fluid. The ejection fraction that does not exceed 35% at up to 30 min after cholecystagogue challenge is considered abnormal, which represents biliary tract dyskinesia (Table 9.2).

Postcholecystectomy complications such as bile leak (Fig. 9.4), cystic duct remnant, biliary ductal strictures, and stenosis are among the other

Table 9.2.   Affecting factors in reducing GBEF.

Drug	Disease or Condition
Opioids	Diabetes mellitus
Atropine	Pregnancy
Calcium channel antagonists	Sprue
Octreotide	Exocrine dysfunction of pancreas
Progesterone, oral pills	Vagotomy

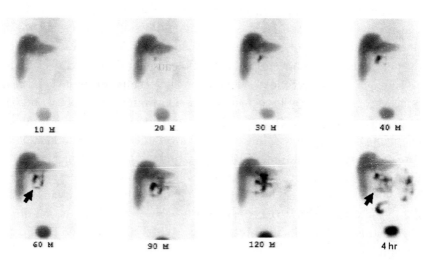

Fig. 9.4.   Bile leak. Hepatobiliary scintigraphy exhibits an abnormal linear activity near the gallbladder fossa at 60 min after injection of Tc-99m DISIDA, which shows increase of radioactivity and geometric distribution until the 4 h following delay-images. This patients underwent total gastrectomy due to stomach cancer and complained of severe abdominal pain after surgery. Arrows show the bile leaking in the localized peritoneal cavity of operation site.

clinical indication of hepatobiliary scintigraphy. Hepatobiliary scintigraphy is also useful to differentiate biliary atresia from neonatal hepatitis and to evaluate the complications associated with liver transplantation.

9.2.4. *Liver scintigraphy*

Various kinds of focal or diffuse disorder in liver can occur. Liver scintigraphy is a simple procedure to detect or differentiate space-occupying lesions and to evaluate diffuse liver disease.

After IV injection of Tc-99m sulfur colloid, the colloid particles are phagocytized by reticuloendothelial cells, which are normally distributed in liver (85% by Kupffer cells), spleen (10%), and bone marrow (5%). Normal findings shows homogenous distribution of radioactivity in liver, spleen, and bone marrow within the normal size according to the distribution ratios of reticuloendothelial system, i.e., the liver has relatively more uptake than the spleen. Functional disorder causes the decreased uptake of colloid in liver with diffuse and mottled appearance, which is caused by the decrease of hepatic blood flow or the dysfunction of Kupffer cells. Reduced extraction of radiolabeled colloid in liver results in relatively greater uptake in spleen, marrow, and sometimes lungs (referred to as "colloid shift").

Space-occupying lesions in the liver are indicated as areas of reduced or absent radioactivity in liver scintigraphy because the corresponding space-occupying lesions has little of reticuloendothelial cells compared to normal parenchyme (Fig. 9.5). The etiologic origins vary from congenital (cyst), infectious (abscess), trauma (hematoma, radiation), degenerative (cirrhosis), benign neoplasm (adenoma, hemangioma), and malignant neoplasm (hepatoma, metastasis). (Table 9.3)

9.3. Oncologic Imaging in GI Tumors

9.3.1. *GI tracts*

The gold standard method for the diagnosis of carcinoma of the GI tracts is endoscopy. It offers both direct visualization of the tumor and the ability to acquire a histologic diagnosis. Although endoscopy provides good visualization of the mucosa, it is not the best method for determination of the

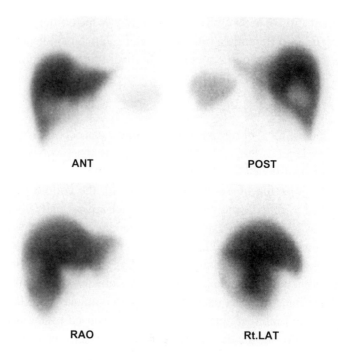

ANT   **POST**

RAO   **Rt.LAT**

Fig. 9.5. A cold space-occupying lesion on liver scintigraphy. Various kinds of benign and malignant lesions in liver can be presented as cold space–occupying lesions in liver scintigraphy. In this case, a simple cyst in right lobe of liver was detected.

depth of invasion by tumor or extent of metastatic involvement. Computed tomography (CT) is currently the most frequently used initial staging tool for investigating tumor extent with respect to tumor invasion to the adjacent organs and also distant metastases. There are limitations of anatomical findings such as lymph node enlargement or indeterminant small nodules in the liver and lung to be determined as benign or malignant by CT. The recent progress of diagnostic and therapeutic methods has made a change in the clinical management of oncologic patients. FDG-PET currently plays no established role in oncologic diagnosis of esophagus and stomach. The detection is dependent on signal intensity based on metabolically active tissue on FDG-PET compared to the lesion size by conventional methods. FDG-PET, tumor metabolic imaging, can provide the supplement information in conjunction with anatomical imaging.[6]

Table 9.3. Correlative imaging scintigraphy in space-occupying lesions in liver.

Disease	Colloid Scan	Initial Flow	Hepatobiliary Scan	Blood Pool Scan (RBC)	FDG PET
Hepatoma	Cold	Increase	Cold or mild uptake	Normal or decrease	Hyper metabolic or isometabolic
Hemangioma*	Cold	Decrease	Cold	Increase	Hypometabolic
Adenoma	Cold or normal	Increase or normal	Normal or mild uptake with delayed excretion	Normal	Isometabolic
Focal nodular hyperplasia	Normal or increase	Increased	Normal or mild uptake with delayed excretion	Normal	Isometabolic
Metastasis	Cold	Increase or normal	Cold	Normal or decrease	hypermetabolic
abscess	Cold	Increase or decrease ("rim effect")	Cold	Normal or decrease	Hypometabolic or hypermetabolic
Focal fatty metamorphosis	Normal	Normal	Normal	Normal or decrease	Isometabolic

*perfusion–blood pool mismatch

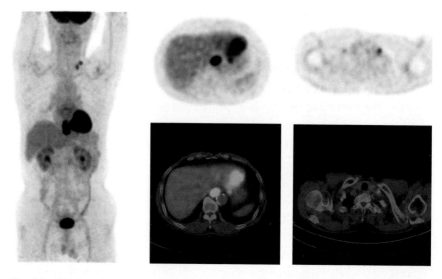

Fig. 9.6. Esophageal carcinoma with cervical lymph node metastases. PET-CT images show a markedly increased uptake of F-18 FDG at the lower chest in lower esophageal carcinoma and a regional lymph node. Additionally, there are two foci of FDG uptake in left lower cervical lymph nodes on PET and PET-CT images. Metastatic cancer cells were proven in the cervical lymph node on ultrasonography-guided biopsies.

9.3.2. *Esophagus and stomach*

Diagnosis and Staging. The role of FDG-PET in the primary diagnosis of esophageal cancer (Fig. 9.6) has not been well established. Studies have consistently demonstrated a high sensitivity for the detection of the primary lesions in patients with known esophageal cancer.[7,8] Flamen *et al.*[8] reported a sensitivity of 95% for the primary tumor visualization in a cohort of 74 patients, whereas, the false-negative results were associated with small T1 lesions. However, benign causes of FDG uptake, which may lead to false positive results include infections esophagitis, Barret's esophagus without malignancy, inflammatory esophagitis caused by reflux esophagitis, and post-procedural changes.[9] No significant correlation has been found between the standardized uptake value (SUV) and depth of tumor invasion. Endoscopic ultrasonography (EUS) has been proved to be the most accurate tool for T staging.[8,10]

PET-CT has a higher specificity than either CT or EUS for lymph node metastases. The presence of discrete focal metabolic activity in periesophageal or regional lymph node is highly indicative of nodal metastases. FDG-PET alone has similar sensitivity but lower specificity and accuracy for the detection of locoregional lymph node metastases than the combined PET-CT imaging (sensitivity, 96% versus 96%; specificity, 59% versus 81%; accuracy, 83% versus 90%, respectively), owing to difficulties in differentiating uptake in periesophageal lymph nodes from that of the lesion.[11] This was ascribed to the poor spatial resolution of PET and problematic attenuation in the chest. Even after taking this into consideration, Block *et al.* reported that PET was almost twice as accurate as CT in predicting involvement of adjacent lymph nodes.[12]

The identification of distant metastasis is one of the most important steps in the preoperative determination of whether the patient has resectable or unresectable disease. The M stage denotes lymphadenopathy that is just beyond locoregional lymph node as *M1a* disease and distant organ metastases as *M1b*. In a comparison study, PET was found to be 86% accurate in the evaluation of *M1a* nodal metastases with a specificity of 90%, whereas the accuracy and specificity for combined CT and EUS assessment were 62% and 69%, respectively.[13] Moreover, PET has been easily demonstrated to accurately show sites of distant metastases, *M1b* disease, with the sensitivity and specificity higher than those for CT and EUS. Thus, in clinical practice, disease staging should be determined using a multimodal approach including information from EUS, PET, and CT.[9]

Restaging and Response Assessment. PET-CT appears to have an important role in response assessment. In a prospective study evaluating CT, EUS, and PET-CT to assess therapeutic response to neoadjuvant chemoradiation, complete response was predicted accurately by EUS in 67% and better by PET-CT in 89%.[14] Weber *et al.*[15] suggested that PET could differentiate responding from non-responding tumors early in the course of therapy, which could help to potentially avoid ineffectual and harmful treatment. However, increased FDG uptake secondary to radiation therapy and postprocedural inflammation can limit the specificity in assessing response on FDG-PET. PET-CT also has a high sensitivity, specificity, and accuracy of 93%, 76% and 87%, respectively, for the detection of recurrence at all sites in patients with treated esophageal carcinoma.[16]

In gastric cancer, PET-CT has not been proven to be highly accurate in the local staging of gastric cancer. Probably one of the reasons is that a physiological FDG uptake in the stomach is observed frequently and its contour of the tracer uptake is variable, which are impossible to differentiate from gastric cancer.[6] The physiological gastric uptake of FDG may be partly due to the smooth muscle activity, but the detailed mechanism is still unknown. T staging of gastric carcinoma is typically assessed with EUS, and multidetector CT has become the standard for N and M staging. However, it is generally expected that PET-CT may a valuable role in the detection of distant metastases.[17] In addition, FDG-PET may also be helpful in the follow-up evaluation of patients undergoing chemotherapy to identify the responder to treatment earlier than the conventional methods.[18]

9.3.3. *Colon and rectum*

Approximately 70% of these patients undergo a radical surgical resection of primary lesions but only two-thirds are cured. After the initial surgical resection of colorectal cancer, the accurate and early detection of potentially respectable metastatic tumors localized in the liver and lung is important in patient management. About one-thirds of patients who underwent curative surgical resection of primary lesion recur, usually within 18 to 24 months after the initial treatment.[19] After the initial surgical resection of colorectal cancer, accurate and early detection of potentially respectable metastatic tumors localized in the liver and lung is important in patient management. CT is sensitive for intraabdominal and pelvic lesions, but there are substantial difficulties differentiating benign fibrosis from malignant recurrence. A scar formation after resection of rectal cancer which mimics the local recurrence on CT/MRI may make it difficult to accurate diagnosis for local recurrence. More accurate preoperative re-staging including FDG-PET would reduce the frequency of surgery for non-resectable recurrence, and more sensitive detection of tumor recurrence may increase the rate of resectability at re-staging. Currently, the main role of PET-CT (Fig. 9.7) is in detecting nodal and organ metastasis, and evaluation postoperative changes and/or residual tissue.

Diagnosis and Staging. Similar to other GI tumors, PET scanners lack the resolution required to evaluate the depth of tumor penetration through the bowel wall and pericolonic lymph nodes anatomically close to the primary tumor. Because of the same reason, microscopic disease cannot be detected

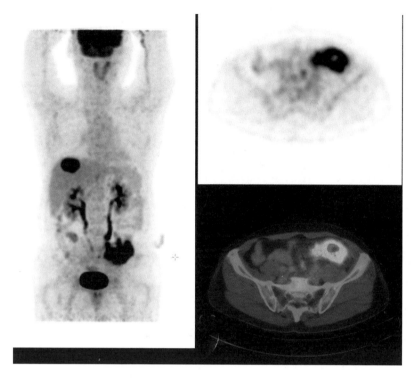

Fig. 9.7. Selected projection and transverse PET images of the whole body show markedly increased uptake of F-18 FDG in the colon carcinoma in descending colon and highly increased uptakes in the metastatic lesion involving liver dome.

by PET. Basically the main diagnostic tool for the detection of primary colorectal cancer is a colonoscopy with biopsy or barium enema. Local lymph node metastases are evaluated as part of the surgical procedure. The sensitivity of FDG-PET for the diagnosis of primary lesions and local lymph node metastases at initial diagnosis and initial preoperative staging is of limited clinical importance.

Despite the superiority of surgery and histopathology at T and local N stages, PET-CT has an advantage at M stage assessment. Imaging to detect nodal or organ metastases is important in directing the general therapeutic approach.[9] Chua *et al.*[20] recently compared PET-CT with standard contrast-enhanced multidetector CT for the evaluation of patients with hepatic metastases and found PET-CT had 94% sensitivity and 75% specificity compared to lower values of 91% and 25% for CT, respectively. PET-CT

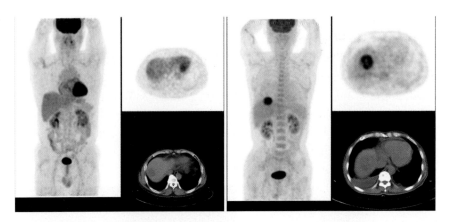

Fig. 9.8. (A) F-18 FDG-PET images of the whole body show different patterns of hepatocellular carcinoma. (A) A low attenuated mass in right lobe of liver on CT show similar FDG uptake as the surronding normal liver parenchyme. Well-differentiated hepatocellular carcinoma was diagnosed at resection on histopathology. (B) Poorly differentiated hepatocellular carcinoma shows markedly increased uptake of F-18 FDG in the hepatocellular carcinoma in liver dome on FDG-PET.

has the ability to directly affect patient management by guiding biopsies or directing surgical resections of liver metastases.

Although PET has high sensitivity for detection of a number of abdominal cancerous lesions, some kinds of neoplasms such as mucinous adenocarcinoma, carcinoid tumors, neuroendocrine tumors, and so on are not FDG avid, so does not show hypermetabolism on FDG PET.[21]

Recurrence Assessment. The differentiation of the treatment sequelae is particularly problematic with distal tumors, in which presacral scarring and pelvic changes are common. In case of PET, as anatomical changes do not affect the metabolism unless there is a leak with persistent inflammation, the presence of metabolic activity in the presacral space generally is indicative of tumor recurrence. FDG-PET was found to be more accurate than CT and carcinoembryonic antigen (CEA) for the detection of recurrent colorectal cancer. The accuracy, sensitivity, and specificity of FDG-PET for the detection of local recurrent tumors were more than 90%.[22] Ito *et al.*[23] compared findings of FDG-PET and MRI with histopathological findings, and FDG-PET could differentiate the scar from the local recurrent tumor. False-negative results on T2-weighted images, which the lesion is not shown as high intense area, may be due to the pathological characteristic of recurrence as fibrotic changes with less tumor cell density. A meta-analysis of

Wiering *et al.*[24] reported pooled sensitivity and specificity of 88% and 96%, respectively, for FDG-PET in detection of hepatic metastases compared with lower values of 83% and 84% for CT. With regard to extrahepatic disease, pooled sensitivity and specificity for PET was 92% and 95%, respectively, in comparison with 61% and 91% for CT. Thus, PET findings resulted in the alteration of clinical management in 32% of patients.

Although FDG-PET is essentially needed to evaluate in patients with suspected recurrent colorectal cancers, we must interpret carefully a FDG uptake in the abdomen. It is often found that the intestinal physiologic FDG uptakes on the PET images which mimic a colorectal lesion. In general, normal intestinal tracer uptake can be differentiated from abnormal uptake by the visible distribution of activity which is linear and can be shown to follow the expected pattern on the coronal/sagittal view. Since PET/CT imaging can increase accuracy and certainty of lesion localization in colorectal cancer,[25] the differentiation of physiological intestinal uptake and pathological uptake would be more accurate if PET-CT can be available or if two-time point PET can be obtained.

9.3.4. *GI stromal tumor*

The role of PET in GI stromal tumor (GIST) is not defined clearly because of there appears to be variable FDG uptake by primary lesion, most likely a reflection of the varied nature of the tumor.[9] Although surgical resection is the best chance for cure, Imatinib is the current treatment of choice for local and distant metastatic disease. Currently, FDG-PET is tried and successfully used to assess the response to Imatinib and to provide prognostic information.[26]

9.3.5. *Hepatobiliary tumors*

Cancers of the liver may arise in the parenchymal cells (hepatocellular cancers), or from the intrahepatic bile ducts (cholangiocarcinomas), or metastasize from other organ tumors. The studies on FDG-PET in primary hepatobiliary tumors were not so many to establish clear indications. It was probably due to relatively low sensitivity, but FDG-PET can afford to be used in the differentiation of malignant hepatic lesions from benign ones, prediction of prognosis by non-invasive grading of differentiation, and the detection of distant metastases. Nevertheless, further studies are necessary for determining the exact role of FDG-PET in the evaluation and management of the patients with hepatobiliary tumors.

Metastatic Disease. Metastatic tumor of the liver is common. Its size, high rate of blood flow, double perfusion by the hepatic artery and portal vein, and its Kupffer cell filtration function combine to make it the next most common site of metastases after the lymph nodes. The most common primary tumors are those of the GI tract, lung, and breast, as well as melanomas. Less common are metastases from tumors of the thyroid, prostate, and skin. PET has been shown to be superior to abdominal ultrasound and CT but not magnetic resonance imaging in the evaluation of both primary and secondary hepatic metastases from multiple primary malignancies.[27]

Hepatocellular Carcinoma. FDG-PET has low sensitivity for detection of hepatocellular carcinoma (HCC), compared to the contrast-enhanced CT (Fig. 9.9). The well-differentiated HCC may retain the properties of normal hepatocytes, and the enzyme activities of glycolytic pathway resemble that of normal hepatocytes. A decrease in differentiation increases glycolytic enzymes levels and decreases glucose-6-phosphatase levels. Well-differentiated and low-grade HCC show lower FDG activity than higher-grade tumors, which can be helpful to assess tumor grade.[28]

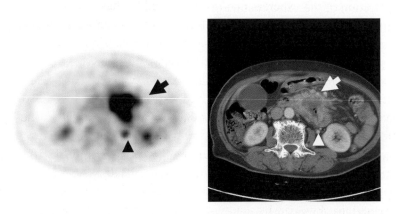

Fig. 9.9. Selected transeverse PET and CT images in uncinate process of pancreas show markedly increased uptake of F-18 FDG in the pancreatic cancer (arrow) and also a regional lympn node metastasis (arrowhead).

Conversely, PET may be better than CT at detecting extrahepatic disease and a recent study highlighted the use of PET at detecting extrahepatic HCC recurrence.[29] Liver transplantation may be considered as a therapeutic option, but tumor recurrence and/or metastasis are the major problems. Kim *et al.*[30] reported the use of FDG-PET for patients with HCC after liver transplatation. The most common sites of recurrence were extrahepatic (60%) and the most common extrahepatic sites were the lungs and bone (31.3% each). The detection rate of FDG-PET–CT was 92.9% for extrahepatic metastases of the tumor size with more than 1 cm.

Recently, Park *et al.*[31] reported that the additional use of C-11 acetate to FDG-PET–CT increases the overall sensitivity for the detection of primary HCC (FDG, 60.9%; C-11 acetate, 75.4%; dual tracers, 82.7%, respectively) but not for the detection of extrahepatic metastases (FDG, 85.7%; ^{11}C acetate, 77.0%; dual tracers, 85.7%, respectively). FDG-PET–CT was more sensitive in the detection of poorly differentiated HCC and FDG-PET–CT has a relatively high sensitivity for the detection of extrahepatic metastases of HCC.

Cholangiocarcinoma. FDG PET–CT and contrast-enhanced CT were found to have comparable accuracy for detection of the primary intrahepatic and extrahepatic cholangiocarcinoma, but FDG-PET showed a poor sensitivity in the detection of locoregional lymph node metastases.[32] However, in relation to metastasis, PET-CT is superior with a sensitivity of 100% for distant metastasis whereas contrast-enhanced CT has a sensitivity of 25%. Petrowsky *et al.*[33] reported that PET-CT staging has an important impact on selection of adequate therapy, resulted in a change of management in 17% of patients deemed resectable after conventional work-up.

Pancreatic Carcinoma. Pancreatic carcinoma is a rather rare disease, but account for more than 4% of all cancer death in the United State.[6] The poor prognosis is related to the fact that symptoms occur only in advanced stages. Contrast-enhanced CT is the most commonly used imaging modality in pancreatic carcinoma with the histologic confirmation. To date, there have been relatively few studies assessing the role and usefulness of PET in the diagnosis and staging of patients with pancreatic carcinoma. Bang *et al.*[34] reported that FDG-PET has a diagnostic accuracy of 95% in the diagnosis and staging of patients with suspected pancreatic carcinoma as compared with 77% accuracy for CT. They also found that FDG-PET was not only superior to CT in the detection of liver metastasis but also detected treatment response in 5 out of 15 cases after chemoradiation therapy, whereas CT could not detect any treatment response. In a meta-analysis of all data, PET and PET-CT had a sensitivity between 90% and 95% with a specificity between 82% and 100% for detection of pancreatic carcinoma, and had a wider sensitivity between 61% and 100% with a specificity between 67% and 100% for overall pancreatic staging.[35] They concluded that PET and PET-CT are best at diagnosis and staging pancreatic carcinoma but are relatively inefficient in the detection of local nodal disease and that further evidence is required before PET-CT could be considered as a first-line imaging modality.

Serial measures of tumor marker levels (CA 19-9) are a sensitive indicator of disease recurrence. However, differentiating recurrent disease from post-surgical/radiotherapy changes with CT or MRI is difficult. Molecular imaging, on the other hand, can detect focal tracer accumulation regardless of morphology. Ruf *et al.*[36] showed that in 31 patients with suspected recurrent disease, 96% of local recurrences were detected with FDG as compared with 23% with CT or MRI. There are therefore indications that FDG-PET may be useful in differentiating fibrosis from recurrent disease, in whole-body restaging of the patient and in identifying the focus of recurrence, where there is an increase in tumor marker levels in the face of a negative or equivocal finding by conventional imaging.

References

1. Habibian MR, Shar C. (2008) Gastrointestinal and correlative abdominal nuclear medicine imaging. In: Habibian MR, Delbeke D, Martin WH, Vitola JV, Sandler MP (eds), *Nuclear Medicine Imaging* 2nd edition. Lippincott, Philadelphia, pp. 202–258.
2. Basu S, Torigian D, Alavi A. (2008) The role of modern molecular imaging techniques in gastroenterology. *Gastroenterology* **135**: 1055–1078.
3. Ryu JS, Park SK. (2008) Gastrointestinal imaging. In: Chung JK, Lee MC (eds), *Nuclear Medicine*. 3rd edition. Korea Medicine, Seoul, pp. 573–628. [in Korean]
4. Urbain JLC, Johnson CL, Vekemans MC. (2000) Gastrointestinal nuclear medicine. In: Schiepers C (ed), *Diagnostic Nuclear Medicine*. Springer, Heidelberg, pp. 123–134.
5. Maurer AH, Urbain JL, Krevsky B, Knight LC, Revesz G, Brown K. (1998) Effects of *in vitro* versus *in vivo* red cell labeling on imaging quality in gastrointestinal bleeding studies. *J Nucl Med Technol* **26**: 87–90.

6. Francis DL, Arulampalam TAH, Costa DC, Ell PJ. (2003) PET and PET/CT of cancers of the esophagus, stomach, and large intestine. In: Von Schulthess GK (ed), *Clinical Molecular Anatomic Imaging*. Lippincott, Philadelpia, pp. 318–333.

7. Fukunaga T, Okazumi S, Koide Y, Isono K, Imazeki K. (1998) Evaluation of esophageal cancers using fluorine-18-fluorodeoxyglucose PET. *J Nucl Med* **39**: 1002–1007.

8. Flamen P, Lerut A, Van Cutsem E, De Wever W, Peeters M, Stroobants S, *et al.* (2000) Utility of positron emission tomography for the staging of patients with potentially operable esophageal carcinoma. *J Clin Oncol* **18**: 3202–210.

9. Cronin CG, Moore M, Blake MA. (2009) Positron emission tomography/computerized tomography for the gastroenterologist and hepatologist. *Clin Gastroenterol Hepatol* **7**: 20–26.

10. Zuccaro G, Sivak MV, Rice TW. (2002) Endoscopic ultrasound and the staging of esophageal and gastric cancer. *Gastrointest Endosc Clin North Am* **2**: 625–636.

11. Bar-Shalom R, Guralnik L, Tsalic M, Leiderman M, Frenkel A, Gaitini D, *et al.* (2005) The additional value of PET/CT over PET in FDG imaging of oesophageal cancer. *Eur J Nucl Med Mol Imaging* **32**: 918–924.

12. Block MI, Patterson GA, Sundaresan RS, Bailey MS, Flanagan FL, Dehdashti F, *et al.* (1997) Improvement in staging of esophageal cancer with the addition of positron emission tomography. *Ann Thorac Surg* **64**: 770–776.

13. Lerut T, Flamen P, Ectors N, Van Cutsem E, Peeters M, Hiele M, *et al.* (2000) Histopathologic validation of lymph node staging with FDG-PET scan in cancer of the esophagus and gastroesophageal junction: A prospective study based on primary surgery with extensive lymphadenectomy. *Ann Surg* **232**: 743–752.

14. Cerfolio RJ, Bryant AS, Ohja B, Bartolucci AA, Eloubeidi MA. (2005) The accuracy of endoscopic ultrasonography with fine-needle aspiration, integrated positron emission tomography with computed tomography, and computed tomography in restaging patients with esophageal cancer after neoadjuvant chemoradiotherapy. *J Thorac Cardiovasc Surg* **129**: 1232–1241.

15. Weber WA, Ott K, Becker K, Dittler HJ, Helmberger H, Avril NE, *et al.* (2001) Prediction of response to preoperative chemotherapy in adenocarcinomas of the esophagogastric junction by metabolic imaging. *J Clin Oncol* **19**: 3058–3065.

16. Guo H, Zhu H, Xi Y, Zhang B, Li L, Huang Y, Zhang J, *et al.* (2007) Diagnostic and prognostic value of 18F-FDG PET/CT for patients with suspected recurrence from squamous cell carcinoma of the esophagus. *J Nucl Med* **48**: 1251–1258.

17. Shoda H, Kakugawa Y, Saito D, Kozu T, Terauchi T, Daisaki H, *et al.* (2007) Evaluation of 18F-2-deoxy-2-fluoro-glucose positron emission tomography for gastric cancer screening in asymptomatic individuals undergoing endoscopy. *Br J Cancer* **97**: 1493–1498.

18. Lim JS, Yun MJ, Kim MJ, Hyung WJ, Park MS, Choi JY, *et al.* (2006) CT and PET in stomach cancer: Preoperative staging and monitoring of response to therapy. *Radiographics* **26**: 143–156.

19. Galandiuk S, Wieand HS, Moertel CG, Cha SS, Fitzgibbons RJ Jr, Pemberton JH, *et al.* (1992) Patterns of recurrence after curative resection of carcinoma of the colon and rectum. *Surg Gynecol Obstet* **174**: 27–32.

20. Chua SC, Groves AM, Kayani I, Menezes L, Gacinovic S, Du Y, *et al.* (2007) The impact of 18F-FDG PET/CT in patients with liver metastases. *Eur J Nucl Med Mol Imaging* **34**: 1906–1914.

21. Blake MA, Singh A, Setty BN, Slattery J, Kalra M, Maher MM, *et al.* (2006) Pearls and pitfalls in interpretation of abdominal and pelvic PET-CT. *Radiographics* **26**: 1335–1353.

22. Huebner RH, Park KC, Shepherd JE, Schwimmer J, Czernin J, Phelps ME, *et al.* (2000) A meta-analysis of the literature for whole-body FDG-PET detection of recurrent colorectal cancer. *J Nucl Med* **41**: 1177–1189.

23. Ito K, Kato T, Tadokoro M, Tadokoro M, Yamada T, Ikeda M, *et al.* (1992) Recurrent rectal cancer and scar: Differentiation with PET and MR imaging. *Radiology* **182**: 549–552.

24. Wiering B, Krabbe PF, Jager GJ, Oyen WJ, Ruers TJ. (2005) The impact of fluor-18-deoxyglucose-positron emission tomography in the management of colorectal liver metastases. *Cancer* **104**: 2658–2670.

25. Cohade D, Osman M, Leal J, Wahl RL. (2003) Direct comparison of FDG-PET and PET-CT imaging in colorectal cancer. *J Nucl Med* **44**: 1797–1803.

26. Goerres GW, Stupp. R, Barghouth G, Hany TF, Pestalozzi B, Dizendorf E, *et al.* (2005) The value of PET, CT and in-line PET/CT in patients with gastrointestinal stromal tumours: Long-term outcome of treatment with imatinib mesylate. *Eur J Nucl Med Mol Imaging* **32**: 153–162.

27. Chua SC, Groves AM, Kayani I, Menezes L, Gacinovic S, Du Y, *et al.* (2007) The impact of 18F-FDG PET/CT in patients with liver metastases. *Eur J Nucl Med Mol Imaging* **34**: 1906–1914.

28. Khan MA, Combs CS, Brunt EM, Lowe VJ, Wolverson MK, Solomon H, *et al.* (2000) Positron emission tomography scanning in the evaluation of hepatocellular carcinoma. *J Hepato* **32**: 792–797.

29. Sun L, Guan YS, Pan WM, Chen GB, Luo ZM, Wu H. (2007) Positron emission tomography/computer tomography in guidance of extrahepatic hepatocellular carcinoma metastasis management. *World J Gastroentero* **13**: 5413–5415.

30. Kim YK, Lee KW, Cho SY, Han SS, Kim SH, Kim SK, *et al.* (2010) Usefulness ^{18}F-FDG positron emission tomography/computed tomography for detecting recurrence of hepatocellular carcinoma in posttransplant patients. *Liver Transpl* **16**: 767–772.

31. Park JW, Kim JH, Kim SK, Kang KW, Park KW, Choi JI, *et al.* (2008) A prospective evaluation of ^{18}F-FDG and ^{11}C-acetate PET/CT for detection of primary and metastatic hepatocellular carcinoma. *J Nucl Med* **49**: 1912–1921.

32. Sun L, Wu H, Guan YS. (2007) Positron emission tomography/computer tomography: Challenge to conventional imaging modalities in evaluating primary and metastatic liver malignancies. *World J Gastroenterol* **13**: 2775–2783.

33. Petrowsky H, Wildbrett P, Husarik DB, Hany TF, Tam S, Jochum W, *et al.* (2006) Impact of integrated positron emission tomography and computed tomography on staging and management of gallbladder cancer and cholangiocarcinoma. *J Hepatol* **45**: 43–50.

34. Bang S, Chung HW, Park SW, Chung JB, Yun M, Lee JD, *et al.* (2006) The clinical usefulness of F-18 fluorodeoxyglucose positron emission tomography in the differential diagnosis, staging, and response evaluation after concurrent chemoradiotherapy for pancreatic cancer. *J Clin Gastroenterol* **40**: 923–929.

35. Pakzad F, Groves AM, Ell PJ. (2006) The role of positron emission tomography in the management of pancreatic cancer. *Semin Nucl Med* **36**: 248–256.
36. Ruf J, Hänninen EL, Oettle H, Plotkin M, Pelzer U, Stroszczynski C, *et al.* (2005) Detection of recurrent pancreatic cancer: Comparison of FDG-PET with CT/MRI. *Pancreatol* **5**: 266–272.

Chapter 10
Nuclear Imaging of Esophageal, Gastric, and Pancreatic Cancers

Hirofumi Shibata, Ukihide Tateishi
and Tomio Inoue

10.1. Esophageal Cancer

10.1.1. *Introduction*

The most common malignant tumor in the proximal two-thirds of the esophagus is squamous cell carcinoma; adenocarcinoma is the most common in the distal one third. About 8,000 cases of squamous cell carcinoma occur annually in the US. It is more common in parts of Asia and in South Africa. In the US, it is four to five times more common among blacks than whites, and two to three times more common among men than women. The primary risk factors are alcohol ingestion and tobacco use (in any form). Other factors include achalasia, human papilloma virus, lye ingestion (resulting in stricture), sclerotherapy, Plummer–Vinson syndrome, irradiation of the esophagus, and esophageal webs. Genetic causes are unclear, but 50% of patients with tylosis (hyperkeratosis palmaris et plantaris), an autosomal dominant disorder, have esophageal cancer by age 45 years, and 95% have it by age 55 years. Adenocarcinoma occurs in the distal esophagus. The incidence of adenocarcinoma is increasing and it accounts for 50% of esophageal carcinoma in whites. It is four times more common among whites than blacks. Alcohol is not an important risk factor, but smoking is contributory to the disease development. Adenocarcinoma of the distal esophagus is difficult to distinguish from adenocarcinoma of the gastric cardia invading the distal esophagus. Most adenocarcinomas arise in Barrett's esophagus, which results from chronic gastroesophageal reflux disease and reflux esophagitis.

In Barrett's esophagus, a metaplastic, columnar, glandular, intestine-like mucosa with brush border and goblet cells replaces the normal stratified squamous epithelium of the distal esophagus during the healing phase of acute esophagitis when healing takes place in the continued presence of stomach acid.

10.1.2. *Discussion*

10.1.2.1. *Staging*

The recent progress in diagnostic and therapeutic methods has changed the clinical management of patients with esophageal cancer. In the field of diagnosis of esophageal cancer, the endoscopic technique using dye or endoscopic ultrasonography (EUS) has increased the diagnostic sensitivity for early esophageal cancer. The prognosis in patients with esophageal cancer has been improved by introducing the lymph node resection of three regions or the superior mediastinum. However, surgery in patients with esophageal cancer is an invasive procedure, and the post-surgical complications are still severe. It requires a cautious treatment decision in patients with esophageal cancer even if the perioperative management has been advanced.[1] Anatomic imaging such as computed tomography (CT), magnetic resonance imaging (MRI), and ultrasonography (US), is the standard examination for investigating tumor extent, tumor invasion to the adjacent organs, and distant metastases. Fluorodeoxyglucose positron emission tomography (FDG-PET) and tumor metabolic imaging can provide supplemental information in conjunction with anatomic imaging.

In stage 0, abnormal cells are found in the innermost layer of tissue lining the esophagus. These abnormal cells may become cancer and spread into nearby normal tissue. Stage 0 is also called carcinoma *in situ*. In stage I, cancer has formed and spread beyond the innermost layer of tissue to the next layer of tissue in the wall of the esophagus. Stage II esophageal cancer is divided into stage IIA and stage IIB, depending on where the cancer has spread. In Stage IIA, the cancer has spread to the layer of esophageal muscle or to the outer wall of the esophagus. In Stage IIB, the cancer may have spread to any of the first three layers of the esophagus and to nearby lymph nodes. In stage III, cancer has spread to the outer wall of the esophagus and may have spread to tissues or lymph nodes near the esophagus. Stage IV esophageal cancer is divided into stage IVA and stage IVB, depending on where the cancer has spread.

10.1.2.2. *T stage*

To study the extent of the primary tumor, we investigated the relationship between T grade in the tumor node metastasis TNM classification of the International Union Against Cancer and the tumor standard uptake value (SUV) of FDG in primary lesions. About 50% of primary lesions of esophageal cancer in the early stage estimated as pT1 (tumor localized within the submucosal layer) were visible on FDG-PET images, while all primary lesions estimated as pT2, pT3, and pT4 were visible. The mean SUV of FDG in pT1 primary lesions was significantly lower than those in pT2, pT3, and pT4. There was a significant linear correlation between the longitudinal diameter of the primary lesion and the SUV of FDG.[2] Several studies have shown that the vast majority of primary esophageal cancers that are first diagnosed by other methods are detectable by FDG-PET, with sensitivities in 90% to 100% range for T2 to T4 tumor. When PET results have been reported to be falsely negative in esophageal cancers, this was usually due to small tumor volume, such as stage T1 primary lesion.[3–7] Moreover, the role of endoscopy in the initial evaluation of the primary tumor is well established, particularly as it is readily accessible, provides histological confirmation of tumor type, and may even prove to be therapeutic in the resection of small tumors. By comparison, PET/CT is not an appropriate first-line investigation given its greater cost and limited availability. Kato *et al.*[8] showed that FDG-PET could be used to identify the primary tumor in only 119 of 149 (80%) patients with esophageal cancer, largely due to a reduced sensitivity of 43% for T1 tumors. Furthermore, false-positive results may also occur due to FDG uptake in the normal esophagus, possibly because of smooth muscle activity or gastroesophageal reflux disease. PET, on the contrary, is limited in its ability to demonstrate the depth of tumor invasion into the esophageal wall due to its intrinsically reduced spatial resolution. Although some authors have attempted to show a relationship between the SUV within the primary tumor and the

T-stage, this has not been corroborated by others. The CT component of integrated PET/CT can suggest the presence of T4 disease when there is a convincing loss of the peri-esophageal fat planes as well as a large arc of contact with major adjacent structures, such as the aorta, left atrium or diaphragmatic crus, but PET/CT has little role otherwise in determining the T-stage.[9]

10.1.2.3. *N stage*

Accurate diagnosis of the extent and number of lymph node metastases is important for the management of patients with esophageal cancer, because it relates to the patients' prognosis. In our study, the diagnostic sensitivity, specificity, and accuracy of FDG PET versus CT for the lymph node metastases were 55% versus 45%, 98% versus 94%, 92% versus 87%, respectively.[2] The sensitivity of FDG-PET and CT was not so high because of the existence of microscopic metastasis. Either intense FDG uptake in the primary lesions or physiologic FDG uptake in the myocardium and stomach may also obscure tracer uptake in the metastatic lesion of the adjacent lymph nodes. The detection by CT of lymph node metastases in the border zone area between the cervical region and the upper mediastinum, such as the supraclavicular and infraclavicular lymph nodes, was difficult in some esophageal cancer cases. In these cases FDG-PET could facilitate the visual interpretation of lymph node metastases. The detection of nodal metastasis with PET is dependent on the volume of tumor in metastasis, the intensity of tracer uptake in the lesion, the background tracer activity, and interpretation criteria. Lesions smaller than 5 mm are not usually detected on PET with FDG, which is consistent with other detection challenges encountered with current FDG-PET technology. In general PET is not exceptionally sensitive, but it has a high specificity for the detection of locoregional lymph node metastases (typical sensitivities of 30% to 80%, but with specificities of 80% to 90%). A meta-analysis evaluating data from 421 patients reported a pooled sensitivity and specificity of FDG PET of 51% and 84%, respectively.[8,10–12] In a recent study, Yuan *et al.* evaluated the role of integrated PET/CT in assessing the extent of nodal disease. In 45 patients with esophageal cancer, and pathological evidence of disease in 82 of 397 excised nodal groups, the sensitivity, specificity, and accuracy of PET/CT in detecting nodal disease were 94%, 92%, and 92%, respectively, compared with 82%, 87%, and 86%, respectively, for PET with side-by-side comparison with CT ($p = 0.032$, 0.067, and 0.006, respectively).[10] PET/CT has relatively limited utility for detection of metastatic dissemination to locoregional lymph nodes. FDG uptake within periesophageal lymph nodes that are anatomically close to the primary tumor is difficult to differentiate from uptake within the esophagus itself owing to the limited spatial resolution of PET. Furthermore, microscopic metastatic disease within lymph nodes may not demonstrate sufficient FDG uptake for detection with PET. In addition, FDG uptake within lymph nodes can occur in benign disease such as granulomatous infection (particularly in regions of endemic histoplasmosis or tuberculosis) or sarcoidosis.[13] In a recent meta-analysis of 12 studies that examined the diagnostic accuracy of PET/CT in preoperative staging of esophageal cancer, PET/CT had a sensitivity of 51% and specificity of 84% for detection of nodal metastases. EUS is superior to PET/CT in detection of locoregional nodal metastases and is the primary modality used in this regard; in one recent prospective study, the combination of EUS and CT had a reported sensitivity of 83% for local nodal metastases. EUS has the added advantage over PET/CT of allowing biopsy of suspicious lymph nodes at the time of detection.[13]

10.1.2.4. *M stage*

In almost all studies to date, FDG-PET has been more accurate than other conventional diagnostic methods in detecting organ or non-regional lymph node metastases. A skip metastasis beyond the adjacent lymph node area is a characteristic phenomenon of esophageal cancer. If the range of the field of view of CT or MRI was not sufficient to observe skip lesions, whole-body FDG-PET would be helpful in detecting these skip lesions. FDG-PET, CT, and EUS are probably equivalent in TNM staging accuracy when used independently. When there is nodal FDG uptake in the upper abdomen, differentiating regional lymph node N1 from celiac lymph node M1a is difficult. In these cases, PET/CT would be quite helpful to obtain the accurate TNM staging classification.[14] Metastases from esophageal cancer are frequently found in the liver, lung, and bone. Lowe *et al.* reported that the greatest contributors to false-positive CT results were non-specific lesions in the liver and local nodal findings.[15] PET and CT added important M staging information that could not be obtained by EUS. A recent meta-analysis of FDG-PET for detection of M1 disease of 67% at a specificity of 97%. The main incremental value of FDG-PET/CT in the evaluation of esophageal cancer lies in its ability to identify unsuspected metastatic disease, which is present in up to 30% of patients at initial diagnosis. Integrated FDG-PET/CT has been shown to have superior accuracy in the staging and re-staging of esophageal cancer compared with PET and CT performed separately. In a study of 32 patients with esophageal cancer with 115 sites suspicious for malignancy, FDG-PET/CT was prospectively compared with PET reviewed side-by-side with CT, for detection, accurate localization and characterization of malignant sites. PET/CT had an incremental value over PET for interpretation of 25 of 115 sites (22%). PET/CT provided better specificity and accuracy than PET (81 and 90% versus 59 and 83%, respectively, $p < 0.01$), proving especially of value in the interpretation of disease sites in the neck, locoregional lymph nodes, and in regions of postoperative anatomical distortion. PET/CT upstaged two patients by detecting nodal metastases (9). In addition, synchronous neoplastic disease can be present in 1.5%–5.5% of patients with esophageal cancer at initial presentation, most commonly in the stomach, head and neck, and colon.[13]

10.1.2.5. *Detection of recurrent disease*

The high sensitivity of PET for detection of recurrent esophageal cancer was confirmed by Kato *et al.*[16] In this study, the sensitivity, specificity, and accuracy of FDG-PET for recurrent esophageal cancer were 96%, 68%, and 82%, respectively. PET had a higher sensitivity for detection of bony metastases than CT but it was less sensitive for detection of pulmonary metastases. Hongbo *et al.*[17] reported 56 patients with previously treated esophageal cancer underwent PET/CT scans. Of these, 45 (80.4%) patients had recurrence in 72 (66.1%) malignant sites. On PET/CT, there were nine false-positive and five false-negative results. The overall sensitivity, specificity, and accuracy of PET/CT for detecting recurrence at all sites were 93.1% (67/72), 75.7% (28/37), and 87.2% (95/109), respectively.

PET/CT was highly sensitive, specific, and accurate at regional and distant sites. At local sites, sensitivity was high but specificity was lower (50%) because of a high incidence of false-positive findings. PET/CT is highly effective for detecting recurrent esophageal cancer. The relatively low specificity at local sites is associated primarily with a high rate of false-positive interpretations at anastomosis. PET/CT can also provide noninvasive and independent prognostic information using SUV and recurrent disease pattern on PET/CT images for previously treated esophageal cancer (Fig. 10.1).

10.1.2.6. *Monitoring of therapeutic response*

Wieder *et al.*[18] investigated the time course of tumor glucose utilization in patients with esophageal cancer undergoing preoperative chemoradiotherapy. They measured the SUV of primary lesions prior to chemoradiotherapy at a radiation dose of 14 to 20 Gy, as well as 30 Gy, and 3 weeks after the completion of chemoradiotherapy. At a radiation dose of 14 to 20 Gy, the SUV was already significantly decreased. The decrease in tumor SUV at this point was 39.6% in patients with a histopathologic response, whereas it was only 22.3% in patients without a histopathologic response. These results suggest that FDG-PET may be used for early identification of non-responding tumors and therapy modification. However, a single post-treatment PET/CT scan is sufficient for assessing therapeutic response because persistent FDG uptake within the primary tumor site correlates with residual viable macroscopic tumor and poor survival after esophagectomy. Weber *et al.* have shown that PET/CT performed after only two cycles of induction chemotherapy allows prediction of the pathologic response to neoadjuvant therapy and the long-term outcome with a sensitivity and specificity of 93% and 95%, respectively.[19] PET/CT has a high diagnostic accuracy for detection of recurrent or metastatic esophageal malignancy; for example, Flamen *et al.*[6] reported a sensitivity of 94%, specificity of 82%, and accuracy of 87% for detection of recurrent esophageal cancer and found that PET provided information that was additional to that obtained with conventional surveillance methods in 27% of patients. Such information influences palliative management decisions and may result in improved patient survival.

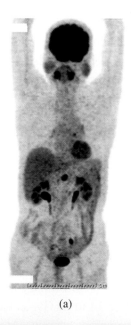

(a)

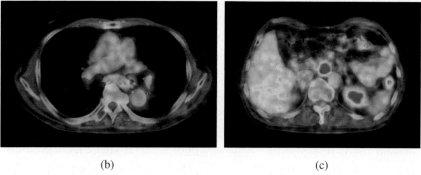

(b)   (c)

Fig. 10.1. (a–c) A 36-year-old man who underwent thoracotomy for esophageal carcinoma. On follow-up PET/CT, abnormal uptake is found in the enlarged subcarinal lymphnode. The SUV_{max} of this lesion is 13.1. This is consistent with recurrent disease. This patient received subsequent radiotherapy.

10.1.3. *Conclusion*

PET/CT with FDG has a role in assessing the effect of neoadjuvant therapy, and potentially in determining the need for adjuvant treatment. Its role as a prognostic marker for patient outcome and as an aid to intensity modulated radiation therapy still requires further investigation.

10.2. Gastric Cancer

10.2.1. *Introduction*

Stomach cancer accounts for an estimated 21,000 cases and over 11,000 deaths in the US annually. Etiology of stomach cancer is multi-factorial, but *Helicobacter pylori* plays a significant role. Gastric adenocarcinoma accounts for 95% of malignant tumors of the stomach; less common are localized gastric lymphomas and leiomyosarcomas. Stomach cancer is the second most common cancer worldwide, but the incidence varies widely; incidence is extremely high in Japan, China, Chile, and Iceland. In the US, incidence has declined in recent decades to the seventh most common cause of death from cancer. In the US, it is most common among blacks, Hispanics, and American Indians. Its incidence increases with age; > 75% of patients are > 50 years.

10.2.2. *Discussion*

10.2.2.1. *Staging*

In stage 0, abnormal cells are found in the inside lining of the mucosal layer of the stomach wall. These abnormal cells may become cancer and spread into nearby normal tissue. Stage 0 is also called carcinoma *in situ*. In stage I, cancer has formed. Stage I is divided into stage IA and stage IB, depending on where the cancer has spread. In Stage IA, cancer has spread completely through the mucosal layer of the stomach wall. In Stage IB, cancer has spread completely through the mucosal layer of the stomach wall and is found in up to six lymph nodes near the tumor; or to the muscularis layer of the stomach wall. In stage II gastric cancer, cancer has spread completely through the mucosal layer of the stomach wall and is found in 7 to 15 lymph nodes near the tumor; or to the muscularis layer of the stomach wall and is found in up to 6 lymph nodes near the tumor; or to the serosal layer of the stomach wall but not to lymph nodes or other organs. Stage III gastric cancer is divided into stage IIIA and stage IIIB depending on where the cancer has spread. In Stage IIIA, the cancer has spread to the muscularis layer of the stomach wall and is found in 7 to 15 lymph nodes near the tumor or the serosal layer of the stomach wall and is found in 1 to 6 lymph nodes near the tumor; or organs next to the stomach but not to lymph nodes or other parts of the body. In Stage IIIB, cancer has spread to the serosal layer of the stomach wall and is found in 7 to 15 lymph nodes near the tumor. In stage IV, cancer has spread to organs next to the stomach and to at least one lymph node; or more than 15 lymph nodes; or other parts of the body.

10.2.2.2. *Primary tumor*

Standard diagnostic tools in the assessment of gastric carcinomas are EUS and CT or staging laparoscopy. The role of FDG-PET in gastric carcinoma is controversial.[20] FDG-PET has been widely used in oncology Diagnosis, but little in the diagnosis of gastric cancer probably because physiological FDG uptake in the stomach is observed frequently and its contour on tracer uptake is variable and impossible to different from gastric cancer.[21] Physiologic gastric uptake of FDG may be due partly to smooth muscle activity, but the details of the mechanism are still unknown.[22] Yoshioka *et al.* found that FDG-PET demonstrated whole lesions in 42 gastric cancer patients with a sensitivity of 71%, specificity of 74%, and accuracy of 73%.[23] Uptake was high in the primary lesions, liver, lymph node, and lung metastases, but low in the bone metastases, ascites, peritonitis carcinomatosa, and pleuritis carcinomatosa.

FDG uptake seems to be strongly dependent on the histologic subtype of the tumor and inversely correlates with the content of mucus.[24−26] Mochiki *et al.*[27] found FDG PET to be superior to CT in identifying the primary tumor in advanced disease. Another study showed that FDG-PET is not an accurate imaging technique for the primary diagnosis of a gastric primary tumor, combining high specificity with low sensitivity. About 20% of patients with gastric cancer are non-assessable by FDG-PET. Sensitivity rate for detecting the primary tumor varies between 58% and 94% among studies (median 81.5%).[25−32] Specificity ranges from 78% to 100% (median 100%). Detection of gastric carcinoma by FDG-PET is partly complicated by background uptake, partly due to high physiological uptake of FDG in the normal gastric wall as a result of its dense blood flow. Moreover, variable and sometimes intense uptake is observed in the normal gastric wall, resembling false-positive pathological uptake.[27,28] Sensitivity of primary tumor identification by FDG-PET is influenced by several other determinants.

The location of the tumor (i.e., proximal/middle/lower one third) is shown to influence the sensitivity of FDG-PET.[25,27,30,33] A second determinant is tumor size or T-stage. The sensitivity of FDG-PET ranges from 26% to 63% in early gastric cancer (EGC; median 43.5%, SUV range 2.1 to 2.8) to 93% to 98% in locally advanced gastric cancer (AGC; median 94%; SUV range 4.3 to 7.9).

10.2.2.3. *Lymph node metastases*

Mochiki *et al.* reported that the sensitivity of PET in detecting nodal metastases was inferior to that of CT, but PET appeared to provide additional information on tumor aggressiveness and prognosis in patients with gastric cancer.[27] Yeung *et al.* found FDG-PET to be highly sensitive in detecting the primary tumor and distant metastases inferior in detecting intra-abdominal lymph node metastases.[31] Five more studies investigated the value of FDG-PET in detecting lymph node metastasis.[27–29,31,32] Sensitivity for metastasis to N1 lymph nodes was very low, ranging from 17.6% to 46.4% (median 27.5%) compared to CT. This could be explained by the relative low spatial resolution of FDG-PET (5 to 7 mm). The perigastric lymph nodes, therefore, cannot be distinguished from the primary tumor or the normal stomach wall. FDG-PET and CT both have a low sensitivity of, respectively, 33% to 46.2% and 44% to 63.1% in detecting metastases at N2 and N3 lymph nodes stations. Specificity, on the contrary, was higher in N1 and N2 lymph node stations with FDG PET, ranging between 91% and 100% (median 96%), compared to CT. PET/CT fusion images have proven to result in better detection of metastatic lymph nodes in esophageal cancer. In a study comparing PET/CT with PET, sensitivity, specificity and accuracy for diagnosing lymph node metastasis were higher for PET/CT.[33]

10.2.2.4. *Peritoneal carcinomatosis*

The diagnosis of intra-abdominal dissemination in patients with gastric cancer is important for determining the indication for surgical resection. Nodules in intra-abdominal cavity can be shown on FDG-PET images, but the differentiation from physiologic intestinal FDG uptake is difficult. This diagnostic dilemma may be resolved by the fusion imaging technique of PET/CT. Three studies investigated the role of FDG PET in detecting peritoneal carcinomatosis.[26,29,34] PET has little value in detecting peritoneal carcinomatosis. It has a low sensitivity (range 9% to 50%; median 32.5%), however, there is a relatively high specificity (63% to 99%; median 88.5%).

10.2.2.5. *Distant metastases*

Kinkel *et al.*[35] found FDG-PET to be the most sensitive non-invasive imaging modality for the diagnosis of hepatic metastases not only from gastric cancers but also from colorectal and gastric carcinomas. Another study in gastric cancer showed that a sensitivity and specificity of 85% and 74% for the detection of liver metastasis; 67% and 88% for lung metastasis; 24% and 76% for ascites; 4% and 100% for pleural carcinomatosis, and 30% and 82% for bone metastasis, respectively.[36]

10.2.2.6. *Monitoring tumor response*

Stahl *et al.*[36] investigated the predictability of FDG-PET for response to neoadjuvant chemotherapy in patients with gastric cancer. They conducted FDG-PET studies in advanced gastric cancer patients at baseline and 14 days after initiation of cisplatinum-based polychemotherapy. When a reduction of tumor FDG uptake by more than 35% was employed as a criterion for subsequent tumor response, the positive and negative predictive value (NPV) of FDG-PET for histopathologic response was 77% and 90%, respectively. Two, relative small studies (44 and 22 patients, respectively) showed that the fractional change in glucose consumption can be assessed by FDG-PET immediately following the first cycle of chemotherapy.[37,38] Moreover, FDG-PET has been shown to be not only a predictor of neoadjuvant chemotherapy-induced clinical and histopathological response, but also, particularly, overall survival. Patients with a metabolic response had a two-year survival of 90%, in contrast to 40% in non-responders.

10.2.2.7. *Local recurrence*

FDG-PET lacks diagnostic accuracy in the early detection of recurrence with sensitivity and NPV of, respectively, 70% and 60% (Fig. 10.2). The high physiological gastric remnant uptake and the low spatial resolution of current hardware unable FDG-PET to detect early recurrence.[39,40]

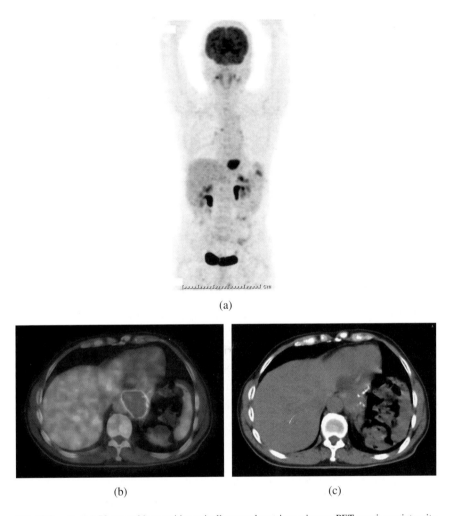

(a)

(b)   (c)

Fig. 10.2. (a–c) A 70-year-old man with surgically treated gastric carcinoma. PET–maximum intensity projection (MIP) image shows abnormal uptake in the left upper abdomen adjacent to left kidney (Fig. 10.2[a]). PET/CT reveals abnormal uptake in the edge of surgical margin (Fig. 10.2[b] and [c]). Corresponding CT images show thickened gastric wall. This patient was diagnosed as having a recurrent disease by endoscopy.

10.2.3. *Conclusion*

FDG-PET has no role in primary tumor detection due to its low sensitivity. FDG-PET has, however, slightly better positive predictive value (PPV) for the detection of lymph node metastasis in comparison to CT in N1 and N2 stations; furthermore, it has a reasonable sensitivity for liver and lung metastases. FDG-PET could have a significant role in monitoring tumor response during neoadjuvant chemotherapy. It adequately detects therapy responders at an early stage. Furthermore, FDG-PET is accurate in predicting the histopathological response and even long term prognosis.[41] The results of PET in the evaluation and monitoring of gastric cancer may improve in the near future. The use of PET/CT fusion imaging has improved imaging in several cancer types.

10.3. Pancreatic Cancer

10.3.1. *Introduction*

Pancreatic cancer, primarily ductal adenocarcinoma, accounts for an estimated 37,000 cases and 33,000 deaths in the US annually. Prognosis is poor because disease is often advanced at the time of diagnosis. Adenocarcinomas of the exocrine pancreas arise from duct cells 9 times more often than from acinar cells; 80% occur in the head of the gland. Adenocarcinomas appear at the mean age of 55 years and occur 1.5 to 2 times more often in men. Prominent risk factors include smoking, a history of chronic pancreatitis, and possibly long-standing diabetes mellitus (primarily in women). Heredity plays some role. Alcohol and caffeine consumption do not seem to be risk factors.

10.3.2. *Discussion*

10.3.2.1. *Tumor Detection*

CT is currently is the most common diagnostic imaging modality. Application of dual-phase CT protocols has been reported to demonstrate 97% sensitivity and 92% PPV for pancreatic tumor detection, 75% sensitivity for hepatic metastasis, 54% sensitivity for nodal metastasis, with an overall 91% accuracy for determining non-resectability.[42] Recent studies have demonstrated NPV of 100% for detection of vascular invasion and 87% NPV for overall resectability.[43] The diagnostic performance of MRI remains similar to that of CT.[44–47] Even with the latest technology improvements, MRI demonstrates sensitivity of 86% and specificity of 89% for detection of pancreatic tumors.[48]

FDG-PET is one of the diagnostic modalities expected to improve the diagnostic accuracy for pancreatic tumors, especially in the differentiation between benign and malignant lesions (Fig. 10.3). FDG-PET reveals high uptake of primary and metastatic lesions of pancreatic cancer, while lower

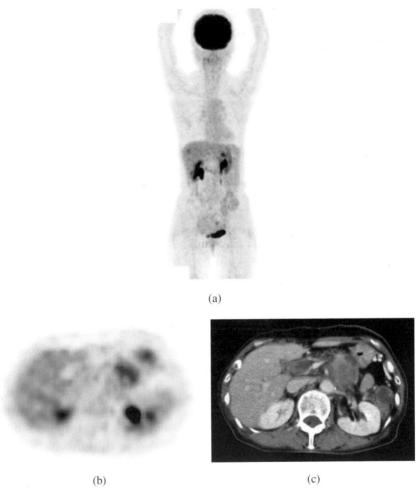

(a)

(b)   (c)

Fig. 10.3. (a–f) A 44-year-old man with pancreatic carcinoma. PET/CT revealed abnormal uptake within the mass of pancreatic body (Fig. 10.3[a–d]). The maximum diameter is 70 mm. Tumor invades adjacent fatty tissue and vascular structures including splenic vein and portal vein (Fig. 10.3[e] and [f]). The SUV$_{max}$ of the main tumor is 10.6. Multiple hepatic metastases are also found. Additionally, multiple abdominal lymphadenopathies and abnormal uptake of adrenal gland and spine are noted. This patient has clinical T4N1M1 disease.

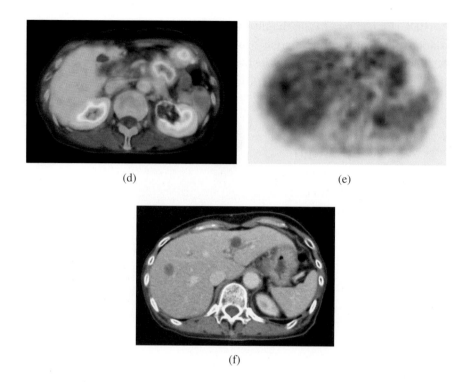

(d)　　　　　　　　　　(e)

(f)

Fig. 10.3. (*Continued*)

FDG uptake occurs in the benign pancreatic lesion such as chronic pancreatitis. Overexpression of the glucose transporter (GLUT) and increased permeability of tumor vessels contributed to the increased FDG uptake in pancreatic cancer.[49,50] Among the subtypes of GLUT, GLUT-1 is especially over expressed in pancreatic cancer.[49,50] Differential diagnosis in cases of chronic pancreatitis, a post-inflammatory mass resulting from formulating pancreatitis mimics malignant pancreatic disease. It is difficult to have an accurate differential diagnosis between the two diseases. The utility of FDG-PET for the differential diagnosis between benign and malignant disease was reported in a comparative study using CT.[51,52] The sensitivity and the specificity of FDG PET ranged from 85% to 100% and 77% to 88%, respectively. Overall accuracy ranged from 85% to 95%. These diagnostic results of FDG-PET were superior to those of CT. Recently, in 10 studies the performance of FDG-PET to differentiate benign form malignant

lesions ranged from 85% to 100% for sensitivity, 67% to 99% for specificity, and 85% to 93% for accuracy. In most of these studies, the accuracy
of FDG-PET imaging was superior to that of CT.[53−61] Moreover, FDG-
PET/CT to differentiate benign form malignant lesions 89% for sensitivity,
69% for specificity. PET/CT had a high PPV (91%) but low NPV (64%)
for cancer.[62] Early detection of pancreatic cancer is still difficult despite
the recent development of imaging technology such us multi-raw detector CT, fast spin echo MRI, and Doppler US. Higashi *et al.*[63] presented a
favorable result for diagnostic sensitivity (74%) of FDG-PET in patients
with pancreatic cancers of less than 2 cm in diameter, with a comparative
study using other imaging modalities as CT, MRI, endoscopic retrograde
cholangiopancreatography (ERCP), and EUS. Many patients with pancreatic diseases suffer from diabetes mellitus, which is a cause of decrease in
FDG tumor uptake. Another study reported that in patients with pancreatic
adenocarcinoma ($n = 65$), PET/CT had a sensitivity and specificity of 89%
and 88%, respectively, for detecting the primary tumor. PET/CT had a PPV
and NPV (NPV) of 97% and 68%, respectively.[64]

10.3.2.2. *Staging*

In stage I, cancer has formed and is found in the pancreas only. Stage I is
divided into stage IA and stage IB, based on the size of the tumor. Stage IA:
The tumor is 2 cm or smaller. Stage IB: The tumor is larger than 2 cm. In
stage II, cancer may have spread to nearby tissue and organs and may have
spread to lymph nodes near the pancreas. Stage II is divided into stage IIA
and stage IIB, based on where the cancer has spread. In Stage IIA, cancer
has spread to nearby tissue and organs but has not spread to nearby lymph
nodes. In Stage IIB, cancer has spread to nearby lymph nodes and may
have spread to nearby tissue and organs. In stage III, cancer has spread to
the major blood vessels near the pancreas and may have spread to nearby
lymph nodes. In stage IV, cancer may be of any size and has spread to distant
organs, such as the liver, lung, and peritoneal cavity. It may have also spread
to organs and tissues near the pancreas or to lymph nodes.

Functional imaging modalities cannot replace anatomic imaging in
the assessment of local tumor resectability. Even fusion imaging with
FDG-PET/CT may not significantly improve local staging given the limited

intrinsic PET resolution, but this has not been fully resolved. The identification of primary tumor extent and regional lymph node metastasis with FDG-PET alone is not clinically sufficient because of a lack of spatial resolution. Physiologic intestinal FDG uptake and intense FDG uptake in the primary lesion obscures the faint FDG uptake in adjacent small lymph node lesions. Fusion images of CT/US and FDG-PET help in the interpretation of tumor extent and regional lymph node metastasis. Reported FDG-PET sensitivity and specificity for lymph node staging is 49% and 63%, respectively.[65-67] The addition of PET/CT to both CT and EUS marginally increased detection of suspicious lymphadenopathy to 53% patients.[64]

FDG-PET is useful for the detection of metastatic hepatic lesions from pancreatic cancer. In certain cases of pancreatic cancer, metastatic lesions in the liver invisible on CT/MRI could be visible on FDG-PET. Delbeke *et al.* reported PET demonstrated hepatic metastases not identified or equivocal on CT and/or distant metastases unsuspected clinically in 33% additional patients.[61] PET/CT improved the detection of distant metastases compared with standard staging alone (81% versus 56%; $p = 0.22$, McNemar test). Standard staging followed by PET/CT further improved the detection of metastases to 88% ($p = 0.06$, McNemar test).[62] Another study about PET/CT reported that the sensitivity of detecting metastatic disease for PET/CT alone, standard CT alone, and the combination of PET/CT and standard CT were 61%, 57%, and 87%, respectively. PET/CT alone had specificity for detection of metastatic disease of 100% with a PPV and NPV of 100% and 91%, respectively. The combination of PET/CT with standard CT had specificity of 92% with a PPV and NPV of 80% and 93%, respectively.[64]

10.3.2.3. *Monitoring the Therapeutic Effect*

FDG-PET in patients with colorectal cancer and head or neck cancer is useful for clinical follow-up and the diagnosis of recurrent disease since a good prognosis in patients with these cancers requires long-term follow-up after the initial treatment. On the other hand, recurrent or metastatic lesions in patients with pancreatic cancer occur earlier than those in patients with colorectal and head or neck cancers. There are few reports describing the utility of FDG-PET for the detection of recurrent disease in patients with pancreatic cancer. However, FDG PET may be useful for the detection of recurrent lesions after the initial surgical treatment, since post-surgical scars, which interfere with the accurate diagnosis of recurrent disease on CT/MRI, may show faint or no FDG uptake. In recent report, FDG-PET reliably detected local and non-locoregional recurrences, whereas CT-MRI was more sensitive for detection of hepatic metastases. Of 25 patients with local recurrences on follow up, initial imaging suggested relapse in 23 patients. Of these, FDG PET detected 96% and CT-MRI 39%. Among 12 liver metastases, FDG-PET detected 42% and CT-MRI 92% correctly.[66] The change of tumor FDG uptake derived from PET imaging before and after treatment may be used as an index of therapeutic effect. Patients with higher FDG uptake in a pancreatic tumor tend to have a poor prognosis. A pilot study by Rose *et al.* determined that FDG-PET imaging might be useful for assessment of tumor response to neoadjuvant therapy.[67] FDG-PET successfully predicted histological evidence of chemoradiation-induced tumor necrosis in 4 of 9 patients who demonstrated at least 50% reduction in tumor SUV after chemoradiation. Another pilot study suggests that the absence of FDG uptake at 1 month after chemotherapy is an indicator of improved survival versus patient in whom persistent up take is present. However, pancreatic cancer tend to have a poor prognosis, evaluation in FDG-PET, PET/CT has a little meaning.

10.3.3. Conclusion

FDG PET/CT has high sensitivity, specificity, PPV, and NPV in evaluating small solid pancreatic lesions in comparison to clinically established imaging modalities. Additional clinical diagnoses can be derived from the whole body by PET/CT. Further studies are required to define the role of FDG-PET/CT in the stratification and clinical management of patients with suspected pancreatic cancer.

References

1. Kuwano H, Sumiyoshi K, Sonoda K, *et al.* (1998) Relationship between preoperative assessment of organ function and postoperative morbidity in patients with esophageal cancer. *Eur J Surg* **164**: 581–586.

2. Kato H, Kuwano H, Nakajima M, *et al.* (2002) Comparison between positron emission tomography and computed tomography in the use of the assessment of esophageal carcinoma. *Cancer* **94**: 921–928.

3. Fukunaga T, Enomoto K, Okazumi S, *et al.* (1994) Analysis of glucose metabolism in patients with esophageal cancer by PET: Estimation of hexokinase activity in the tumor and usefulness for clinical assessment using 18F-fluorodeoxyglucose. *Nippon Geka Gakkai Zasshi* **95**(5): 317–325.

4. Block MI, Patterson GA, Sundaresan RS, *et al.* (1997) Improvement in staging of esophageal cancer with the addition of positron emission tomography. *Ann Thorac Surg* **64**(3): 770–776; discussion 776–777.

5. Kole AC, Plukker JT, Nieweg OE, *et al.* (1998) Positron emission tomography for staging of esophageal and gastresophageal malignancy. *Br J Cancer* **78**(4): 521–527.

6. Flamen P, Lerut A, Van Cutsem E, *et al.* (2000) Utility of positron emission tomography for the staging of patients with potentially operable esophageal carcinoma. *J Clin Oncol* **18**(18): 3202–3210.

7. Meltzer CC, Luketich JD, Friedman D, *et al.* (2000) Whole-body FDG positron emission tomographic imaging for staging esophageal cancer comparison with computed tomography. *Clin Nucl Med* **25**(11): 882–887.

8. Kato H, Miyazaki T, Nakajima M, *et al.* (2005) The incremental effect of positron emission tomography on diagnostic accuracy in the initial staging of esophageal carcinoma. *Cancer* **103**(1): 148–156.

9. Chowdhury FU, Bradley KM, Gleeson FV, *et al.* (2008) The role of 18F-FDG PET/CT in the evaluation of esophageal carcinoma. *Clinical Radiol* **63**: 1297–1309.

10. Yuan S, Yu Y, Chao KS, *et al.* (2006) Additional value of PET/CT over PET in assessment of locoregional lymph nodes in thoracic esophageal squamous cell cancer. *J Nucl Med* **47**(8): 1255–1259.

11. Kneist W, Schreckenberger M, Bartenstein P, *et al.* (2003) Positron emission tomography for staging esophageal cancer: Does it lead to a different therapeutic approach? *World J Surg* **27**(10): 1105–1112.

12. Heeren PA, Jager PL, Bongaerts F, *et al.* (2004) Detection of distant metastases in esophageal cancer with (18)P-FDG PET. *J Nucl Med* **45**(6): 980–987.

13. John F. Bruzzi, Reginald F. Munden, Mylene T. Truong, *et al.* (2007) PET/CT of esophageal cancer: Its role in clinical management. *RadioGraphics* **27**: 1635–1652

14. van Westreenen HL, Westerterp M, Bossuyt PM, *et al.* (2004) Systematic review of the staging performance of 18F-fluorodeoxyglucose positron emission tomography in esophageal cancer. *J Clin Oncol* **22**(18): 3805–3812.

15. Lowe VJ, Mullan BP, Wiersema M, *et al.* (2002) Prospective comparison of PET, CT and EUS in the initial staging of esophageal cancer patients: Preliminary results. *J Nucl Med* **43**: 66.

16. Kato H, Miyazaki T, Nakajima M, *et al.* (2004) Value of positron emission tomography in the diagnosis of recurrent esophageal carcinoma. *Br J Surg* **91**(8): 1004–1009.

17. Hongbo G, Hui Z, Yan X, *et al.* (2007) Diagnostic and prognostic value of 18F-FDG PET/CT for patients with suspected recurrence from squamous cell carcinoma of the esophagus. *J Nucl Med* **48**: 1251–1258.

18. Wieder H, Zimmermann K, Becker K, *et al.* (2002) Time course of tumor glucose utilization in patients with squamous cell carcinomas of the esophagus undergoing preoperative chemoradiotherapy. *J Nucl Med* **43**: 66.

19. Weber WA, Ott K, Becker K, *et al.* (2001) Prediction of response to preoperative chemotherapy in adenocarcinomas of the esophagogastric junction by metabolic imaging. *J Clin Oncol* **19**: 3058–3065.

20. Rosenbaum SJ, Stergar IH, Antoch IG *et al.* (2006) Staging and follow-up of gastrointestinal tumors with PET/CT. *Abdominal Imaging* **31**: 25–35.

21. Shreve PD, Anzai Y, Wahl RL. (1999) Pitfalls in oncologic diagnosis with FDG PET imaging: Physiologic and benign variants. *Radiograph* **19**: 61–77.

22. Cook GJR, Fdgelman I, Maisey M. (1996) Normal physiological and benign pathological variants of 18-fluoro-2-deoxyglucose positron emission tomography scanning: Potential for error in interpretation. *Semin Nucl Med* **24**: 308–314.

23. Yoshioka K, Yamaguchi K, Kubota K, *et al.* (2002) FDG PET in gastric cancer with metastases or recurrence. *J Nucl Med* **43**: 67.

24. Ott K, Weber WA, Fink U, *et al.* (2003) Fluorodeoxyglucose positron emission tomography in adenocarcinomas of the distal esophagus and cardia. *World J Surg* **27**: 1035–1039.

25. Stahl A, Ott K, Weber WA, *et al.* (2003) FDG PET imaging of locally advanced gastric carcinomas: Correlation with endoscopic and histopathological findings. *Eur J Nucl Med Mol Imaging* **30**: 288–295

26. Yoshioka T, Yamaguchi K, Kubota K, *et al.* (2003) Evaluation of 18F-FDG PET in patients with a, metastatic, or recurrent gastric cancer. *J Nucl Med* **44**: 690–699.

27. Mochiki E, Kuwano H, Katoh H, *et al.* (2004) Evaluation of 18F-2-deoxy-2-fluoro-D-glucose positron emission tomography for gastric cancer. *World J Surg* **28**: 247–253.

28. Yun M, Lim JS, Noh SH, *et al.* (2005) Lymph node staging of gastric cancer using (18) F-FDG PET: A comparison study with CT. *J Nucl Med* **46**(10): 1582–1588.

29. Chen J, Cheong JH, Yun MJ, *et al.* (2005) Improvement in preoperative staging of gastric adenocarcinoma with positron emission tomography. *Cancer* **103**(11): 2383–2890.

30. Mukai K, Ishida Y, Okajima K, Isozaki H, Morimoto T, Nishiyama S. (2006) Usefulness of preoperative FDG PET for detection of gastric cancer. *Gastric Cancer* **9**(3): 192–196.

31. Yeung HW, Macapinlac H, Karpeh M, Finn RD, Larson SM. (1998) Accuracy of FDG PET in gastric cancer. Preliminary experience. *Clin Positron Imaging* **1**(4): 213–221.

32. Kim SK, Kang KW, Lee JS, *et al.* (2006) Assessment of lymph node metastases using 18F-FDG PET in patients with advanced gastric cancer. *Eur J Nucl Med Mol Imaging* **33**(2): 148–55.

33. Yuan S, Yu Y, Chao KS, *et al.* (2006) Additional value of PET/CT over PET in assessment of locoregional lymph nodes in thoracic esophageal squamous cell cancer. *J Nucl Med* **47**(8): 1255–1259.

34. Lim JS, Kim MJ, Yun MJ, *et al.* (2006) Comparison of CT and 18F-FDG PET for detecting peritoneal metastasis on the preoperative evaluation for gastric carcinoma. *Korean J Radiol* **7**(4): 249–56.

35. Kinkel K, Lu Y, Both M, *et al.* (2002) Detection of hepatic metastases from cancers of the gastrointestinal tract by using noninvasive imaging methods (US, CT, MR imaging, PET): A meta-analysis. *Radiology* **224**: 748–756.

36. Stahl A, Ott K, Becker K, *et al.* (2002) Prediction of response to neoadjuvant chemotherapy in patients with gastric cancer by FDG PET. *J Nucl Med* **43**: 67.

37. Ott K, Fink U, Becker K, *et al.* (2003) Prediction of response to preoperative chemotherapy in gastric carcinoma by metabolic imaging: Results of a prospective trial. *J Clin Oncol* **21**(24): 4604–4610.

38. Di FF, Pinto C, Rojas Llimpe FL, *et al.* (2007) The predictive value of 18F-FDG PET early evaluation in patients with metastatic gastric adenocarcinoma treated with chemotherapy plus cetuximab. *Gastric Cancer* **10**(4): 221–227.

39. Yun M, Choi HS, Yoo E, Bong JK, Ryu YH, Lee JD. (2005) The role of gastric distention in differentI,Ating recurrent tumor from physiologic uptake in the remnant stomach on 18F-FDG PET. *J Nucl Med* **46**(6): 953–957.

40. De PT, Flamen P, Van CE, *et al.* (2002) Whole-body PET with FDG for the diagnosis of recurrent gastric cancer. *Eur J Nucl Med Mol Imaging* **29**(4): 525–529.

41. Dassen AE, Lips DJ, Hoekstra CJ, *et al.* (2009) FDG PET has no definite role in preoperative imaging in gastric cancer. *EJSO* 1–7.

42. Diehl SI, Lehman I, Sadiek M, *et al.* (1998) Pancreatic cancer: Value of dual phase helical CT in assessing resectability. *Radiology* **206**: 373–378.

43. Vargas R, Nino-Murcia M, Trueblood W, *et al.* (2004) MDCT in pancreatic adenocarcinoma: Prediction of vascular invasion and respectability using a multiphasic technique with curved planar reformations. *AJR Am J Roentgenol* **182**: 419–425.

44. Bluemke DA, Fishman EK. (1998) CT and MR evaluation of pancreatic cancer. *Surg Oncol Clin North Am* **7**: 103–124.

45. Catalano C, Pavone P, Laghi A, *et al.* (1998) Pancreatic adenocarcinoma: Combination of MR angiography and MR cholangiopancreatography for the diagnosis and assessment of resectability. *Bur Radiol* **8**: 428–434.

46. Irie H, Honda H, Kaneko K, *et al.* (1997) Comparison of helical CT and MR imaging in detecting and staging small pancreatic adenocarcinoma. *Abdom Imaging* **22**: 429–433.

47. Trede M, Rumstadt B, Wendl, *et al.* (1997) Ultrafast magnetic resonance imaging improves the staging of pancreatic tumors. *Ann Surg* 226393–226405.

48. Birchard KR, Semelka RC, Hyslop WB, *et al.* (2005) Evaluation of pancreatic cancer by MRI. *AJR Am J Roentgenol* **185**: 700–703.

49. Higashi T, Tamaki N, Honda T, *et al.* (1997) Expression of glucose transporters in human pancreatic tumors compared with increased FDG accumulation in PET study. *J Nucl Med* **38**: 1337–1344.

50. Reske SN, Grillenberger KG, Glatting G, *et al.* (1997) Overexpression of glucose transporter 1 and increased FDG uptake in pancreatic carcinoma. *J Nucl Med* **38**: 1344–1348.

51. Inokuma T, Tamaki N, Torizuka T, *et al.* (1995) Evaluation of pancreatic tumors with positron emission tomography and F-18 fluorodeoxyglucose: Comparison with CT and US. *Radiology* **195**: 345–352.

52. Delbeke D, Rose DM, Chapman WC, *et al.* (1999) Optimal interpretation of FDGPET in the diagnosis, staging and management of pancreatic carcinoma. *J Nucl Med* **40**: 1784–1791.

53. Bares R, Klever P, Hauptmann S, *et al.* (1994) F-18-fluorodeoxyglucose PET in vivo evaluation of pancreatic glucose metabolism for detection of pancreatic cancer. *Radiology* **192**: 79–86.

54. Stollfuss JC, Glatting G, Friess H, *et al.* (1995) 2-(Fluorine-18)-fluoro-2deoxy D-glucose PET in detection of pancreatic cancer: Value of quantitative image interpretation. *Radiology* **195**: 339–344.
55. Kato T, Fukatsu H, Ito K, *et al.* (1995) Fluorodeoxyglucose positron emission tomography in pancreatic cancer: An unsolved problem. *Eur J Nucl Med* **22**: 32–39.
56. Friess H, Langhans J, Ebert M, *et al.* (1995) Diagnosis of pancreatic cancer by 2[F-18]-fluoro-2-deoxy-D-glucose positron emission tomography. *Gut* **36**: 771–777.
57. Ho CL, Dehdashti F, Griffeth LK, *et al.* (1996) FDG PET evaluation of indeterminate pancreatic masses. *Comput Assisted Tomograph* **20**: 363–369.
58. Zimny M, Bares R, Fass J, *et al.* (1997) Fluorine-18 fluorodeoxyglucose positron emission tomography in the differential diagnosis of pancreatic carcinoma: A report of 106 cases. *Bur J Nucl Med* **24**: 678–682.
59. Keogan MT, Tyler D, Clark 1, *et al.* (1998) Diagnosis of pancreatic carcinoma: Role of FDG PET. *AJR AmJ Roentgenol* **171**: 1565–1570.
60. Imdahl SA, Nitzsche E, Krautmann F, *et al.* (1999) Evaluation of positron emission tomography with 2-[18F]fluoro-2-deoxy-D-glucose for the differentiation of chronic pancreatitis and pancreatic cancer. *Br J Surg* **86**(2): 194–199.
61. Delbeke D, Chapman WC, Pinson CW, *et al.* (1999) F-18 fluorodeoxyglucose imaging with positron emission tomography (FDG PET) has a significant impact on diagnosis and management of pancreatic ductal adenocarcinoma. *J Nucl Med* **40**: 1784–1792.
62. Stefan H, Goerres GW, Markus S, *et al.* (2005) Positron emission tomography/computed tomography influences on the management of resectable pancreatic cancer and its cost-effectiveness. *Ann Surg* **242**: 235–243.
63. Higashi T, Nakamoto Y, Saga T, *et al.* (2000) Clinical contribution of FDG PET in evaluating small pancreatic tumors 20mmin diameter or smaller. *Gut* United European Gastroenterology Week [abstract].
64. Jeffrey MF, Alfredo AS, Marcovalerio M, *et al.* (2008) PET/CT fusion scan enhances ct staging in patients with pancreatic neoplasms. *Ann Surg Oncol* **15**(9): 2465–2471.
65. Diederichs CG, Staib I, Vogel J, *et al.* (2000) Values and limitations of FDG PET with preoperative evaluations of patients with pancreatic masses. *Pancreas* **20**: 109–116.
66. Ruf J, Lopez HE, Oettle H, *et al.* (2005) Detection of recurrent pancreatic cancer: Comparison of FDG-PET with CT/MRI. *Pancreatology* **5**(2–3): 266–272.
67. Rose DM, De1beke D, Beauchamp RD, *et al.* (1999) 18-Fluorodeoxyglucosepositron emission tomography (18FDG PET) in the management of patients with suspected pancreatic cancer. *Ann Surg* **229**: 729–738.

Chapter 11
Nuclear Urology

Ukihide Tateishi and E. Edmund Kim

11.1. Introduction

Despite technical advances in CT, MRI, and ultrasonography, nuclear medicine has maintained its crucial role in the functional assessment of the urinary tract, particularly the kidneys. Nuclear renal imaging plays an important role in providing an estimate of relative renal function. Absolute renal function such as glomerular filtration rate can be measured by blood sample–based methods. Nuclear renogram plays important roles in the diagnosis of renovascular hypertension and renal transplant complications. Recently, the usefulness of the positron emission tomography (PET) with ^{18}F-fluorodeoxyglucose (FDG), which reflects the glucose metabolism in some cells, has been established in clinical oncology. However, there are some limitations in the utilization of ^{18}F-FDG-PET for the genitourinary imaging. FDG is excreted in the urine after intravenous injection. So, the activity in the urine can mask the abnormal activity in genitourinary structures or occasionally be mistaken for active tumor foci. Although some reports proposed methods to decrease the activity in the urine such as bladder irrigation,[1] forced diuresis by furosemide,[2] and retrograde filling with sterile saline after bladder irrigation,[3] it may be difficult to use them routinely in clinical practice. Combined PET/computed tomography (CT) imaging may be helpful for anatomical assessment around urinary tracts.

Some reports have suggested the utility of ^{18}F-FDG-PET for the patients with primary genitourinary cancers. ^{18}F-FDG-PET is often useful for the detection of unexpected distant metastases that were not identified by conventional imaging methods such as CT or magnetic resonance imaging

267

(MRI). Furthermore, ^{18}F-FDG-PET has some potential for treatment monitoring and outcome prediction as well as other cancers. This chapter focuses on the utility and limitation of ^{18}F-FDG-PET as a genitourinary imaging method.

In addition, different PET tracers (e.g., ^{11}C-choline, ^{18}F-choline, and ^{11}C-acetate) have been introduced and successfully reported as a useful tool for assessment of genitourinary tumors, particularly prostate cancers. These tracers will be arbitrarily referred to in this chapter.

11.2. Renal Anatomy and Physiology

The kidneys are located in the lumbar region at a depth of about 6 cm from the surface of the back. Their upper and lower poles lie between 12th thoracic vertebra and 3rd lumbar vertebra, respectively. Each kidney is about 12 cm long, 6 cm wide, 3 cm thick, and weighs about 150 g. The renal parenchyma consists of pale outer cortex and inner darker medulla. The cortex has a relatively homogeneous appearance, but the medulla consists of radially striated cones called renal pyramids, the apices of which form papillae which project into the renal sinus and interface with a calyx. The renal artery divides into several interlobar arteries at the renal hilum which themselves branch to form arcuate arteries, running between the cortex and medulla. Smaller interlobular arteries branch off, and finally afferent arterioles supply blood to the glomerular capillaries. The renal functional unit, the nephron, consists of glomerulus and its attached tubule. The proximal convoluted tubule and Henle's loop are collectively called as the proximal tubule, and the distal convoluted tubule and collecting duct as the distal tubule. The main function of kidneys is to conserve substances that are essential to life, and the kidneys are helpful to maintain the constancy of the extracellular fluid. The kidneys consume about 20% of all oxygen used by the body at rest. About 20% of cardiac output (1,100 ml/min) is required to provide energy for the blood cleansing process. The glomeruli have a huge surface area, and thus only modest glomerular perfusion pressure (GPP) (about 8 mm Hg) is needed for filtration. However, a drop in GPP of only 15% stops filtration. Renal plasma flow (RPF), component of blood available for filtration, is around 600 ml/min [(1−hematocrit) × RPF]. Normal glomerular filtration rate (GFR) is about 120 ml/min, and thus filtration fraction (FF = GFR/RPF) is about 20%. The proximal convoluted tubule is the site for reabsorption of 90% filtered sodium and 75% filtered water. Although nuclear renal imaging agents are cleared from the blood by different renal mechanisms with different extraction efficiencies, they can be used to measure relative renal function from gamma camera imaging based on glomerulotubular balance, which ensures that a change in GFR is paralleled by a change in proximal tubular reabsorption. Although disease may cause the overall FF to vary, the FF for each kidney will be the same to determine relative renal function.

11.3. Radiopharmaceuticals

Diethylenetriaminepentaacetic acid (DTPA) diffuses rapidly into the extravascular space and is cleared from the plasma purely by glomerular filtration. The plasma clearance is the same as the renal clearance. Dynamic imaging with Tc-99m DTPA reveals rapid transit through renal cortex with the activity appearing in the collecting system within a few minutes. Tc-99m DTPA is used when estimating renal GFR in milliliter per minute from the renogram. Although the renogram curves are noisy when renal function is poor, the relative renal function can still be estimated with acceptable accuracy down to a GFR level of about 20 ml/min. Tc-99m mercaptoacetyl-triglycine (MAG3) is the agent of choice for renographic procedures except for absolute functional measurement. Its extraction efficiency is two to three times higher than Tc-99m DTPA but lower than ^{123}I ortho-iodohippurate (OIH). Tc-99m 2,3-dimercaptosuccinic acid (DMSA) is avidly taken by cells of the proximal tubule, and renal uptake continues to rise for about 6 h after injection. It is useful to evaluate renal cortex in patients with glomeru-lonephritis or renal mass.

11.4. Radionuclide Renography

In basic renography, a continuous series of 10-sec duration digital images of the urinary tract are recorded over about 30 min following injection of radiopharmaceuticals. Imaging processing is performed using computer-generated regions of interest (ROIs) to generate the time–activity curve (Fig.). Diuresis renography is a diagnostic tool for detecting upper urinary tract obstruction. The maximal total diuresis by intravenous furosemide (0.5 mg/kg) in adult patient with normal renal function is around 20 ml/min, which is about 20 times that of normal. Furosemide (1 mg/kg for infants and 5 mg/kg for children and adults) is rapidly injected at around 15–20 min after injection of radionuclide, which allows the effect of the drug on the renogram to be properly appreciated. The renographic response to furosemide depends on many factors, including renal function, urine flow rate, renal pelvic volume, elasticity of the wall of renal pelvis, and degree of ureteric peristalsis. Obstructive and non-obstructive hydronephrosis have a characteristic appearance on the renogram post-furosemide, provided that the affected kidney GFR is above 15 ml/min. The renographic response to furosemide can be called if the fall in the curve is rapid, substantial and has a concave slope with less than 10-min half-time of clearance after injection of furosemide (Fig.). There is a so-called Homsy sign with initial positive renographic response to furosemide, followed by a premature leveling off or a rise due to high flow or intermittent obstruction.

Captopril renography comprises two separate renograms, one to act as baseline and another 1 h after oral administration of 25 mg captopril, angiotensin-converting enzyme (ACE) inhibitor, causing individual renal GFR to fall in patients with renovascular hypertension (functionally significant renal artery stenosis). The main intrarenal effect of ACE inhibition is on GFR, and thus Tc-99m DTPA is the agent in this context. However, the quality of DTPA image falls as renal function decreases. Tc-99m MAG3 is a better choice in that situation.

Transplant renography is simply perfusion renography applied to the renal transplant. The perfusion index is derived from the time–activity curve. Deteriorating perfusion indicates an acute rejection, but renal biopsy and Doppler ultrasound have been more used to diagnose rejection.

11.5. Renal Cell Carcinoma

Some early reports showed a high sensitivity more than 90% of ^{18}F-FDG-PET for detection of primary renal cell carcinoma (RCC).[4,5] However, following studies which examined large number of patients showed a lower sensitivity. Aide *et al.* and Kang *et al.* showed low sensitivity of ^{18}F-FDG PET for detection of primary lesions of 47% and 60%, respectively.[6,7] In both these studies, the sensitivity of ^{18}F-FDG-PET was much lower than CT, whose sensitivity was more than 90%. One of the causes may be that the excretion of FDG via the kidneys masks the uptake to primary RCC. However, because some large tumors with extrarenal development are often either not visualized or showed only slight FDG uptake (Fig. 11.1), the other factors such as an inaccessibility of FDG to the large tumors are probably involved.[6] Therefore, the role of ^{18}F-FDG-PET in the diagnosis of RCC is limited.

However, ^{18}F-FDG-PET may be useful in detection of unexpected distant metastases. The previous report by Aide *et al.*[6] showed high accuracy of 94% for detecting distant metastases. Majhail *et al.*[8] examined 24 patients with suspected distant metastases from histopathologically proven RCC.

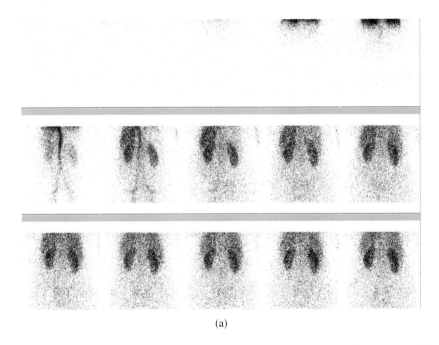

(a)

Fig. 11.1. Normal renal scan using Tc-99m MAG$_3$ with good blood flow (a) as well as prompt uptake and excretion of the activity (b). Renogram curves (c) show normal slopes from bilateral kidneys. Right-to-left renal split functional ratio is approximately 50 to 50.

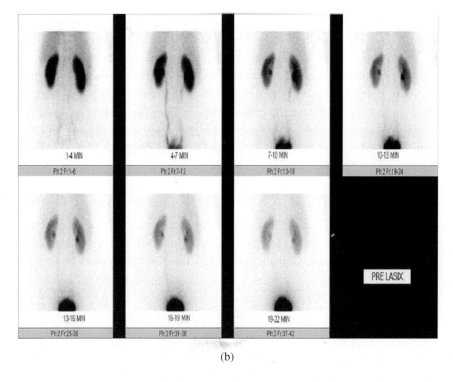

(b)

Fig. 11.1. (*Continued*)

Although their results showed low overall sensitivity of 63.6% for detection of distant metastases, ^{18}F-FDG-PET showed high sensitivity of 92.9% when limited to the lesions more than 2 cm in size. Furthermore, the positive predictive value was 100% in their study and they concluded that positive ^{18}F-FDG-PET may alleviate the need for a biopsy in selected situations. The fact that small metastases in some organs (e.g., retroperitoneal lymph nodes [LN], lung, and bone) may be missed by ^{18}F-FDG PET as well as other malignancies must be considered. The conventional imaging methods should be used complementarily for evaluation of RCC.

11.6. Bladder Cancer

Similar to the other genitourinary malignancies, the excretion of FDG via the urinary tracts represents a significant limitation of ^{18}F-FDG-PET for

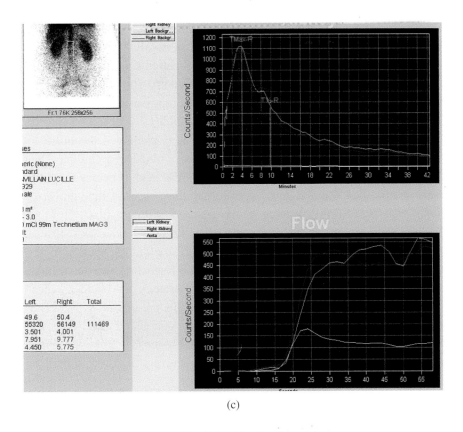

Fr:1 76K 256x256

les

ieric (None)
idard
MLLAIN LUCILLE
329
iale

} m²
- 3.0
} mCi 99m Technetium MAG3
It
)

Left	Right	Total
49.6	50.4	
55320	56149	111469
3.501	4.001	
7.951	9.777	
4.450	5.775	

(c)

Fig. 11.1. *(Continued)*

evaluation of primary bladder cancers. Kosuda *et al.*[9] showed low sensitivity of 66.7% for detecting primary lesions in their preliminary study despite retrograde irrigation of the urinary bladder with saline. However, in their study, ^{18}F-FDG-PET could differentiate viable recurrent bladder cancer from radiation-induced alterations in two patients. This result may indicate the feasibility of ^{18}F-FDG-PET in patients with bladder cancer.

In patients with newly diagnosed bladder carcinoma, LN involvement and the presence of distant metastasis are strong negative determinants of prognosis. Kosuda *et al.* reported that PET imaging identified 17 of 17 patients with metastatic disease (lung, bone, and LN) as well as 2 of 3 patients with localized LN involvement.[9] Drieskens *et al.* examined 55 patients with invasive bladder cancer and found that the sensitivity, specificity, and accuracy of correlative imaging of ^{18}F-FDG-PET with CT (PET-CT) were 60%, 88%, and 78%, respectively.[10] In addition, they demonstrated that median survival time of patients in whom PET-CT showed some metastatic lesions was significantly shorter than patients without positive PET-CT studies. Furthermore, similar results were found in another study by Heicappell *et al.*[11] in which 67% detection rate for local nodal disease was reported. Kibel *et al.*[12] evaluated the utility of ^{18}F-FDG-PET/CT for staging of muscle-invasive bladder carcinoma. Their results (sensitivity of 70%, specificity of 94%, and accuracy of 88%) were better than the previous reports and they showed that the prognosis was significantly poorer in the patients with positive ^{18}F-FDG-PET/CT than in those with negative ^{18}F-FDG PET/CT. Given these results, ^{18}F-FDG-PET may have the potential to detect small or unexpected metastases owing to addition of metabolism-based information and the accurate staging leads to the appropriate therapeutic strategy for bladder cancer. On the other hand, Swinnen *et al.*[13] compared pre-operative ^{18}F-FDG-PET/CT and CT results of 41 patients and concluded that there was no advantage for combined ^{18}F-FDG-PET/CT over CT alone for lymph node staging of invasive bladder cancer or recurrent high-risk superficial disease.

Using other tracers that are not excreted in the urine improves the sensitivity of PET for detecting primary bladder cancer. Ahlstrom *et al.*[14] showed that ^{11}C-methionine PET visualized 18 of 23 primary tumors (78%). Gofrit *et al.* showed that ^{11}C-choline PET/CT successfully detected primary and metastatic transitional cell carcinoma and concluded that ^{11}C-choline PET/CT is a promising tool for preoperative staging of advanced transitional cell carcinoma.[15] In these fields, further studies with larger population are needed to verify the utility.

11.7. Prostate Cancer

11.7.1. [18]*F-FDG-PET*

Some studies have shown that FDG is generally not a suitable PET tracer for diagnosing prostate cancer. Most primary prostate cancers have low FDG uptake and there is a significant overlap in FDG uptake values in benign prostatic hyperplasia (BPH) and prostate cancer.[16,17] Evaluation of local LN metastases is often difficult because of high FDG uptake in urinary bladder. Although bone is the second most common site of metastatic disease after LN in prostate cancer,[18] osteoblastic bone metastases often show minimal FDG uptake, which causes false-negative results of PET (Fig. 11.2). Shreve *et al.* reported low sensitivity (65%) of ^{18}F-FDG-PET in the detection of bone metastases that was lower than bone scintigraphy.[19] However, some bone metastases do not show any morphological changes on CT. ^{18}F-FDG-PET may be useful for detection of these metastases (Fig. 11.3). Hofer *et al.* and Schoder *et al.* showed that ^{18}F-FDG-PET is not useful for the detection of local recurrence after radical prostatectomy.[17,20] On the other hand, there are a few studies that showed the utility of ^{18}F-FDG-PET for monitoring effect of chemotherapy and predicting prognosis.[21,22]

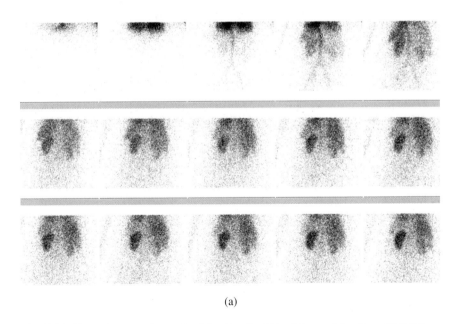

(a)

Fig. 11.2. Obstructive uropathy on the right side. Good blood flow and function of left kidney. Decreased blood flow (a) and continuous uptake of Tc-99m MAG$_3$ in the right kidney even after the injection of lasix (b). Renogram (c) shows normal slopes from the left kidney and rising slope from the right kidney. Right-to-left renal split functional ratio is approximately 24 to 76.

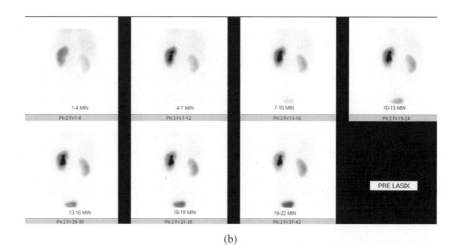

(b)

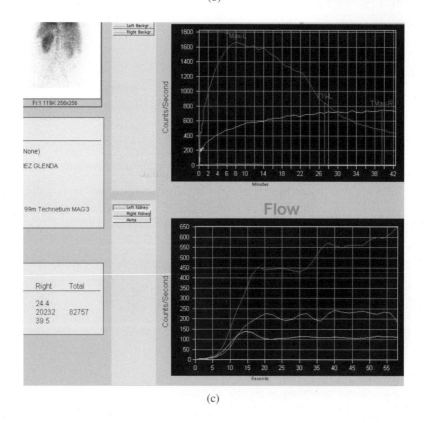

(c)

Fig. 11.2. (*Continued*)

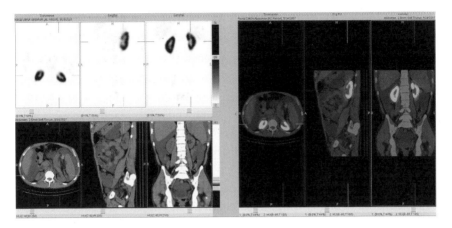

Fig. 11.3. SPECT/CT of kidneys with Tc-99m DMSA shows a good outline of renal cortices of bilateral kidneys.

11.7.2. ^{11}C-choline PET

Choline is one of the components of phosohatidylcholone, an essential element of phospholipids in the cell membrane. ^{11}C-choline uptake in prostate cancers is considered to be based on increased proliferative activity or upregulation of choline kinase. However, Breeuwsma *et al.* were unable to demonstrate a relation between *in vivo* uptake of ^{11}C-choline and cell proliferation by tumor histology and Ki-67 expression, which is a nuclear protein complex that is expressed during cell replication.[23] They suggest that a process other than proliferation is responsible for the uptake of ^{11}C-choline in prostate cancers.

There are many studies that refer to the utility of ^{11}C-choline PET for the evaluation of prostate cancers. Hara *et al.* suggested that ^{11}C-choline PET has advantages over ^{18}F-FDG-PET in the absence of urinary activity and the high uptake in the prostate cancer itself.[24] Kotzerke *et al.* concluded that ^{11}C-choline PET is a promising tool for the detection of LN and bone metastases with high sensitivity and specificity (92% and 90%, respectively) in their early study.[25] However, in the study by Farsad *et al.*,[26] ^{11}C-choline PET/CT showed a low sensitivity (66%) and negative predictive value (55%), and the high rate of false-negative results were considered to be caused by small dimension and low uptake of prostate cancer. They concluded that ^{11}C-choline PET/CT has the feasibility to identify cancer foci within prostate but the routine use of ^{11}C-choline PET/CT as a first-line screening procedure is not recommended.

Reske *et al.* using maximum standardized uptake value (SUV_{max}) threshold of 2.65 reported ^{11}C-choline PET sensitivity, specificity, and accuracy of 81%, 87% and 84%, respectively.[27] And their study showed that SUV_{max} did not correlate significantly with PSA or Gleason score but did correlate with T stage. However, similar to ^{18}F-FDG PET, SUV_{max} has some overlaps between prostate cancer and BPH,[26,28] and various results of the correlation between SUV_{max} and PSA, Gleason score, and pathological stage are reported. Martorana *et al.* reported high sensitivity (83%) of ^{11}C-choline PET/CT for localization of nodules 5 mm or greater, but its sensitivity for the assessment of extraprostatic extension was much lower than MRI (22% versus 63%).[29]

In comparison with magnetic resonance spectroscopy (MRS), Yamaguchi *et al.* reported that ^{11}C-choline PET exhibits higher sensitivity than MRS (100% versus 65%).[30] On the other hand, Testa *et al.* reported the opposite result that ^{11}C-choline PET exhibits lower sensitivity than three-dimensional MRS (55% versus 81%) in their sextant analysis.[31]

It is difficult to determine whether ^{11}C-choline PET is a useful imaging method for the initial diagnosis of prostate cancers. However, there are some reports suggesting that ^{11}C-choline PET is useful for the evaluation of prostate cancer after primary treatment such as a prostatectomy. Giovacchini *et al.* showed a significant negative correlation between SUV_{max} and anti-androgenic therapy and suggested that ^{11}C-choline PET/CT could be used to monitor the response to anti-androgenic therapy.[28] Picchio *et al.* compared ^{11}C-choline PET and ^{18}F-FDG-PET for restaging prostate cancer in a group of 100 patients.[32] They showed that ^{11}C-choline PET was superior to ^{18}F-FDG-PET and complementary to conventional imaging techniques. Recently, Richter *et al.* showed similar results that the sensitivity of ^{11}C-choline PET and ^{18}F-FDG-PET was 60.6% and 31% in all cases, while sensitivity increased to 80% and 40% in PSA levels more than 1.9 ng/ml, respectively.[33] Scattoni *et al.* prospectively evaluated the utility of ^{11}C-choline PET/CT in the diagnosis of LN recurrence in prostate cancer patients with PSA failure after surgery.[34] They showed the high positive predictive value (86%) on a per lesion basis and they concluded that

[11]C-choline PET/CT provides a basis for further treatment decisions such as a LN dissection. Krause *et al.* showed a positive relationship between the detection rate of ^{11}C-choline PET/CT and the serum PSA-level in patients with a biochemical recurrence.[35] In this study, the detection rate was 36% even for a PSA value <1 ng/ml.

11.7.3. *[18]F-choline PET*

[11]C is characterized by a short half-life of only 20 min, which may cause logistic problems when a cyclotron is not available on site. In contrast, ^{18}F-fluorocholine (FCH) can overcome this limitation due to the longer half-life of [18]F (110 min). Although FCH has some urinary excretion at 4 to 5 min after injection, FCH uptake in the prostate bed rises rapidly and reaches a plateau by approximately 3 min after injection.[36]

Price *et al.*[37] compared FCH-PET and FDG-PET for prostate cancers with *in vitro* study and clinical assessment. Their *in vitro* data demonstrated greater FCH than FDG uptake in androgen-dependent and androgen-independent prostate cancer cells, and PET in humans showed that FCH was better than FDG for detecting primary and metastatic prostate cancer. However, some studies suggested that FCH-PET has some limitations as well as FDG-PET, which is difficult to differentiate prostate cancers from BPH and to detect small lesions.[38,39] Although Igerc *et al.* showed similar results, they determined that FCH-PET could contribute useful additional information regarding the detection of the primary tumor in 5 patients (25% of their subjects) with elevated PSA level and negative prostate needle biopsy.[40] Beheshti *et al.* evaluated the potential value of FCH PET/CT in the preoperative staging of prostate cancer with 130 patients who had intermediate or high risk of extracapsular disease.[41] They found a significant correlation between sections with the highest FCH uptake and sextants with maximal tumor infiltration. Furthermore, FCH-PET/CT led to a change in therapy in 15% of all patients due to the detection of LN or bone metastases.

FCH-PET has some potential for the assessment of patients with a biochemical recurrence after primary treatment. Schmidt *et al.* evaluated nine patients who underwent FCH PET/CT for recurrent prostate cancer.[39] They showed that localization of recurrent tumor tissue was possible in all patients and concluded that FCH-PET/CT is a promising imaging modality for detecting local recurrence and LN metastases. Cimitan *et al.* evaluated the potential of FCH PET/CT in the assessment of suspected recurrence of prostate cancer with 100 patients with a persistent increase in serum PSA levels after treatment.[42] In this study, most of negative FCH-PET/CT scans were obtained in patients with serum PSA <4 ng/ml and with a Gleason score <8. Thus, they concluded that FCH-PET/CT helps to exclude distant metastases in selected patients when salvage local treatment is intended.

Recently, Beheshti *et al.* evaluated the utility of FCH-PET/CT for the assessment of bone metastases in prostate cancer.[43] The sensitivity, specificity, and accuracy of FCH-PET/CT in detecting bone metastases was 79%, 97%, and 84%, respectively, and 24% of detected lesions had no detectable morphological changes on CT. They concluded that FCH-PET/CT is promising tool for the early detection of bone metastases in prostate cancer patients.

11.7.4. ^{11}C-Acetate PET

The uptake of ^{11}C-Acetate reflects tissue metabolism through entry into catabolic or anabolic pathways mediated by acetyl-coenzyme A. Yoshimoto *et al.* reported that ^{14}C-Acetate accumulation in four different tumor cell lines was higher than that in the fibroblast cells, and this accumulation in tumor cells was shown to be caused by enhanced lipid synthesis.[44] Furthermore, ^{11}C-Acetate is not excreted via the urinary tract. Therefore, ^{11}C-Acetate PET is considered to be useful for the assessment of prostate cancers than ^{18}F-FDG-PET. Oyama *et al.* reported that ^{11}C-Acetate PET showed higher sensitivity than ^{18}F-FDG-PET for detecting the primary lesions (100% versus 83%), and they also reported that ^{11}C-Acetate PET was more sensitive for detecting of LN or bone metastases.[45]

There are some reports that evaluated the utility of ^{11}C-Acetate PET for detecting of recurrent prostate cancers. Kotzerke *et al.* examined 31 patients with increasing prostate-specific antigen (PSA) following complete prostatectomy and showed high sensitivity (83%) of ^{11}C-acetate PET for detecting local recurrence of prostate cancer.[46] In this study, small recurrent lesions showed false-negative results because of limited resolution of PET. Oyama *et al.* compared the utilities of ^{11}C-acetate PET and ^{18}F-FDG-PET and reported that ^{11}C-Acetate PET could detect more recurrent lesions than ^{18}F-FDG PET (30% versus 9%), limiting the analysis to patients with findings also confirmed by CT, bone scintigraphy, biopsy, or considered highly likely to represent tumor.[47] Fricke *et al.* reported the similar results but their study showed that ^{18}F-FDG-PET was more accurate for detecting bone metastases.[48] Sandblom *et al.*[49] and Albrecht *et al.*[50] examined patients with prostate-specific antigen (PSA) relapse after radical prostatectomy or initial radiotherapy and they showed high sensitivity of ^{11}C-acetate PET (75% and 82%, respectively) for detecting recurrent lesions. These results may suggest that ^{11}C-acetate PET is useful method for early detection and localization of prostate cancer recurrence.

11.7.5. *Other tracers for PET*

Although planar bone scintigraphy with ^{99m}Tc-methylene diphosphonate (MDP) has been used extensively for the evaluation of prostate cancer patients, false-negative bone scans can result from the absence of reactive changes or slow glowing lesions in which reactive bone is not detectable.[18] Recently, ^{18}F-fluoride has been introduced as a new tracer for PET, the uptake of which reflects blood flow and remodeling of bone. Even-Sapir *et al.* compared the detection of bone metastases by ^{99m}Tc-MDP planar bone scintigraphy, single-photon emission computed tomography (SPECT), ^{18}F-fluoride PET, and ^{18}F-fluoride PET/CT in patients with high-risk prostate cancer.[51] They showed that all of the sensitivity, specificity, positive predictive value, and negative predictive value of ^{18}F-fluoride PET/CT were 100%.

For the purpose of imaging androgen receptor expression, a new tracer, 16β-^{18}F-fluoro-5α-dihydrotestosterone (^{18}F-FDHT), was recently developed. Larson *et al.* assessed 7 patients with progressive metastatic prostate cancer who underwent ^{18}F-FDHT-PET and ^{18}F-FDG-PET, and found that ^{18}F-FDHT-PET and ^{18}F-FDG-PET was positive 78% and 97% of the lesions which were identified by conventional imaging, respectively.[52] In this study, treatment with testosterone resulted in diminished FDHT uptake in metastases. Dehdashti *et al.* showed a sensitivity of 86% on a lesion-based analysis in the assessment of ^{18}F-FDHT PET scans of 19 patients with metastatic prostate cancer.[53]

[11]C-methionine PET reflects the metabolism of amino acid in tumor cells. Toth *et al.* evaluated 20 patients with increased serum PSA level and negative repeat biopsies.[54] In their study, ^{11}C-methionine PET was positive in 15 patients, in 7 of whom (47%) the next repeat biopsy vertified carcinoma. Nunez *et al.* reported that ^{11}C-methionine PET had higher sensitivity in detecting metastastic lesions of prostate cancer than ^{18}F-FDG-PET (72% versus 48%) using conventional imaging modalities as standard reference.[55]

11.8. Germ Cell Tumors

11.8.1. *Primary staging*

Germ cell tumors (GCTs) are classified as either non-seminomatous GCTs or seminomas. As well as other malignant tumors, accurate classification of pathology and staging are important to determine the types of treatment.[56]

^{18}F-FDG-PET may be often used for initial staging of GCTs. Although Albers *et al.* showed high sensitivity (91%) and specificity (100%) of ^{18}F-FDG-PET for the initial staging of stage I and II testicular GCTs, they reported that ^{18}F-FDG-PET could not detect small lesions with a maximal diameter less than 0.5cm or mature teratoma at any size.[57] Spermon *et al.* reported similar false-negative cases.[58] De Wit *et al.* concluded that ^{18}F-FDG-PET as a primary staging tool for clinical stage I/II non-seminomatous GCTs yielded only slightly better results than CT from their multicenter prospective study.[59] In 2008, European Germ Cell Cancer Consensus group (EGCCCG) declared that ^{18}F-FDG-PET is not recommended in the primary staging of testicular GCTs.[60]

11.8.2. *Surveillance*

In patients with stage I disease, to avoid unnecessary toxicity from chemotherapy or radiation therapy, surveillance protocols after orchidectomy are frequently adopted. Hain *et al.* evaluated 55 patients who underwent ^{18}F-FDG-PET for detecting residual or recurrent GCTs retrospectively.[61] In patients with residual masses on CT, the positive and negative predictive values of ^{18}F-FDG PET were 96% and 90%, respectively. ^{18}F-FDG-PET effected a management change in 57% of cases, and clinical follow-up was adopted in 52% of them instead of planned therapy before ^{18}F-FDG PET. The other early studies showed high negative predictive value (>90%) of ^{18}F-FDG-PET for detecting metastases.[62,63]

It seems that the patients with negative ^{18}F-FDG PET findings do not require adjuvant treatment and can be monitored with surveillance. However, a recent prospective study, which evaluated large number of patients with high-risk (lymphovascular invasion positive), clinical stage I non-seminomatous GCTs, showed that 33 (38%) of 87 patients with negative ^{18}F-FDG PET findings relapsed, with a median follow up of 12 months.[64] ^{18}F-FDG-PET is not able to identify patients suitable for surveillance by itself.

11.8.3. *Assessment of treatment response*

^{18}F-FDG PET/CT can detect both of morphologic and metabolic changes in tumor cells and has some potentials in monitering therapy of GCTs (Fig. 11.4). To identify residual diseases after chemotherapy is important

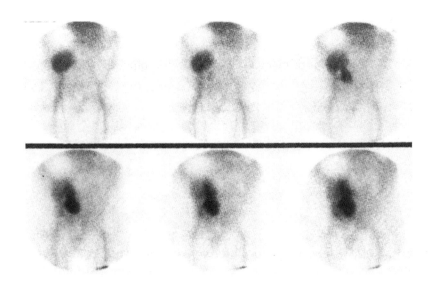

Fig. 11.4. Transplant kidney in the right pelvis shows an accumulation of Tc-99m MAG$_3$ in the urinoma.

for determining the need for additional therapy. There are many reports that assessed the utility of ^{18}F-FDG-PET in the evaluation of post-chemotherapy residual masses in GCTs.

Seminoma is sensitive to chemotherapy and radiation therapy and a residual mass after treatment usually constitutes only fibrosis and necrosis.[56] It is often difficult to distinguish between residual viable tumors and these fibrotic scar tissues by conventional imaging methods. Two early studies showed conflicting results whether ^{18}F-FDG-PET is useful for detecting viable tumor tissue in residual post-chemotherapy masses of seminoma patients.[65,66] However, the results of a large prospective study, the SEM-PET trial, showed that ^{18}F-FDG-PET was more accurate than other modalities for assessment.[67] In this trial, ^{18}F-FDG-PET correctly characterized all patients with residual tumor in masses greater than 3 cm as well as 95% of masses smaller than 3 cm. The specificity and sensitivity was 100% and 80%, respectively, for ^{18}F-FDG-PET and 74% and 70% for CT. In other words, a positive PET scan is a specific predictor for the presence of a viable tumor and a negative PET scan may help to avoid unnecessary surgery particularly in larger lesions (Fig. 11.5). Becherer *et al.* showed similar results and recommended the routine use of ^{18}F-FDG-PET for the evaluation of post-chemotherapy seminoma residuals.[68]

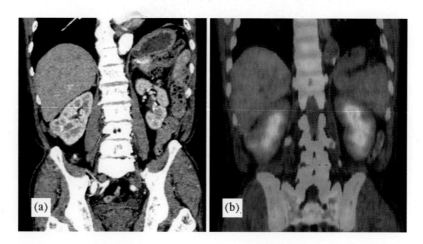

Fig. 11.5. Enhanced CT shows a hypervascular renal clear cell carcinoma in the right kidney. There is a minimal uptake of F-18-FDG in the tumor with 2.8 SUV$_{max}$.

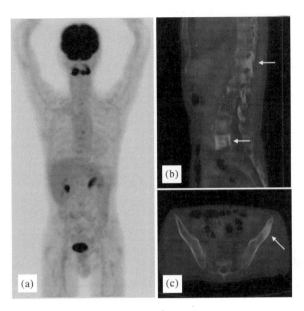

Fig. 11.6. Osteoblastic metastases of prostate cancer in vertebrae and left iliac bone on CT. There is no significant FDG uptake.

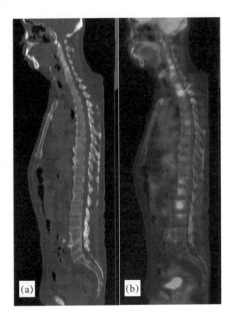

Fig. 11.7. Increased F-18 FDG uptake in vertebral metastases of prostate cancer. CT was essentially negative.

285

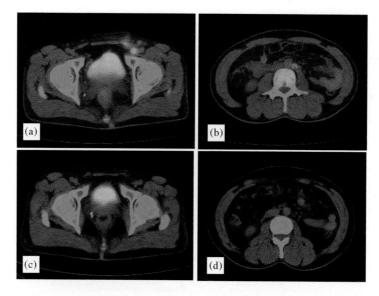

Fig. 11.8. Increased F-18 FDG uptake in left inguinal and paraaortic nodal metastases of seminoma before chemotherapy (a,b). These nodes become smaller, and FDG uptake disappeared, indicating therapeutic response.

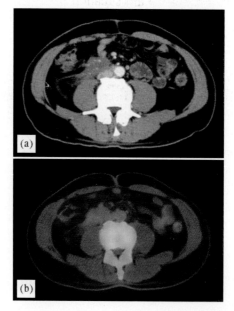

Fig. 11.9. Residual seminoma in the retroperitoneum on contrasted CT, but no significant FDG uptake, suggesting fibrotic therapeutic changes.

As well as seminoma, several studies showed that ^{18}F-FDG PET can be useful for detection of residual viable lesions in post-chemotherapy masses in non-seminomatous GCT patients. Kollmannsberger *et al.* showed high positive predictive value (92%) in their prospective study.[69] Putra *et al.* showed that a positive PET scan was accurate in 16 of 18 non-seminomatous GCT patients.[70] However, Oechsle *et al.* prospectively assessed ^{18}F-FDG-PET of 121 patients with stage IIC or III non-seminomatous GCT and showed poor accuracy of 56% which was not better than the accuracy of CT or serum tumor marker level.[71] Generally, mature differentiated teratoma, which has a risk of malignant transformation, has variable low uptake or no uptake and cannot be distinguished from fibrosis or necrosis.[56] Pfannenberg *et al.* compared ^{18}F-FDG-PET, CT/MRI and tumor marker kinetics in the evaluation of post-chemotherapy residual masses in metastatic germ cell tumor and concluded that ^{18}F-FDG-PET is a valuable diagnostic method to complement CT/MRI or tumor marker. However, on the other hand, they commented that residual masses with negative PET findings still require resection.[72] Although, to decide whether the response requires surgery is important, ^{18}F-FDG-PET use in this situation is limited.

11.8.4. *Prognostic prediction*

Although of the importance of ^{18}F-FDG-PET in improving staging and follow-up has been well established, recently, the use and value of PET as a predictor of outcome is a topic.[73] Bokemeyer *et al.* assessed 23 patients after high-dose salvage chemotherapy for relapsed germ cell cancer. When SUV < 2 after the initial part of treatment was defined as a negative PET scan, the values of the outcome prediction were 91%, 59%, and 48% of ^{18}F-FDG PET, CT, and tumor marker, respectively.[74]

References

1. Koyama K, Okamura T, Kawabe J, *et al.* (2003) Evaluation of ^{18}F-FDG PET with bladder irrigation in patients with uterine and ovarian tumors. *J Nucl Med* **44**: 353–358.
2. Kamel EM, Jichlinski P, Prior JO, *et al.* (2006) Forced diuresis improves the diagnostic accuracy of ^{18}F-FDG PET in abdominopelvic malgnancies. *J Nucl Med* **47**: 1803–1807.

3. Lin WY, Wang KB, Tsai SC, *et al.* (2009) Unexpected accumulation of F-18 FDG in the urinary bladder after bladder irrigation and retrograde filling with sterile saline: A possible pitfall in PET examination. *Clin Nucl Med* **34**: 560–563.
4. Ramdave S, Thomas GW, Berlangieri SU, *et al.* (2001) Clinical role of F-18 fluorodeoxyglucose positron emission tomography for detection and management of renal cell carcinoma. *J Urol* **166**: 825–830.
5. Goldberg MA, Mayo-Smith WW, Papanicolaou N, *et al.* (1997) FDG PET characterization of renal masses: Preliminary experience. *Clin Radiol* **52**: 510–515.
6. Aide N, Cappele O, Bottet P, *et al.* (2003) Efficiency of [^{18}F]FDG PET in characterizing renal cancer and detecting distant metastases: A comparison with CT. *Eur J Nucl Med Mol Imag* **30**: 1236–1245.
7. Kang DE, White Jr RL, Zuger JH, *et al.* (2004) Clinical use of fluorodeoxyglucose F 18 positron emission tomography for detection of renal cell carcinoma. *J Urol* **171**: 1806–1809.
8. Majhail NS, Urbain JL, Albani JM, *et al.* (2003) F-18 fluorodeoxyglucose positron emission tomography in the evaluation of distant metastases from renal cell carcinoma. *J Clin Oncol* **21**: 3995–4000.
9. Kosuda S, Kison PV, Greenough R, *et al.* (1997) Preliminary assessment of fluorine-18 fluorodeoxyglucose positron emission tomography in patients with bladder cancer. *Eur J Nucl Med* **24**: 615–620.
10. Drieskens O, Oyen R, Poppel HV, *et al.* (2005) FDG-PET for preoperative staging of bladder cancer. *Eur J Nucl Med Mol Imag* **32**: 1412–1417.
11. Heicappell R, Muller-Mattheis V, Reinhardt M, *et al.* (1999) Staging of pelvic lymph nodes in neoplasms of the bladder and prostate by positron emission tomography with 2-[(18)F]-2-deoxy-D-glucose. *Eur Urol* **36**: 582–587.
12. Kibel AS, Dehdashti F, Kats MD, *et al.* (2009) Prospective study of [^{18}F]fluorodeoxyglucose positron emission tomography/computed tomography for staging of muscle-invasive bladder carcinoma. *J Clin Oncol* **27**: 4314–4320.
13. Swinnen G, Maes A, Pottel H, *et al.* (2010) FDG-PET/CT for the preoperative lymph node staging of invasive bladder cancer. *Eur Urol* **57**: 641–647.
14. Ahlstrom H, Malmstrom PU, Letocha H, *et al.* (1996) Positron emission tomography in the diagnosis and staging of urinary bladder cancer. *Acta Radiol* **37**: 180–185.
15. Gofrit ON, Mishani E, Orevi M, *et al.* (2006) Contribution of [^{11}C]-choline positron emission tomogramphy/computerized tomography to preoperative staging of advanced transitional cell carcinoma. *J Urol* **176**: 940–944.
16. Effert PJ, Bares R, Handt S, *et al.* (1996) Metabolic imaging of untreated prostate cancer by positron emission tomography with sup 18 fluorine-labeled deoxyglucose. *J Urol* **155**: 994–998.
17. Hofer C, Laubenbacher C, Block T, *et al.* (1999) Fluorine-18-fluorodeoxyglucose positron emission tomography is useless for the detection of local recurrence after radical prostatectomy. *Eur Urol* **36**: 31–35.
18. Beheshti M, Langsteger W, Fogelman I. (2009) Prostate cancer: Role of SPECT and PET in imaging bone metastases. *Semin Nucl Med* **39**: 396–407.
19. Shreve PD, Grossman HB, Gross MD, *et al.* (1996) Metastatic prostate cancer: Initial findings of PET with 2-deoxy-2-[F-18]fluoro-D-glucose. *Radiology* **199**: 751–756.

20. Schoder H, Herrmann K, Gonen M, *et al*. (2005) 2-[^{18}F]fluoro-2-deoxyglucose positron emission tomography for the detection of disease in patients with prostate-specific antigen relapse after radical prostatectomy. *Clin Cancer Res* **11**: 4761–4769.

21. Morris MJ, Akhurst T, Larson SM, *et al*. (2005) Fluorodeoxyglucose positron emission tomography as an outcome measure for castrate metastatic prostate cancer treated with antimicrotubule chemotherapy. *Clin Cancer Res* **11**: 3210–3216.

22. Oyama N, Akino H, Kanamaru H, *et al*. (2002) Prognostic value of 2-deoxy-2-[F-18]fluoro-D- glucose positron emission tomography imaging for patients with prostate cancer. *Mol Imaging Biol* **4**: 99–104.

23. Breeuwsma AJ, Pruim J, Jongen MM, *et al*. (2005) *In vivo* uptake of [^{11}C]choline does not correlate with cell proliferation in human prostate cancer. *Eur J Nucl Med Mol Imag* **32**: 668–673.

24. Hara T, Kosaka N, Kishi H. (1998) PET imaging of prostate cancer using carbon-11-choline. *J Nucl Med* **39**: 990–995.

25. Kotzerke J, Prang J, Neumaier B, *et al*. (2000) Experience with carbon-11 choline positron emission tomography in prostate carcinoma. *Eur J Nucl Med* **27**: 1415–1419.

26. Farsad M, Schiavina R, Castellucci P, *et al*. (2005) Detection and localization of prostate cancer: Correlation of ^{11}C-choline PET/CT with histopathologic step-section analysis. *J Nucl Med* **46**: 1642–1649.

27. Reske SN, Blumstein NM, Neumaier B, *et al*. (2006) Imaging prostate cancer with ^{11}C-choline PET/CT. *J Nucl Med* **47**: 1249–1254.

28. Giovacchini G, Picchio M, Coradeschi E, *et al*. (2008) [^{11}C]choline uptake with PET/CT for the initial diagnosis of prostate cancer: Relation to PSA levels, tumour stage and anti-androgenic therapy. *Eur J Nucl Med Mol Imaging* **35**: 1065–1073.

29. Martorana G, Schiavina R, Corti B, *et al*. (2006) ^{11}C-choline positron emission tomography/computerized tomography for tumor localization of primary prostate cancer in comparison with 12-core biopsy. *J Urol* **176**: 954–960.

30. Yamaguchi T, Lee J, Uemura H, *et al*. (2005) Prostate cancer: A comparative study of ^{11}C-choline PET and MR imaging combined with proton MR spectroscopy. *Eur J Nucl Med Mol Imaging* **32**: 742–748.

31. Testa C, Schiavina R, Lodi R, *et al*. (2007) Prostate cancer: Sextant localization with MR imaging, MR spectroscopy, and ^{11}C-choline PET/CT. *Radiology* **244**: 797–806.

32. Picchio M, Messa C, Landoni C, *et al*. (2003) Value of [^{11}C]choline-positron emission tomography for re-staging prostate cancer: A comparison with [^{18}F]fluorodeoxyglucose-positron emission tomography. *J Urol* **169**: 1337–1340.

33. Richter JA, Rodriguez M, Rioja J, *et al*. (2010) Dual tracer ^{11}C-choline and FDG-PET in the diagnosis of biochemical prostate cancer relapse after radical treatment. *Mol Imaging Biol* **12**: 210–217.

34. Scattoni V, Picchio M, Suardi N, *et al*. (2007) Detection of lymph-node metastases with integrated [^{11}C]choline PET/CT in patients with PSA failure after radical retropubic prostatectomy: Results comfirmed by open pelvic-retroperitoneal lymphadenectomy. *Eur Urol* **52**: 423–429.

35. Krause BJ, Souvatzoglou M, Tuncel M, *et al*. (2008) The detection rate of [^{11}C]choline-PET/CT depends on the serum PSA-value in patients with biochemical recurrence of prostate cancer. *Eur J Nucl Med Mol Imaging* **35**: 18–23.

36. DeGrado TR, Baldwin SW, Wang S, *et al.* (2001) Synthesis and evaluation of (18)F-labeled choline analogs as oncologic PET tracers. *J Nucl Med* **42**: 1805–1814.

37. Price DT, Coleman RE, Liao RP, *et al.* (2002) Comparison of [18F]fluorocholine and [18F]fluorodeoxyglucose for positron emission tomography of androgen dependent and androgen independent prostate cancer. *J Urol* **168**: 273–280.

38. Kwee SA, Coel MN, Lim J, *et al.* (2005) Prostate cancer localization with 18fluorine fluorocholine positron emission tomography. *J Urol* **173**: 252–255.

39. Schmid DT, John H, Zweifel R, *et al.* (2005) Fluorocholine PET/CT in patients with prostate cancer: Initial experience. *Radiology* **235**: 623–628.

40. Igerc I, Kohlfurst S, Gallowitsch HJ, *et al.* (2008) The value of 18F-choline PET/CT in patients with elevated PSA-level and negative prostate needle biopsy for localization of prostate cancer. *Eur J Nucl Med Mol Imaging* **35**: 976–983.

41. Beheshti M, Imamovic L, Broinger G, *et al.* (2010) 18F choline PET/CT in the preoperative staging of prostate cancer in patients with intermediate or high risk of extracapsular disease: A prospective study of 130 patients. *Radiology* **254**: 925–933.

42. Cimitan M, Bortolus R, Morassut S, *et al.* (2006) [18F]fluorocholine PET/CT imaging for the detection of recurrent prostate cancer at PSA relapse: Experience in 100 consecutive patients. *Eur J Nucl Med Mol Imaging* **33**: 1387–1398.

43. Beheshti M, Vali R, Waldenberger P, *et al.* (2010) The use of F-18 choline PET in the assessment of bone metastases in prostate cancer: Correlation with morphological changes on CT. *Mol Imaging Biol* **12**: 98–107.

44. Yoshimoto M, Waki A, Yonekura Y, *et al.* (2001) Characterization of acetate metabolism in tumor cells in relation to cell proliferation: Acetate metabolism in tumor cells. *Nucl Med Biol* **28**: 117–122.

45. Oyama N, Akino H, Kanamaru H, *et al.* (2002) 11C-acetate PET imaging of prostate cancer. *J Nucl Med* **43**: 181–186.

46. Kotzerke J, Volkmer BG, Neumaier B, *et al.* (2002) Carbon-11 acetate positron emission tomography can detect local recurrence of prostate cancer. *Eur J Nucl Med* **29**: 1380–1384.

47. Oyama N, Miller TR, Dehdashti F, *et al.* (2003) 11C-acetate PET imaging of prostate cancer: Detection of recurrent disease at PSA relapse. *J Nucl Med* **44**: 549–555.

48. Fricke E, Machtens S, Hofmann M, *et al.* (2003) Positron emission tomography with 11C-acetate and 18F-FDG in prostate cancer patients. *Eur J Nucl Med Mol Imaging* **30**: 607–611.

49. Sandblom G, Sorensen J, Lundin N, *et al.* (2006) Positron emission tomography with 11C-acetate for tumor detection and localization in patients with prostate-specific antigen relapse after radical prostatectomy. *Urology* **67**: 996–1000.

50. Albrecht S, Buchegger F, Soloviev D, *et al.* (2007) 11C-acetate PET in the early evaluation of prostate cancer recurrence. *Eur J Nucl Med Mol Imaging* **34**: 185–196.

51. Even-Sapir E, Mester U, Mishani E, *et al.* (2006) The detection of bone metastases in patients with high-risk prostate cancer: 99mTc-MDP planar bone scintigraphy, single- and multi-field-of-view SPECT, 18F-fluoride PET, and 18F-fluoride PET/CT. *J Nucl Med* **47**: 287–297.

52. Larson SM, Morris M, Gunther I, *et al.* (2004) Tumor localization of 16β-^{18}F-fluoro-5α-dihydrotestosterone versus ^{18}F-FDG in patients with progressive, metastatic prostate cancer. *J Nucl Med* **45**: 366–373.

53. Dehdashti F, Picus J, Michalski JM, *et al.* (2005) Positron tomographic assessment of androgen receptors in prostatic carcinoma. *Eur J Nucl Med Mol Imaging* **32**: 344–350.

54. Toth G, Lengyel Z, Balkay L, *et al.* (2005) Detection of prostate cancer with ^{11}C-methionine positron emission tomography. *J Urol* **173**: 66–69.

55. Nunez R, Macapinlac HA, Yeung HW, *et al.* (2002) Combined ^{18}F-FDG and ^{11}C-methionine PET scans in patients with newly progressive metastatic prostate cancer. *J Nucl Med* **43**: 46–55.

56. Sohaib SA, Koh D, Husband JE. (2008) The role of imaging in the diagnosis, staging, and management of testicular cancer. *Am J Roentgenol* **191**: 387–395.

57. Albers P, Bender H, Yilmaz H, *et al.* (1999) Positron emission tomography in the clinical staging of patients with stage I and II testicular germ cell tumors. *Urology* **53**: 808–811.

58. Spermon JR, Geus-Oei LF, Kiemeney LA, *et al.* (2002) The role of [18]fluoro-2-deoxyglucose positron emission tomography in initial staging and re-staging after chemotherapy for testicular germ cell tumours. *BJU Int* **89**: 549–556.

59. De Wit M, Brenner W, Hartmann M, *et al.* (2008) [18F]-FDG-PET in clinical stage I/II non-seminomatous germ cell tumours: Results of the German multicentre trial. *Ann Oncol* **19**: 1619–1623.

60. Krege S, Beyer J, Souchon R, *et al.* (2008) European consensus on diagnosis and treatment of germ cell cancer: A report of the second meeting of the European Germ Cell Cancer Consensus group (EGCCCG) part I. *Eur Urol* **53**: 473–496.

61. Hain SF, O'Doherty MJ, Timothy AR, *et al.* (2000) Fluorodeofyglucose positron emission tomography in the evaluation of germ cell tumours at relapse. *Br J Cancer* **83**: 863–869.

62. Cremerius U, Wildberger JE, Borchers H, *et al.* (1999) Does positron emission tomography using 18-fluoro-2-deoxyglucose improve clinical staging of testicular cancer? Results of a study in 50 patients. *Urology* **54**: 900–904.

63. Lassen U, Daugaard G, Eigtved A, *et al.* (2003) Whole-body FDG-PET in patients with stage I non-seminomatous germ cell tumours. *Eur J Nucl Med* **30**: 396–402.

64. Huddart RA, O'Doherty MJ, Padhani A, *et al.* (2007) [18]Fluorodeoxyglucose positron emission tomography in the prediction of relapse in patients with high-risk, clinical stage I nonseminomatous germ cell tumors: Preliminary report of MRC Trial TE22 – the NCRI Testis Tumour Clinical Study Group. *J Clin Oncol* **25**: 3090–3095.

65. Ganjoo KN, Chan RJ, Sharma M, *et al.* (1999) Positron emission tomography scans in the evaluation of postchemotherapy residual masses in patients with seminoma. *J Clin Oncol* **17**: 3457–3460.

66. De Santis M, Bokemeyer C, Becherer A, *et al.* (2001) Predictive impact of 2-[18]fluoro-2-deoxy-D-glucose positron emission tomography for residual postchemotherapy masses in patients with bulky seminoma. *J Clin Oncol* **19**: 3740–3744.

67. De Santis M, Becherer A, Bokemeyer C, *et al.* (2004) 2-[18]fluoro-deoxy-D-glucose positron emission tomography is a reliable predictor for viable tumor in postchemotherapy seminoma: An update of the prospective multicentric SEMPET trial. *J Clin Oncol* **22**: 1034–1039.

68. Becherer A, De Santis M, Karanikas G, *et al.* (2005) FDG PET is superior to CT in the prediction of viable tumour in post-chemotherapy seminoma residuals. *Eur J Rad* **54**: 284–288.

69. Kollmannsberger C, Oechsle K, Dohmen BM, *et al.* (2002) Prospective comparison of [18F]fluorodeoxyglucose positron emission tomography with conventional assessment by computed tomography scans and serum tumor markers for the evaluation of residual masses in patients with nonseminomatous germ cell carcinoma. *Cancer* **94**: 2353–2362.

70. Putra LJ, Lawrentschuk N, Ballok Z, *et al.* (2004) ^{18}F-fluorodeoxyglucose positron emission tomography in evaluation of germ cell tumour after chemotherapy. *Urology* **64**: 1202–1207.

71. Oechsle K, Hartmann M, Brenner W, *et al.* (2008) [18F]fluorodeoxyglucose positron emission tomography in nonseminomatous germ cell tumors after chemotherapy: The German multicenter positron emission tomography study group. *J Clin Oncol* **26**: 5930–5935.

72. Pfannenberg AC, Oechsle K, Bokemeyer C, *et al.* (2004) The role of [18F] FDG-PET, CT/MRI and tumor marker kinetics in the evaluation of postchemotherapy residual masses in metastatic germ cell tumors-prospects for management. *World J Urol* **22**: 132–139.

73. Lucignani G and Larson SM. (2010) Doctor, what does my future hold? The prognostic value of FDG-PET in solid tumours. *Eur J Nucl Med Mol Imaging* **37**: 1032–1038.

74. Bokemeyer C, Kollmannsberger C, Oechsle K, *et al.* (2002) Early prediction of treatment response to high-dose salvage chemotherapy in patients with relapsed germ cell cancer using [18F]FDG PET. *Br J Cancer* **86**: 506–511.

Chapter 12
Bone and Joint Nuclear Imaging

Seok-ki Kim

12.1. Introduction

Skeletal nuclear imaging (NI) is the most common procedure performed among the diagnostic nuclear medicine imaging techniques. Skeletal NI shares most of the characteristics of the radionuclide imaging technique. It is very sensitive and can detect subtle metabolic and functional changes at an early stage. It is a technically easy and inexpensive modality that can cover the whole body. It is non-invasive and a safe technique and is generally has no side effects. There are no major contraindications when using a relatively low dose of radiation.

Skeletal NI has been assumed to be less specific because of the limited anatomical resolution and the less selective characteristics of some of the radiopharmaceuticals. The spatial resolution of the imaging equipment has recently improved, and the fusion technology with CT gives additional anatomical information, which improves the specificity of skeletal NI. Moreover, the new skeletal radiopharmaceuticals are more selective in nature than the conventional skeletal radiopharmaceuticals such as the technetium-labeled phosphate agents and it is also helpful that we interpret NI taking into account the clinical context.

Technetium-labeled phosphate agents such as ^{99m}Tc-methylene diphosphonate (MDP) and the dual-head gamma camera have made skeletal nuclear medicine imaging the most common clinical procedure since the 1970s. Other radiopharmaceuticals such as ^{18}F-fluorodeoxy glucose (FDG), radiolabeled white blood cells (WBCs), and ^{18}F-NaF (NaF) have since enriched skeletal NI.

12.2. Agents for Skeletal NI

12.2.1. *Agents for osteoblastic activity*

The typical agents that depict osteoblastic activity are phosphate analogues and fluoride agents. First, phosphate analogues are the most commonly used radiopharmaceuticals for osteoblastic activity. Although pyrophosphate and polyphosphate agents were initially introduced, ^{99m}Tc-diphosphonate radiopharmaceuticals such as MDP and ^{99m}Tc hydroxyl-methylene diphosphonate (HDP) have been adopted as the standard agents for skeletal NI because of their higher skeletal uptake, faster blood-pool clearance, and better *in vivo* stability. MDP is administered through intravenous injection. It circulates in the vascular system for a short time and then it subsequently rapidly accumulates in the bone. The residual MDP is excreted via the urine. Approximately half of the administered dose is eliminated within about 4 h (Fig. 12.1).

NaF can be used as an alternative to diphosphate agents. ^{18}F-fluoride diffuses through the capillaries into the extracellular fluid and this is followed by a relatively slow exchange of hydroxyl ions in the hydroxyapatite crystal, and mainly at the surface of the skeleton.[1] The uptake of ^{18}F-fluoride is approximately two-fold higher and its blood clearance is significantly faster

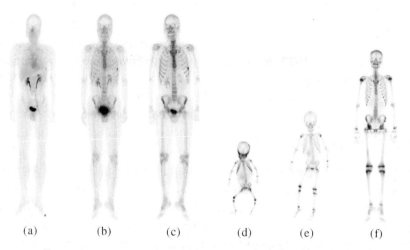

(a)   (b)   (c)   (d)   (e)   (f)

Fig. 12.1. ^{99m}Tc-MDP bone scan images were performed in 36-year-old man at (a) 5 min, (b) 1 hour, and (c) 2 hours after injection. The focal uptake of right rib was caused by fracture. Bone scans of children shows typical uptakes of the epiphyseal plate and the costochondral junction. Children were aged (d) 1 year, (e) 3 years, and (f) 13 years.

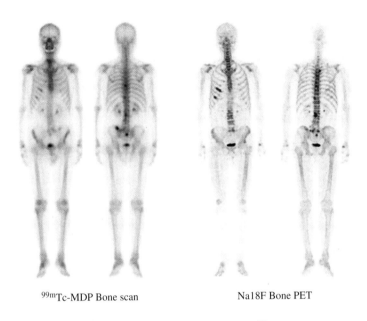

99mTc-MDP Bone scan   Na18F Bone PET

Fig. 12.2.   99mTc-MDP bone scan and Na18F PET.

compared with that of MDP. High-quality skeletal images can be obtained less than 1 h after the intravenous administration of NaF (Fig. 12.2). As a result, NaF-PET has higher spatial resolution and substantially greater sensitivity. NaF was approved for clinical use by the U.S. Food and Drug Administration in 1972, but it was not an attractive radiopharmaceutical because of the technical limitations at that time. The recent fast modern PET scanner and NaF logistic system have caused an increase in NaF imaging.

12.2.2. *Selective skeletal agent*

FDG is established and used as an oncological agent. It is also readily taken up in various infectious and inflammatory conditions. FDG is transported into cells by glucose transporters, is phosphorylated by hexokinase inside the cell to form fluorodeoxyglucose-6-phosphate, and then it accumulates. Metastasis or primary bone tumor cells take up more FDG than normal tissue. FDG accumulates in sites of infection because it accumulates in activated lymphocytes, neutrophils, and macrophages, with a minimal decrease over time.[2,3] These characteristics make FDG suitable for imaging skeletal metastasis, primary bone tumor, and various inflammatory and infectious diseases.

^{67}Ga-citrate has been used for imaging of infection and inflammation ever since the early 1970s. ^{67}Ga-citrate accumulates both in acute and chronic infection and in non-infectious inflammation with very good sensitivity. But the specificity and spatial resolution are not good. Because of slow excretion, it takes a long time until imaging after injection, and the dose of radiation exposure is high. Although ^{67}Ga-citrate is now less frequently used, it has been used mainly to diagnose or to exclude osteomyelitis with reasonable sensitivity (73%) and relatively low specificity (61%).[4]

Radiolabeled leukocytes can be used for diagnosing skeletal infection. Both ^{111}In-labeled and ^{99m}Tc-labeled WBCs (^{99m}Tc-WBCs) have excellent performance for their diagnostic accuracy. But ^{99m}Tc-WBCs have more favorable imaging characteristics and are more convenient to use for most indications. The main drawbacks of ^{111}In-WBC and ^{99m}Tc- WBC are their laborious preparation, the requirement of specialized equipment, and the handling of potentially infectious blood. Unlike ^{111}In-WBCs, ^{99m}Tc-WBCs are relatively unstable and ^{99m}Tc-hexamethylpropylene amine oxime can elute from the WBC, and this can subsequently be excreted through the kidneys, the gallbladder, and the intestine.[5]

12.3. Imaging Technique and New Scanners

Skeletal NI is scanned mostly as planar image using ^{99m}Tc-based diphophonate agents, ^{99m}Tc-WBCs, and ^{111}In-WBCs. Although the anterior and posterior planar images give sufficient information in most cases, additional views or tomography are needed due to superimposed images. Examples of additional views are as follows: oblique views for the lateral ribs, scapula, and ribs, and the squat views of the pelvis for separating bladder activity and the pubic bones. For small structures, magnification views may be useful for improving the visualization of the hands and wrists in the adult and for the hip joints in pediatric patients.

Tomographic nuclear NI, SPECT, and PET are favorable for complex structures such as the lumbar spine, knees, the base of the skull, and the facial bones. For example, SPECT imaging is essential to identify abnormalities

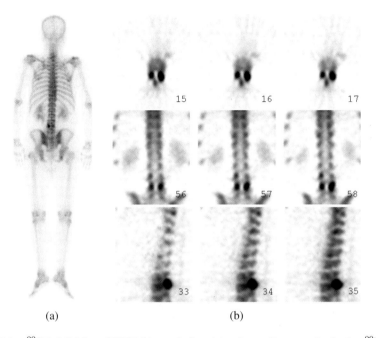

(a)   (b)

Fig. 12.3. ^{99m}Tc-MDP bone SPECT (b) reveals facet joint abnormality more clearly than ^{99m}Tc-MDP bone scan (a).

in the facet joints (Fig. 12.3). Planar imaging alone cannot separate activity in the facet joints from associated activity in the vertebral body caused by fracture. Tomography improves the detection and anatomical localization of lesions and it is more readily available compared with other tomographic imaging such as CT and MRI. In this context, NaF-PET might give extra information compared to a planar bone scan.

Fusion technology such as PET/CT and SPECT/CT can improve the specificity of planar imaging or tomographic imaging alone. Although software fusion, which was developed earlier, is conceptually fascinating, it was too slow and cumbersome to use practically. But a hardware-based fusion technique is sufficiently convenient to apply to the everyday clinical activities. From a different view, multimodality imaging raises questions about the additional radiation burden and the need for an optimal protocol.

Generally, skeletal NI is acquired a couple of hours after the injection of radiopharmaceuticals. The images at the early phase after injection can convey other information. A short period after injection, usually 1 min, is proper for blood flow information. Following 2 to 5 min post-injection, the blood pool can be depicted. Increased accumulation of MDP on the blood flow and blood pool images accounts for the combination of increased vascularity and vascular permeability of bone tumors, healing trauma and inflammatory and infected conditions. We call it the triple phase; collecting these two phases and the delayed phase, and the blood flow and blood pool phase images can be obtained combined for practical convenience.

12.4. Normal Appearance and the Perception and Interpretation of Abnormal Findings

12.4.1. *Normal variants and perception of abnormal findings*

The main components of bone are hydroxyapatite crystals and collagen. Bone is highly vascularized living tissue. The osteoclasts perform bone resorption and removal, and the osteoblasts form new bone. These two types of cells coordinate closely for bone remodeling, which is finely balanced and continues for life. Bone remodeling diffusely occurs in the whole skeleton and this accounts for the background low uniform uptake of radionuclide on skeletal NI.

In order to perceive abnormal findings on skeletal NI, we should be familiar with the normal findings and normal variants. There are some normal variants and non-specific findings that can mislead investigators and some incidental findings that are not directly related to skeletal lesion and can provide unexpected information. A patient's age, gender, any history of trauma or surgery, and other clinical information are vital and helpful to avoid false interpretation. In addition, the images should be interpreted keeping the clinical context in mind. Previous imaging and other types of images should be compared and referred if they are available.

Normally, the skeletal system represents diffuse mild symmetrical uptake about the midline. Some background soft tissue uptake is observed with variable intensities, which are influenced by obesity and the renal function. As skeletal radiopharmaceuticals are excreted through the urinary system, normal variants in the urinary tract and urinary obstruction can be incidentally revealed. Renal insufficiency, renal agenesis, and horseshoe kidney are all well visualized if the renal function is adequate. In some clinical situation, a ruptured urinary system might be visualized. MDP can accumulate in soft tissues, which may be incidental or significant depending on the clinical setting. The common causes of extraosseous uptake includes normal breast tissue, breast carcinoma, liver metastases, osteosarcoma metastases, soft tissue sarcomas, tumoral calcinosis, pleural effusion, ascites, calcified uterine fibroids, injection sites, surgical scars, and old hematomas.

Various artifacts can be noted. The metallic materials of a pacemaker and a Halter monitor, orthopedic devices, and small objects such as coins, belt buckles, and zippers can create a subtle photopenic area, which can lead to misinterpretation. The injection site can be superimposed on bone uptake and misinterpreted as pathology, although this is rare.

Contamination by spillage or urine is usual and this is easily detected by reimaging after undressing or cleaning. In some cases, the camera can be directly contaminated and then a similar pattern of abnormal findings are seen for all the patients. The patient's posture, such as the subtle rotation of the pelvis, can be interpreted as apparent asymmetry without pathology.

In the normal immature skeleton, the highest uptake of MDP occurs at the epiphyseal plates, which are the sites of active bone growth (Fig. 12.1). This uptake fades when the epiphyses fuse and growth ceases. This phenomenon can be useful when early or delayed epiphyseal closure is suspected. In children, the epiphyseal growth plate normally shows intense uptake. Metastases adjacent to the epiphyseal growth plate can be masked and so close comparison with the contralateral limb and alternative imaging strategies are recommended.

12.4.2. *Disease-specific patterns and characteristics*

Before discussing the specific imaging patterns and characteristics of skeletal disease, it is very useful and practical to consider and categorize the commonly encountered imaging findings and clinical situations.

Multiple versus solitary lesions: In the setting of a metastatic work-up, the number and distribution of focal uptakes are important. Multiple uptake lesions in most cancers strongly suggests multiple skeletal metastases, and especially if they are distributed randomly and asymmetrically in the axial skeleton, which includes the bones of the spine, ribs, and sternum; the skull and facial bones; and the pelvis, with sparing the appendicular skeleton.[6] But this is not an absolute rule and some tumors, and especially non–small cell carcinoma, can metastasize to form metastatic distal appendicular lesions.

If multiple hot spots are randomly distributed regionally, then the interpretation may be problematic. A case with multiple spinal hot spots cannot be assumed to be metastases because of a high prevalence of benign lesions such as degenerative disease, which cannot be easily distinguished from tumor. A linear array of multiple hot spots of the ribs and a recent history of trauma with or without osteoporosis certainly indicate traumatic lesions (Fig. 12.4).

Solitary focal abnormality is much more problematic than multiple uptakes. Solitary metastasis is uncommon but can be suspected according to the type of primary tumor and the tumor site. A solitary asymmetric sternal lesion in a patient with breast cancer has a very high chance of being bony invasion from parasternal breast cancer. Single rib lesions and

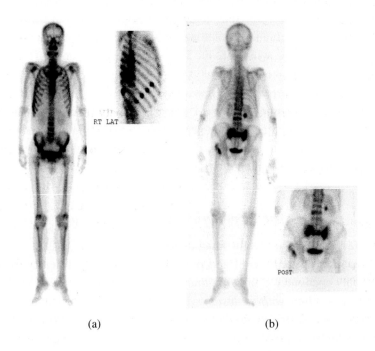

(a)   (b)

Fig. 12.4. Rib fracture (a) and posterior view of sacral insufficiency fracture (b).

a single spinal hot spot in patients with a known primary tumor are much more likely to be due to simple trauma or benign lesion than metastatic disease[7,8]; vertebral body fractures have a characteristic linear pattern of hot uptake on bone scans. However, it is not possible to completely differentiate solitary focal lesions. Sequential follow-up scans are extremely helpful; multiple metastatic lesions usually increase in size, number, and intensity of uptake without treatment. A follow-up bone scan after a few months that shows reduced activity at a previous hot uptake site suggests a benign cause. For further evaluation, complementary imaging should be considered and MRI is probably the best current method for differentiating benign from malignant causes. If necessary, histologic confirmation may be required in some cases for the precise diagnosis.

Photopenic lesions: Some bone lesions present as less uptake than the surrounding normal activity. If these photopenic lesions are small, then they are obscured and perceiving them is difficult. Photopenic lesions can be seen in avascular lesions, in the presence of rapidly growing pure osteolytic metastases with no reactive increased osteoblastic activity and in lesions with low bone turnover. Multiple myeloma is purely osteoblastic and it shows as photopenic lesion on scans. Unless large in size or number, photopenic areas are more difficult to detect than hot uptake. However, associated pathologic fracture and the healing process shows hot uptake. Highly aggressive tumors often destroy neighboring bones and associated bone resorption overwhelms the osteoblastic activity for bone repair. This results in loss of bone tissue and replacing it with non-skeletal tumor tissues. Although bony involvement in this setting is apparent, it is often difficult to locate this photopenic area. Fortunately, the photopenic area may exhibit thin peripheral hot uptake at the edge of bone involvement in some cases.

Diffuse uptakes in the axial skeleton with reduced renal visualization: We rarely encounter the case that shows diffuse bone uptake in the axial skeleton; the distribution of bone uptake seems symmetric, but it is a little inhomogeneous. Renal visualization is reduced. This has been called a "superscan" and occurs when nearly all the bones are involved by tumor. It is most common in patients with carcinoma of the prostate or breast. As the bony uptake is much higher than the normal background uptake, the kidney is relatively poorly visualized. Because the uptake seems symmetric, misinterpretation as normal uptake is possible.

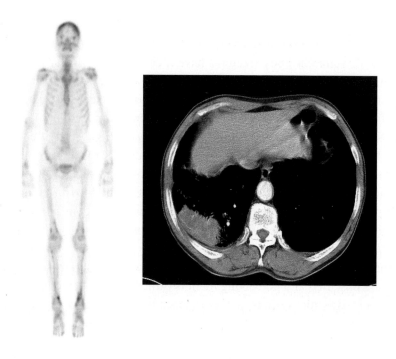

Fig. 12.5. Hypertrophic pulmonary osteoarthropathy affecting femora and tibiae with lung lesion.

Other abnormal findings: Tram-like increased uptake along the cortex of the long bones may be seen in the patients with thoracic or gastrointestinal disease, including malignancies of the lung and pleura. This is called as hypertrophic pulmonary osteoarthropathy and might be a non-metastatic manifestation of the primary tumor (Fig. 12.5). Elderly women who had received external radiation to the pelvic bone often present with a horizontal linear uptake in the sacrum. This is unlikely to be metastasis and it turns out to be insufficiency fracture in many cases.

Complementary imaging: If there is any doubt about the significance of an abnormality on skeletal NI, then other imaging procedures can be invaluable, and these studies should be viewed alongside the skeletal NI to gain the maximum benefit. If it is necessary to further investigate with other imaging modalities, then plain imaging is still the most important and the first candidate. When the findings from the skeletal NI are interpreted with these plain images, it is advantageous to characterize a lesion to explain the findings. In view of the increased sensitivity of the skeletal NI over plain film, if the radiographs are normal, then CT or MRI should be considered. The choice of modality will depend on the area of the body in question and the suspected pathology.

12.5. Clinical Applications

12.5.1. *Skeletal metastasis*

12.5.1.1. *Breast cancer*

Breast cancer is the most common cause of skeletal involvement in women. Bone metastases affect 8% of all patients with breast cancer, but this incidence can reach 30%–85% in patients with advanced disease.[9,10] Breast cancer initially metastasizes as intramedullary lesion, so the skeletal metastases from the breast cancer are mainly located in the axial skeleton and they are most commonly in the spine and pelvis followed by the ribs, skull, and femora (Fig. 12.6). Although breast cancer can metastasize

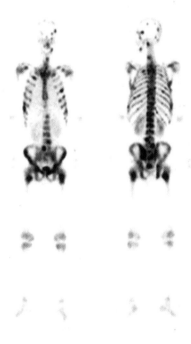

Fig. 12.6. Extensive skeletal metastases from breast cancer.

as osteolytic, osteoblastic, or mixed lesions, most lesions present as osteoblastic metastases.

Bone scan is the first method for detecting skeletal metastasis in breast cancer patients. The reported sensitivity and specificity of a bone scan for the detection of bone metastases have ranged between 62%–100% and 78%–100%, respectively.[10] The detection rate of bone metastases by bone scan in patients with early-stage breast cancer is very low (0.82% and 2.55% in patients with stages I and II, respectively), and this increases to 16.75% in patients with stage III disease and 40.52% in patients with stage IV disease. Routine screening with bone scan is recommended only for patients with advanced stage disease and it is not recommended for a patient with early stage disease if there is no clinical suspicion of bony metastasis, such as new musculoskeletal symptoms, biochemical abnormalities, rising tumor markers, and abnormal radiographic findings.[11,12]

Several groups have compared FDG-PET and bone scan for breast cancer.[13-17] Their reports show a little incongruity but overall, bone scan and FDG-PET showed similar sensitivity. FDG-PET was a little superior to a bone scan in terms of the specificity. FDG-PET for detecting skeletal metastases has demonstrated a sensitivity of 56%–100%.[19,20] According to lesion-by-lesion analysis, osteoblastic lesions were more apparent on the bone scan than on FDG-PET, whereas osteolytic lesions were more discernible on FDG-PET.[16] FDG-PET showed more intense FDG accumulation in osteolytic lesions than that in the mixed or osteoblastic lesions. Discrepancies between the findings on a bone scan and FDG-PET can be explained by the different uptake mechanisms of these tracers. Although the uptake of MDP is related to the osteoblastic response of the bone to the tumor, the uptake of FDG is related to the metabolic activity of the tumor itself. FDG is more likely to detect metastases at an earlier stage than a bone scan, when the tumor is still confined to the bone marrow, before an osteoblastic reaction that can be visualized on bone scan occurs (Fig. 12.7).

NaF is a non-specific PET tracer that is used for assessment of bone metastases. NaF and ^{99m}Tc-diphosphonate share the same uptake mechanism. NaF-PET shows focally increased uptake in both osteolytic and osteoblastic skeletal metastases. The overall sensitivity and specificity of ^{18}NaF-PET for the detection of metastases were assumed to be higher than that for a bone scan. Although few published reports have compared

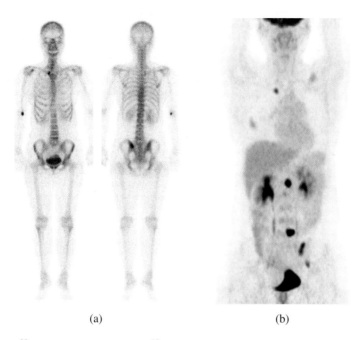

(a)   (b)

Fig. 12.7. ^{99m}Tc-MDP bone scan (a) and ^{18}F-FDG-PET (b) were performed at the same time. ^{18}F-FDG-PET shows spinal lesions which are occult in bone scan.

NaF-PET with FDG-PET in patients with breast cancer, NaF-PET can be sensitive for osteoblastic skeletal metastasis in patients with breast cancer. As the spine, which is structurally complex, is a common site of skeletal metastases in breast cancer patients, the tomographic images from SPECT and other fusion technologies are helpful for interpretation.

Monitoring after treatment is indicated for breast cancer, but bone scanning has many pitfalls for this indication. A bone scan might be insensitive. The increased bone turnover by the healing process and by persistent bony metastasis cannot be inherently differentiated. Therefore, a partial response to therapy may not be depicted on a bone scan, despite the evidence of clinical improvement and prolonged survival. This situation is called the "flare phenomenon," and it is most commonly encountered with breast and prostate cancer (Fig. 12.8). This is characterized by increased tracer uptake during the first few months after the initiation of treatment. Existing metastases show an increase of activity and the visual extent of tumor. Previously faint lesions become apparent and even previously undetected lesions might

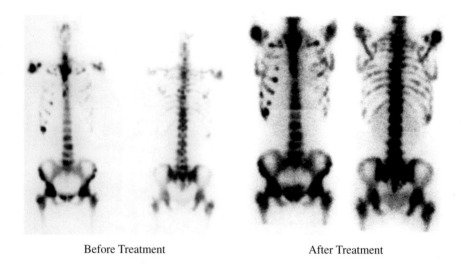

Before Treatment   After Treatment

Fig. 12.8. Flare phenomenon in breast cancer patient.

newly appear. A repeat bone scan performed after six months of treatment will demonstrate a gradual decrease in the degree of tracer uptake associated with the flare phenomenon.[20]

FDG-PET is also of value for assessing the response to treatment. The FDG accumulation on skeletal metastatic lesion mostly decreases after treatment in both osteolytic and osteoblastic lesion. After treatment, 81% of the osteolytic FDG-avid lesions became osteoblastic on CT and FDG-negative, suggesting the presence of a healing process.[21] This increased attenuation on CT and a decrease in the SUV of bone metastases after treatment were associated with a response to therapy.

12.5.1.2. *Lung cancer*

Skeletal metastatic disease from lung cancer is present in 20%–30% of patients at the time of the initial diagnosis.[22] Evaluation for metastases has conventionally been performed using MDP bone scan. Bone scan is useful to exclude patients who are potentially incurable by surgery and to prevent unnecessary surgery or neoadjuvant therapy. The new guidelines for non–small cell lung cancer mandates FDG-PET, which means that it has now largely replaced bone scan as a staging tool where it is available.

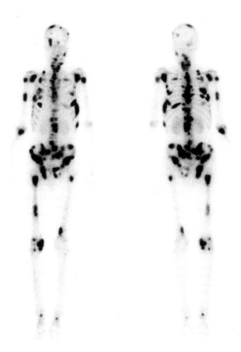

Fig. 12.9. Multiple skeletal metastases from lung cancer. Some appendigeal bony metastases are noticed.

Skeletal metastases from lung cancer are usually well visualized on a bone scan. Unlike other tumor, appendigeal metastases are not rare and there is also solitary appendigeal metastasis (Fig. 12.9). Usually, the metastatic site seems osteolytic and clinically aggressive. A planar bone scan alone has lower sensitivity for detecting osteolytic and vertebral column metastases.[23] The spine is the most commonly affected region in patients with lung cancer metastases. Vertebral metastases are especially liable to be undetected by a planar bone scan. Bone SPECT is advantageous for detecting lesions in complex structures, such as the spine, which would overlap on the planar images. Extension of an area of increased uptake from the vertebral body into the pedicle was found to be a useful sign for predicting malignancy.[24] Metastases virtually always begins within the vertebral body, so that lesions confined to the pedicle without involvement of the vertebral body proper are seldom malignant (this appearance is more commonly produced by fractures or osteoid osteoma).[25] Fractures may be presented as horizontal linear increased uptake within the vertebral body. MRI remains of particular value at this location for detecting a tumor extension to the intervertebral neural foramina and the spinal cord primarily because of its higher contrast resolution than CT. Bone SPECT and FDG-PET have been recently recommended for newly diagnosed lung cancer. Both are cost-effective and have improved accuracy. Bone SPECT and FDG-PET even change the clinical management in around 9% and 11% of the cases, respectively.[25]

FDG-PET may enable earlier detection of metastatic foci than a bone scan.[26] In a direct comparative study, the accuracy of PET and bone scanning for the detection of bony metastases in patients with newly diagnosed lung cancer were 94% and 85%, respectively, with sensitivity values of 91% and 75% and specificity values of 96% and 95%, respectively.[27] Few studies have addressed the role of NaF-PET in lung cancer. Despite insufficient data, NaF-PET was shown to be significantly more accurate than bone scanning for the evaluation of bone metastases in patients with lung cancer. It changes the management in 9.7% of the patients, albeit at a higher cost.[28] FDG-PET has high accuracy and convenience for whole body imaging, if it is clinically available. FDG-PET is likely to dominate the evaluation of skeletal metastases from lung carcinoma in the near future. NaF-PET/CT is likely to be more advantageous that bone scanning. Bone scanning may play a more minor role.

The vast majority of bony metastases from all types of lung carcinomas show a lytic pattern, and this usually makes them readily detectable on both the CT and PET. It has been noted that CT-positive but PET-negative lesions are significantly more prevalent after therapy.[16] These lesions may appear osteoblastic, which presumably reflects a reparative effect after treatment.

12.5.1.3. *Thyroid cancer*

Bone metastases from differentiated thyroid cancer (papillary and follicular carcinomas) occur in 2%–13% of the patients.[29] They are more frequent in patients with follicular carcinoma (7%–28%) as compared with that of patients with papillary carcinoma (1.4%–7%).[30] When bone metastases are present, the overall 10-year survival rate is around 13%–21%,[29] which compares with an overall 10-year survival rate of more than 80% for these cancers.

Metastatic lesions from these cancers are typically osteolytic, and a relatively high proportion of false-negative results occur on the bone scanning of patients with differentiated thyroid cancer.[31] A radioiodine whole-body scan (^{131}I or ^{123}I) is a more specific and sensitive technique than MDP but is only effective for well-differentiated thyroid tumors. The radioiodine whole-body scan shows bone metastases specifically, but simultaneously, many physiological or non-specific findings are also depicted and it lacks anatomical references. So the interpretation must be done cautiously. These may include ectopic foci of normal thyroid tissue, physiological uptake by the salivary glands or stomach, and by a variety of inflammatory and infectious processes in various organs. Sometimes there is unexplained uptake by the liver, breast, or thymus. SPECT/CT is helpful for equivocal foci.

Unlike differentiated thyroid cancer, less differentiated thyroid cancer frequently does not uptake radioiodine, which is quite common in the cases of multiple skeletal metastases. FDG-PET is likely to be valuable for cases with elevated thyroglobulin levels, and negative diagnostic or post-therapy radioiodine WBS.[32,33] Thyrotropin (TSH) stimulates thyroid metabolism, glucose transport, and glycolysis. Several studies have demonstrated that TSH stimulation improved the detection of occult thyroid metastases with FDG-PET, as compared with the scans performed with TSH suppression. The positron-emitting radioisotope [124]I, for instance, has shown promising results in one study in which PET with using this tracer detected more small bone metastases as compared with that of ^{131}I-WBS.[34]

12.5.1.4. *Renal cell cancer*

Up to 20% of patients with renal cell carcinoma have metastatic disease at presentation, of which 30%–40% of the cases involve the skeleton,[35] and up to 35% of all patients will develop bone metastases at some point during the course of their disease.[36] Bone metastases from renal cell carcinoma are typically expansile, osteolytic, and often highly vascular lesions that may give rise to severe bone pain and debilitating complications such as pathologic fractures and spinal cord compression. Most bone metastases are symptomatic, hence a bone scan is usually undertaken only when patients show suggestive symptoms.

Bone scanning has demonstrated a low yield of finding skeletal metastasis. Bone metastases show a variable, often low, degree of uptake on bone scanning owing to their osteolytic nature. The sensitivity of a bone scan is relatively low, varying from 10% to 60% and even among patients with a high probability of skeletal involvement.[37] Bone scanning also underestimated the extent of metastatic involvement. The most commonly affected sites are the pelvis and ribs (48% of patients in each case) and the vertebral column (42% of patients).[36] Unfortunately, these areas have some scintigraphic difficulty and the evaluation of bony uptake can be particularly challenging. Additional SPECT would be expected to significantly improve the diagnostic capability of bone scanning. A bone scan is also not capable of detecting an accompanying soft-tissue extension, which is relatively common in this disease and it is often neurologically significant. Correlation with the plain radiography is therefore helpful for the interpretation.

FDG-PET appears to offer improved accuracy for the detection of bone metastases as compared with that of bone scan. FDG-PET had good sensitivity (77.3%–100%) and accuracy (100%), compared with 77.5% and 59.6%, respectively, for bone scan and 93.8% and 87.2%, respectively, for combined CT and bone scan.[38,39] As bone metastasis in renal cell carcinoma is accompanied by non-osseous pathologies such as spinal cord compression, FDG PET/CT seems to be of value. Although little published data is available, combined NaF-PET/CT may well be an excellent means of evaluating for bony metastases of renal cell carcinoma.

12.5.1.5. *Multiple myeloma*

Multiple myeloma, in which monoclonal plasma cells proliferate, primarily involves the bone marrow and presents with multiple, well-defined, intramedullary osteolytic lesions. Bone scan may significantly underestimate the skeletal involvement, especially in newly diagnosed patients. Therefore, a main indication of bone scanning here is identification of pathologic fractures.

Another agent, which has a different mechanism of accumulation with a phosphate agent, has been tried in multiple myeloma. ^{99m}Tc-MIBI is a lipophilic radiotracer whose uptake appears to parallel the cellular mitochondrial activity[40] so that it is increased in neoplastic cells, including those of myeloma. The degree of ^{99m}Tc-MIBI uptake correlates with the extent of myelomatous involvement as well as the serologic markers of disease activity, such as lactate dehydrogenase, C-reactive protein and beta-2 microglobulin.[41] A negative ^{99m}Tc-MIBI scan has a high negative predictive value for excluding myeloma in patients with monoclonal gammopathy of an unknown significance. ^{11}C-methionine may be of value as this tracer reflects amino acid metabolism and transport, and protein synthesis.[42]

The clinical experience with FDG-PET for multiple myeloma is also insufficient. The FDG uptake for tumors with low proliferation is low and multiple myeloma shows variable degrees of FDG accumulation. FDG-PET may detect active foci of marrow involvement in patients with plasmacytoma, and this enables making a correct diagnosis of myeloma.[43] According to a recent study that compared FDG-PET/CT and MRI, the former performed better in detecting focal lesions throughout the body. MRI outperformed FDG-PET/CT for detecting more diffuse lesions.[44] FDG-PET/CT is likely to be most helpful in the further evaluation of ambiguous lytic lesions that are detected on a skeletal survey, and especially in the appendicular skeleton, and also for the investigation of suspected extramedullary disease. A consensus report from the Scientific Advisors of the International Myeloma Foundation suggests that whole-body FDG-PET imaging may be helpful for clarification of the disease classification or the prognostic categorization.[42]

12.5.1.6. *Prostate cancer*

Prostate cancer is one of the commonest cancers in men. Bone is the second most common site of metastatic disease after lymph nodes. Bone metastasis is related to a poor prognosis. The early detection of metastatic bone disease and the definition of its extent, pattern, and aggressiveness are crucial for proper staging and restaging; it is particularly important for patients with high-risk primary disease before initiating radical prostatectomy or radiation therapy.

The majority of bone metastases are osteoblastic and they appear sclerotic on X-ray. Because of the osteoblastic nature of the bone metastases, a bone scan is very sensitive for detecting bone metastasis from prostate cancer; the predilection of the bone metastases for the pelvis and lower spine is explained by the metastasis that occurs via the low-pressure paravertebral venous plexus.

Using the prostate specific antigen (PSA) level, the Gleason score, and the clinical stage, it is possible to estimate a patient's risk. This information can help decide which patients require a bone scan for staging and also for the interpretation of equivocal lesions. Although bone scanning has been routinely used for the evaluation of prostate cancer patients, bone metastasis is rare in the low risk patients. Although there is some uncertainty whether a PSA level of 10 or 20 ng/ml should be used as an upper threshold for performing a scan, a level less than 10 ng/ml is very rarely associated with bone metastases at presentation.[45] Bone scanning is also the preferred investigation in patients with suspected recurrent disease.

There is convincing evidence that FDG-PET is not useful for the evaluation of bone metastasis in prostate cancer patients because it is less sensitive than a bone scan, although there are some data to suggest that FDG-PET may be of value for assessing therapy in well-defined clinical groups. Because of the low uptake of FDG, other agents with different uptake mechanisms have been tried; cell membrane proliferation as assessed by radiolabeled phospholipids (^{11}C and ^{18}F choline), fatty acid synthesis (^{11}C acetate), amino acid transport and protein synthesis (^{11}C methionine), the androgen receptor expression (^{18}F-FDHT), and osteoblastic activity (^{18}F-fluoride). There is currently insufficient data for their clinical results.

12.5.2. *Primary bone tumors: Benign and malignant*

The role of bone scanning in diagnosing and managing primary malignant bone tumors has decreased, but a few specific clinical applications still remain.

Although the imaging features of primary bone tumor on a bone scan are not specific, it can be valuable when the plain radiographs have been unhelpful for localizing an abnormality. The predominant role of a bone scan for primary malignant bone tumors is to detect skeletal metastases. Although a bone scan cannot be relied on to detect soft-tissue metastases, some soft-tissue metastasis are occasionally seen, especially in patients with osteosarcoma. A three-phase bone scan may add information about the vascularity of a lesion.

Osteogenic tumors usually shows increased uptake on a bone scan. Benign osteogenic tumors (osteoma, osteoid osteoma, osteoblastoma) and malignant osteosarcoma all show hot uptake. The hot uptake itself is limitedly helpful for making the differential diagnosis. MDP highly accumulates in some cartilaginous tumors like growing osteochondroma, chondroblastoma and chondrosarcoma.

Among the fibrous tumors, fibrous dysplasia, malignant fibrous histiocytoma, and fibrosarcoma all show hot uptakes. Among them, fibrous dysplasia can be incidentally encountered on a bone scan. It is a developmental anomaly of bone formation and it presents as an expansile lytic medullary lesion. Its common location is the long bones, ribs, skull, and facial bones. In case of long bones, it involves the meta-diaphysis and spares the epiphysis. The monostotic form is more common than the polyostotic form.

Giant cell tumor is a locally aggressive neoplasm that is composed of osteoclast-like giant cells that involve the epiphyses in skeletally mature patients and it shows intense uptake around the periphery with little activity in the central portion (the "doughnut sign"). Aneurysmal bone cyst is an expansile lesion of bone and it contains of thin-walled blood filled cystic cavities. It represents a purely lytic reaction without a periosteal reaction and there are fluid-fluid levels. It is common in long tubular bones and usually presents with a deficit area on a bone scan. Intraosseous hemangioma is benign lesion composed of newly formed blood vessels with moderate uptake or photopenia on a bone scan. Enostosis (a bone island) does not accumulate agent on a bone scan.

In contrast to the restricted indications for bone scanning, a larger role is expected for FDG-PET/CT for imaging primary bone tumor. FDG-PET has been shown to be more accurate than a bone scan for detecting bone metastases in some tumor such as Ewing's sarcomas.[46,47] But the sensitivity of FDG-PET for staging primary bone tumors appears to vary between different types of tumor and the location of metastasis, and FDG-PET has limited sensitivity for detecting small pulmonary metastases compared with that of CT. Generally, it is assumed that FDG-PET has good specificity. However, it has been reported that some giant cell tumors and fibrous dysplasia may show uptake that's equivalent to osteosarcomas and that some other benign bone lesions may show high FDG accumulation.[48] A cautious approach is required when interpreting FDG-PET.

Although several studies have reported the ability of a bone scan to predict the histologic response to preoperative chemotherapy, the accuracy seems moderate and it is unlikely to be superior to that of contrast-enhanced MRI.[49] Several studies have reported that serial ^{18}F-FDG-PET assessment of osteosarcomas and Ewing's sarcomas is a good non-invasive method to predict the pathologic neoadjuvant chemotherapy response.[50,51] A high baseline uptake of FDG in osteosarcoma has been reported to show an inverse correlation with the prognostic indicators and it is associated with a poor outcome with similar results for the patients with high post-treatment FDG activity.[52]

12.5.3. *Metabolic bone diseases*

Metabolic bone disorders are heterogeneous and they have global or focal changes in bone metabolism. When metabolic bone disorders or their complications are associated with biochemical and microscopic changes, plain X-ray or anatomical imaging cannot detect the abnormalities. A bone scan is valuable with superior sensitivity for making the diagnosis, detecting complications, and monitoring the treatment response.

Osteoporosis is defined as a systemic skeletal disease that is characterized by increased bone turnover and the resultant low bone density and microarchitectural deterioration of bone tissue, with an increase in bone fragility and susceptibility to fractures. Despite these pathologies, the changes on a bone scan are not apparent because of the subtle symmetric changes over all the body's bones. So a MDP bone scan has no routine clinical role in the diagnosis of osteoporosis, but a bone scan is very sensitive for diagnosing unsuspected osteoporotic fractures at other sites, such as the ribs, pelvis, and hip, which are difficult to image with other imaging modalities. A bone scan is very useful for assessing the timing of fractures. This feature of a bone scan is essential for making the differential diagnosis of pain in the patients with multiple persistent fractures seen on plain X-rays. A bone scan can assess a culprit recent fracture among many old fractures or unsuspected abnormalities other than fractures such as diseased facet joints.

Paget's disease shows characteristic intense uptake on a bone scan (Fig. 12.10). Most patients with Paget's disease have polyostotic disease,

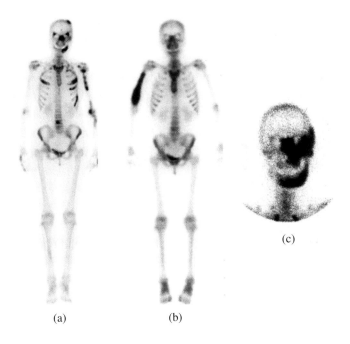

(c)

(a)　　　　　　(b)

Fig. 12.10.　Polyostotic Paget's disease (a) and monostotic Paget's diseases (b) and (c).

which is frequently involved in the pelvis, scapula, and vertebrae. The characteristic feature of Paget's disease is that it often involves the whole extent of the bone. For example, in case of vertebrae, hot uptakes involve the vertebral body and posterior elements, as well as the spinous and transverse processes. A bone scan may occasionally identify accompanying fractures. A bone scan is a convenient way to evaluate the whole skeleton and it has shown greater sensitivity for detecting the affected sites in symptomatic patients with Paget's disease, as compared with other imaging tools. A bone scan can be performed for monitoring the response after successful bisphosphonate treatment. In polyostotic patients, some bones may completely normalize, whereas a small proportion remains unchanged. Persistent active disease that is evident on a bone scan may be an indication for more aggressive therapy. A bone scan may add extra information to simply measuring the alkaline phosphatase levels alone. In patients with monostotic disease, and in whom the alkaline phosphatase levels are relatively normal,[53] a bone scan may be a more valuable method to monitor the treatment response.

A bone scan may also sensitively detect reactivation of Paget's disease after treatment. Some studies have tried quatitation methods with bone scan and NaF-PET to measure the treatment response, and the general finding was good correlation with the other biochemical and clinical markers of disease activity.[53]

Most cases of primary hyperparathyroidism are asymptomatic. In severe cases, there is increased skeletal turnover that is evident on a bone scan. The most important finding is the generalized diffuse increased uptake throughout the skeleton that may be identified because of the increased contrast between bone and soft tissues. This is commonly termed the metabolic superscan to differentiate it from superscans caused by widespread bone metastases. The imaging findings are often helpful to differentiate hypercalcemia due to hyperparathyroidism or widespread skeletal metastases. Other typical features include a prominent calvarium and mandible, beading of the costochondral junctions, and a "tie" sternum.[54] Severe forms of hyperparathyroidism may be associated with ectopic calcification, which can lead to uptake of bone radiopharmaceuticals in the soft tissue, such as microcalcification in the lungs. Associated brown tumors might uncommonly represent focal skeletal uptake.

Patients with osteomalacia usually demonstrate features on a bone scan that are similar to those described in hyperparathyroidism, although in the early stages of the disease the features may appear normal.[55] The tracer avidity may reflect diffuse uptake in the osteoid, although it is more likely due to the degree of secondary hyperparathyroidism that is present. The presence of focal lesions may represent pseudofractures or true fractures. Pseudofractures are characteristically found in the ribs, the scapula, the pubic rami, and the femori. The detection of pseudofracutures with bone scan is more sensitive than that with performing radiography.[56]

Renal osteodystrophy is caused by chronic renal dysfunction and often demonstrates the most severe cases of metabolic bone disease. It has complex features mixed with osteoporosis, osteomalacia, and secondary hyperparathyroidism. The most common bone scan appearance is diffuse homogenous skeletal uptake with little bladder activity. Bone scanning does not have diagnostic meaning for renal osteodystrophy and it has become rare because the frequency of untreated severe renal diseases has decreased.

12.5.4. *Trauma and sports injury*

The response to skeletal damage is characterized by hyperemia, formation of callus, and remodeling. The skeletal radiopharmaceuticals bind with high affinity, thus leading to avid uptake. Radiopharmaceuticals can accumulate in bone bruising and in acute trabecular microfractures that are without frank cortical disruption.[57] Bone scanning has extensive applications for diagnosis and monitoring of bony and soft-tissue trauma. Bone scanning is useful for both acute and sub-acute trauma. The focal uptake of fracture sites reflects the increased vascularity and bone formation of the healing process. Bone scanning has inherently high contrast-resolution, which enables the early detection of bone trauma. Such changes precede structural abnormalities, and therefore, they can be detected earlier than with using conventional radiology. This is detectable as early as 24 hours following fracture. As an injury heals, the accumulation of activity becomes less intense, and the uptake in 90% of fractures sites will have returned to normal by 2 years. A bone scan is not usually employed for the diagnosis of an arthropathy, although the pattern of uptake can help to characterize a disorder in some limited cases. Bone scanning has been used to a limited degree for the seronegative arthorpathies. For example, ankylosing spondylitis or Reiter' syndrome shows sacroiliac joint activity and focal uptake at the site of tendon insertion on a bone scan. As attached soft tissue injury combined with bone fracture is frequent, the acquisition of the three-phase bone scan images is mandatory. Tomographic technique and hybrid imaging makes the identification of the precise site of injury quite obvious. Hybrid imaging devices have allowed the coregistration of a high contrast resolution bone scan with the high spatial resolution of CT.

Occult fractures on plain radiography can be sensitively detected with a bone scan. The strengths of the bone scan are its sensitivity for detecting fracture and its potential to expose associated, but unsuspected, injuries or other diagnoses to explain the symptoms. Although MRI is superior for the anatomical resolution of the fracture site and sensitivity, a bone scan has similar high sensitivity and may be more readily available. The most commonly encountered clinical situation is an elderly patient with a suspected femoral neck fracture. Carpal bone fractures are also notorious for being radiographic occult fractures for some weeks after injury. Unexpected fractures in elderly female patients with osteoporosis or exposure to external bean radiation can be detected with a bone scan. In a woman with a history of cancer, occult fracture with associated periosteal soft-tissue reaction can mimic bone metastasis with soft tissue invasion. This is not uncommon in patients with uterine cervix cancer.

Stress fractures refer to fractures occurring in normal bone that has been subjected to repetitive or prolonged muscular action such as running. These are common in athletes. It is assumed that repeated stress can lead to periosteal resorption and weakening of the bone. Stress fractures can occur at many sites in the skeleton, but they are most common in the lower limb and particularly the tibia, and this may be bilateral. A bone scan has high sensitivity for these stress fractures and the bone scan image is typically abnormal one to two weeks in advance of the radiographic changes. Its sensitivity for this diagnosis approaches 100%.[58] Triple-phase bone scanning is useful for differentiating the spectrum of stress injury. Acute fractures demonstrate local increased MDP uptake on all phases, while injury involving only the soft tissues will be normal on the delayed phase. "Shin splits" is an interesting type of stress injury. Soft tissue disorder is present, but the blood flow and blood pool images are usually normal. However, the delayed images reveal characteristic longitudinally oriented linear areas of increased uptake of varying intensity that involve one-third or more of the posterior tibial cortex, thereby allowing differentiation from tibial stress fracture.[59]

Reflex sympathetic dystrophy is called by many pseudonyms, including algodystrophy, Sudek's atrophy, and complex regional pain syndrome. Reflex sympathetic dystrophy typically occurs in a limb that has been subjected to trauma, but sometimes no cause can be identified. It is characterized by a combination of intense pain, vasomotor disturbance, soft tissue swelling, and skin changes, but its definition is imprecise and this varies from specialty to specialty, with no gold standard for its diagnosis.[60] The bone scan appearances depend on the stage of the disease process, and the appearances are variable, reflecting the complex physiological changes inherent in this condition. The most suggestive pattern of uptake is increased activity on all phases of a triple-phase study, with diffuse uptake and periarticular accumulation on the delayed phase. However, during the late stages of the disease, decreased uptake may be the case in the early phases of the scan. Comparison with the normal side is obviously crucial.

12.5.5. *Inflammation and infection of the skeletal system*

12.5.5.1. *Osteomyelitis*

Childhood osteomyelitis is most commonly caused by hematogenous spread, whereas the organism spreads contiguously and it is inoculated directly in adults. The risk of osteomyelitis from soft tissue infection is high in diabetics, with neuropathic ulceration of the feet and bedridden patients with dependent ulceration. Direct inoculation may be possible due to penetrating injury and as a complication of surgery. Although a plain radiograph is the initial investigation, it cannot discern abnormality for up to three weeks from the time of infection. Although an MDP bone scan is used as a complementary imaging procedure for the evaluation of osteomyelitis, it can diagnose osteomyelitis more sensitively and at an earlier stage. In a diabetic patient, a bone scan is routinely used for the evaluation for osteomyelitis.

Three-phase bone scanning has been reported to have an accuracy of over 90%.[61] The classic appearance of osteomyelitis on three-phase bone scans is localized increased uptake on all phases, which consists of focal hyperperfusion, focal hyperemia, and more focally increased and intense delayed bone uptake (Fig. 12.11). A three-phase bone scan is sensitive for infection, and particularly in the absence of a pre-existing bony abnormality. Unfortunately, fractures, tumors, and joint neuropathy, which are the underlying conditions of osteomyelitis, may also mimic osteomyelitis on a three-phase bone scan, and so this reduces the specificity of the technique.

Labeled WBC imaging is reported to be more sensitive and specific for diagnosing pedal osteomyelitis than that of a bone scan alone.[62]

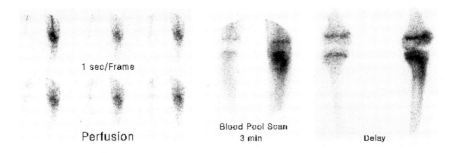

1 sec/Frame

Perfusion

Blood Pool Scan
3 min

Delay

Fig. 12.11.   Three-phase bone scan of acute osteomyelitis.

[99m]Tc-Hexamethylpropyleneamine oxime (HMPAO)-WBC is generally more sensitive for the detection of acute osteomyelitis than for detecting chronic osteomyelitis, which is supposedly due to the enhanced influx of leukocytes in acute osteomyelitis. However, ^{111}In-WBC is preferred for imaging chronic osteomyelitis and low-grade infection as performing 24-h imaging with this technique is feasible. But false-positive WBC scan results are probably attributable to inflammation and hematopoietically active bone marrow. A WBC scan shows the best results when it combines with other skeletal imaging; combined ^{111}In-WBC and ^{99m}Tc-MDP SPECT/CT showed high sensitivity and specificity for ostemyelitis. The diagnosis of spinal osteomyelitis has low sensitivity despite the use of ^{111}In-WBC or ^{99m}Tc-WBC.

12.5.5.2. *Osteomyelitis in patients with diabetes*

A WBC scan can be very useful in diabetic neuropathic joints, which mimic osteomyelitis both clinically and radiologically, but this WBC scan often requires being combined with a bone scan for accurate anatomical localization of abnormalities. However, labeled WBCs also accumulate in normal marrow and the distribution of which is highly variable, and particularly in the presence of systemic disease. This can lead to a false-positive interpretation. The addition of marrow imaging such as ^{99m}Tc-sulfur colloid can identify the location of marrow and detect the lesions of WBC accumulation with the absence of marrow activity, which can be assumed to represent infection. This combined technique has a reported accuracy of over 90%.[61]

It is not clear whether FDG-PET/CT can detect osteomyelitis in the patients with diabetic foot ulcers. Some studies have reported that FDG-PET/CT has a high negative predictive value, whereas another has reported the very low sensitivity of FDG-PET.[63,64] Although FDG-PET and SPECT/CT technology might be feasible and helpful, the reports have been very heterogeneous in their methodology and they all had a small number of subjects.

12.5.5.3. *Orthopedic implant infections*

Differentiation between infection and aseptic loosening of a joint prosthesis is extremely important. On a bone scan, focally increased radionuclide uptake around the prosthesis such as at the tip of the femoral prosthesis is commonly considered to represent loosening, while diffusely increased uptake in the blood pool and on the delayed phase is commonly considered to represent infection.[61]

However, infection may also be present in the prostheses with focal uptake patterns. Without infection or loosening, there is normally increased MDP uptake around the prosthetic components for many months following hip replacement, so a bone scan within 12 months of an arthroplasty procedure may be of limited value in ruling out loosening and infection due to the existing inflammatory changes following surgery.[65] Hip and knee replacements can be cemented or cementless. The phenomenon is even more pronounced with the more recent cementless prostheses, which also cause increased accumulation of white cells.[66] In patients with a cementless hip prosthesis, the persistent uptake is more prevalent beyond 1-year after replacement.[67] The type and location of the prosthesis and the amount of time that elapsed between implantation and imaging must be taken into account during interpretation. While a normal bone scan is therefore very useful, positive findings require that they be taken in context with other features.

Radiolabeled WBC scan is generally good for diagnosing infection in a prosthesis. Implantation of a prosthesis may alter the bone marrow distribution at the site of intervention. However, the inability to distinguish radiolabeled WBC uptake in infection from uptake in the bone marrow is a problem. This issue can be overcome by performing additional bone marrow imaging. Both radiolabeled WBCs and bone marrow agent such as ^{99m}Tc-sulfur colloid accumulate in the bone marrow, whereas only WBCs accumulate in infection. The reported sensitivity, specificity, and accuracy using both imaging modalities are 96%, 97%, and 97%, respectively.[68] An alternative combination of a WBC scan and a ^{67}Ga-citrate scan could be considered. More intense ^{67}Ga uptake is seen in infection, but a ^{67}Ga-citrate scan does not seem to be superior to the others types of scans.

It is still a matter of debate whether satisfactory diagnostic accuracy for diagnosing infection can be obtained with FDG-PET in patients with metallic implants. FDG-PET has shown contradictory results in the studies that consisted of patients with knee and hip prostheses. FDG accumulation at the bone–prosthesis interface, except the head and the tip, represents infection. Although a trade-off of sensitivity and specificity was observed, in general, FDG-PET is highly sensitive with insufficient specificity. If we combine a bone scan and FDG-PET for the interpretation or use fusion technology, the specificity is increased without the loss of sensitivity. In spite of these efforts, combined ^{111}In WBC and ^{99m}Tc-sulfur colloid SPECT/CT seems to be significantly better than FDG-PET.[69]

References

1. Schirrmeister H. (2007) Detection of bone metastases in breast cancer by positron emission tomography. *Radiol Clin North Am* **45**: 669–676.
2. Kubota R, Yamada S, Kubota K, *et al.* (1992) Intratumoral distribution of fluorine-18-fluorodeoxyglucose *in vivo*: High accumulation in macrophages and granulation tissues studied by microautoradiography. *J Nucl Med* **33**: 1972–1980.
3. Kubota R, Kubota K, Yamada S, *et al.* (1994) Microautoradiographic study for the differentiation of intratumoral macrophages, granulation tissues and cancer cells by the dynamics of fluorine-18-fluorodeoxyglucose uptake. *J Nucl Med* **35**: 104–112.
4. Gratz S, Dorner J, Fischer U, *et al.* (2002) 18F-FDG hybrid PET in patients with suspected spondylitis. *Eur J Nucl Med Mol Imaging* **29**: 516–524.
5. Peters AM. (1994) The utility of [99mTc]HMPAO-leukocytes for imaging infection. *Semin Nucl Med* **24**: 110–127.
6. Krasnow AZ, Hellman RS, Timins ME, *et al.* (1997) Diagnostic bone scanning in oncology. *Semin Nucl Med* **27**: 107–141.
7. Tumeh SS, Beadle G, Kaplan WD. (1985) Clinical significance of solitary rib lesions in patients with extraskeletal malignancy. *J Nucl Med* **26**: 1140–1143.
8. Coakley FV, Jones AR, Finlay DB, Belton IP. (1995) The aetiology and distinguishing features of solitary spinal hot spots on planar bone scans. *Clin Radiol* **50**: 327–330.
9. Coleman RE, Rubens RD. (1987) The clinical course of bone metastases from breast cancer. *Br J Cancer* **55**: 61–66.
10. Hamaoka T, Madewell JE, Podoloff DA, *et al.* (2005) Bone imaging in metastatic breast cancer. *J Clin Oncol* **22**: 2924–2953.
11. Coleman RE, Rubens RD, Fogelman I. (1988) Reappraisal of the baseline bone scan in breast cancer. *J Nucl Med* **29**: 1045–1049.
12. Yeh KA, Fortunato L, Ridge JA, *et al.* (1995) Routine bone scanning in patients with T1 and T2 breast cancer: A waste of money. *Ann Surg Oncol* **2**: 319–324.
13. Ohta M, Tokuda Y, Suzuki Y, *et al.* (2001) Whole body PET for the evaluation of bony metastases in patients with breast cancer: Comparison with 99mTc-MDP bone scan. *Nucl Med Commun* **22**: 875–879.
14. Yang SN, Liang JA, Lin FJ, *et al.* (2002) Comparing whole body 18F-2-deoxyglucose positron emission tomography and technetium-99m methylene diphosphonate bone scan to detect bone metastases in patients with breast cancer. *J Cancer Res Clin Oncol* **128**: 325–328.

15. Gallowitsch H-J, Kresnik E, Gasser J, *et al*. (2003) F-18 fluorodeoxyglucose positron-emission tomography in the diagnosis of tumor recurrence and metastases in the follow-up of patients with breast carcinoma. A comparison to conventional imaging. *Invest Radiol* **38**: 250–256.

16. Uematsu T, Yuen S, Yukisawa S, *et al*. (2005) Comparison of FDG PET and SPECT for detection of bone metastases in breast cancer. *Am J Roentgenol* **184**: 1266–1272.

17. Nakai T, Okuyama C, Kubota T, *et al*. (2005) Pitfalls of FDG-PET for the diagnosis of osteoblastic skeletal metastases in patients with breast cancer. *Eur J Nucl Med Mol Imaging* **32**: 1253–1258.

18. Fogelman I, Cook G, Israel O, *et al*. (2005) Positron emission tomography and bone metastases. *Semin Nucl Med* **35**: 135–142.

19. Du Y, Cullum I, Illidge TM, *et al*. (2007) Fusion of metabolic function and morphology: Sequential [18F] fluorodeoxyglucose positron-emission tomography/computed tomography studies yield new insights into the natural history of skeletal metastases in breast cancer. *J Clin Oncol* **25**: 3440–3447.

20. Vogel CL, Schoenfelder J, Shemano I, *et al*. (1995) Worsening bone scan in the evaluation of antitumor response during hormonal therapy of breast cancer. *J Clin Oncol* **13**: 1123–1128.

21. Stafford SE, Gralow JR, Schubert EK, *et al*. (2002) Use of serial FDG PET to measure the response of bone-dominant breast cancer to therapy. *Acad Radiol* **9**: 913–921.

22. Schirrmeister H, Glatting G, Hetzel J, *et al*. (2001) Prospective evaluation of the clinical value of planar bone scans, SPECT, and (18)F-labeled NaF PET in newly diagnosed lung cancer. *J Nucl Med* **42**: 1800–1804.

23. Schirrmeister H, Guhlmann A, Elsner K, *et al*. (1999) Sensitivity in detecting osseous lesions depends on anatomic localization: Planar bone scan versus 18F PET. *J Nucl Med* **40**: 1623–1629.

24. Savelli G, Maffioli L, Maccauro M, *et al*. (2001) Bone scan and the added value of SPECT (single photon emission tomography) in detecting skeletal lesions. *J Nucl Med* **45**: 27–37.

25. De Maeseneer M, Lenchik L, Everaert H, *et al*. (1999) Evaluation of lower back pain with bone scan and SPECT. *Radiographics* **19**: 901–912.

26. Peterson JJ, Kransdorf MJ, O'Connor MI. (2003) Diagnosis of occult bone metastases: Positron emission tomography. *Clin Orthop Relat Res* **415**(suppl): S120–S128.

27. Cheran SK, Herndon JE, Patz EF. (2004) Comparison of whole-body FDGPET to bone scan for detection of bone metastases in patients with a new diagnosis of lung cancer. *Lung Cancer* **44**: 317–325.

28. Hetzel M, Arslandemir C, Konig H-H, *et al*. (2003) F-18 NaF PET for detection of bone metastases in lung cancer: Accuracy, cost-effectiveness, and impact on patient management. *J Bone Miner Res* **18**: 2206–2214.

29. Muresan MM, Olivier P, Leclere J, *et al*. (2008) Bone metastases from differentiated thyroid carcinoma. *Endocr Relat Cancer* **15**: 37–49.

30. Tickoo SK, Pittas AG, Adler M, *et al*. (2000) Bone metastases from thyroid carcinoma: A histopathologic study with clinical correlates. *Arch Pathol Lab Med* **124**: 1440–1447.

31. Ito S, Kato K, Ikeda M, *et al*. (2007) Comparison of 18F-FDG PET and bone scan in detection of bone metastases of thyroid cancer. *J Nucl Med* **48**: 889–895.

32. Grunwald F, Menzel C, Bender H, *et al*. (1997) Comparison of 18FDG-PET with 131iodine and 99mTc-sestamibi scan in differentiated thyroid cancer. *Thyroidology* **7**: 327–335.

33. Schluter B, Bohuslavizki KH, Beyer W, *et al*. (2001) Impact of FDG PET on patients with differentiated thyroid cancer who present with elevated thyroglobulin and negative 131I scan. *J Nucl Med* **42**: 71–76.

34. Freudenberg LS, Antoch G, Jentzen W, *et al*. (2004) Value of (124)I-PET/CT in staging of patients with differentiated thyroid cancer. *Eur Radiol* **14**: 2092–2098.

35. Kollender Y, Bickels J, Price WM, *et al*. (2000) Metastatic renal cell carcinoma of bone: Indications and technique of surgical intervention. *J Urol* **164**: 1505–1508.

36. Zekri J, Ahmed N, Coleman RE, *et al*. (2001) The skeletal metastatic complications of renal cell carcinoma. *Int J Oncol* **19**: 379–382.

37. Staudenherz A, Steiner B, Puig S, *et al*. (1999) Is there a diagnostic role for bone scanning of patients with a high pretest probability for metastatic renal cell carcinoma? *Cancer* **85**: 153–155.

38. Wu HC, Yen RF, Shen YY, *et al*. (2002) Comparing whole body 18F-2-deoxyglucose positron emission tomography and technetium-99m methylene diphosphate bone scan to detect bone metastases in patients with renal cell carcinomas — A preliminary report. *J Cancer Res Clin Oncol* **128**: 503–506.

39. Kang DE, White RL, Zuger JH, *et al*. (2004) Clinical use of fluorodeoxyglucose F 18 positron emission tomography for detection of renal cell carcinoma. *J Urol* **171**: 1806–1809.

40. Chiu ML, Kronauge JF, Piwnica-Worms D. (1990) Effect of mitochondrial and plasma membrane potentials on accumulation of hexakis (2-methoxyisobutylisonitrile) technetium(I) in cultured mouse fibroblasts. *J Nucl Med* **31**: 1646–1653.

41. Alexandrakis MG, Kyriakou DS, Passam FH, *et al*. (2002) Correlation between the uptake of Tc99m-sestamibi and prognostic factors in patients with multiple myeloma. *Clin Lab Hematol* **24**: 155–159.

42. Durie BGM, Kyle RA, Belch A, *et al*. (2003) Myeloma management guidelines: A consensus report from the scientific advisors of the International Myeloma Foundation. *Hematol J* **4**: 379–398.

43. Kato T, Tsukamoto E, Nishioka T, *et al*. (2000) Early detection of bone marrow involvement in extramedullary plasmacytoma by whole-body F-18 FDG positron emission tomography. *Clin Nucl Med* **25**: 870–873.

44. Fonti R, Salvatore B, Quarantelli M, *et al*. (2008) 18F-FDG PET/CT, 99mTc-MIBI, and MRI in evaluation of patients with multiple myeloma. *J Nucl Med* **49**: 195–200.

45. Lee N, Fawaaz R, Olsson CA, Benson MC, Benson MC, Petrylak DP, Schiff PB, Bagiella E, Singh A, Ennis RD. (2000) Which patients with newly diagnosed prostate cancer need a radionuclide bone scan? An analysis based on 631 patients. *Int J Radiat Oncol Biol Phys* **48**: 1443–1446.

46. Franzius C, Sciuk J, Daldrup-Link HE, *et al*. (2000) FDG-PET for detection of osseous metastases from malignant primary bone tumours: Comparison with bone scan. *Eur J Nucl Med* **27**: 1305–1311.

47. Györke T, Zajic T, Lange A, *et al*. (2006) Impact of FDG PET for staging of Ewing sarcomas and primitive neuroectodermal tumours. *Nucl Med Commun* **27**: 17–24.

48. Aoki J, Watanabe H, Shinozaki T, *et al.* (2001) FDG PET of primary benign and malignant bone tumors: Standardized uptake value in 52 lesions. *Radiology* **219**: 774–777.

49. Erlemann R, Sciuk J, Bosse A, *et al.* (1990) Response of osteosarcoma and Ewing's sarcoma to preoperative chemotherapy: Assessment with dynamic and static MR imaging and skeletal scan. *Radiology* **175**: 791–796.

50. Schulte M, Brecht-Krauss D, Werner M, *et al.* (1999) Evaluation of neoadjuvant therapy response of osteogenic sarcoma using FDG PET. *J Nucl Med* **40**: 1637–1643.

51. Hawkins DS, Schuetze SM, Butrynski JE, *et al.* (2005) [18F]Fluorodeoxyglucose positron emission tomography predicts outcome for Ewing sarcoma family of tumors. *J Clin Oncol* **23**: 8828–8834.

52. Franzius C, Bielack S, Flege S, *et al.* (2002) Prognostic significance of (18)FFDG and (99m)Tc-methylene diphosphonate uptake in primary osteosarcoma. *J Nucl Med* **43**: 1012–1017.

53. Patel S, Pearson D, Hosking DJ. (1995) Quantitative bone scan in the management of monostotic Paget's disease of bone. *Arthritis Rheum* **38**: 1506–1512.

54. Fogelman I, Carr D. (1980) A comparison of bone scanning and radiology in the evaluation of patients with metabolic bone disease. *Clin Radiol* **31**: 321–326.

55. Fogelman I, McKillop JH, Bessent RG, *et al.* (1978) The role of bone scanning in osteomalacia. *J Nucl Med* **19**: 245–248.

56. Fogelman I, McKillop JH, Greig WR, *et al.* (1977) Pseudofractures of the ribs detected by bone scanning. *J Nucl Med* **18**: 1236–1237.

57. Mink JH, Deutsch AL. (1989) Occult cartilage and bone injuries of the knee: Detection, classification and assessment with MR imaging. *Radiology* **170**: 823–829.

58. Drubach LA, Connolly LP, D'Hemecourt PA, Treves ST. (2001) Assessment of the clinical significance of asymptomatic lower extremity uptake abnormality in young athletes. *J Nucl Med* **42**: 209–212.

59. Love C, Din AS, Tomas MB, Kalapparambath TP, Palestro CJ. (2003) Radionuclide bone imaging: An illustrative review. *Radiographics* **23**: 341–358.

60. Fournier RS, Holder LE. (1998) Reflex sympathetic dystrophy: Diagnostic controversies. *Semin Nucl Med* **28**: 116–123.

61. Palestro CJ, Torres MA. (1997) Radionuclide imaging in orthopedic infections. *Semin Nucl Med* **27**: 334–345.

62. Palestro CJ. (1994) Musculoskeletal infection. In: Freeman LM (ed) *Nuclear Medicine Annual.* pp. 91–119, Raven Press, New York.

63. Basu S, Chryssikos T, Houseni M, *et al.* (2007) Potential role of FDG PET in the setting of diabetic neuro-osteoarthropathy: Can it differentiate uncomplicated Charcot's neuroarthropathy from osteomyelitis and soft-tissue infection? *Nucl Med Commun* **28**: 465–472.

64. Schwegler B, Stumpe KD, Weishaupt D, *et al.* (2008) Unsuspected osteomyelitis is frequent in persistent diabetic foot ulcer and better diagnosed by MRI than by 18F-FDG PET or 99mTc-MOAB. *J Intern Med* **263**: 99–106.

65. Stumpe KDM, Nötzli HP, Zanetti M, Kamel EM, Hany TF, Gorres GW, von Schulthess GK, Hodler J. (2004) FDG PET for differentiation of infection and aseptic loosening in total hip replacements: Comparison with conventional radiography and three-phase bone scan. *Radiology* **231**: 333–341.

66. Turpin S, Lambert R. (2001) Role of scan inmusculoskeletal and spinal infections. *Radiol Clin North Am* **39**: 169–189.

67. Oswald SG, Van Nostrand D, Savory CG, Anderson JH, Callaghan JJ. (1989) Three-phase bone scan and indium white cell scan following porous coated hip arthroplasty: A prospective study of the prosthetic tip. *J Nucl Med* **30**: 1321–1331.

68. Palestro CJ, Kim CK, Swyer AJ, Capozzi JD, SolomonRW, Goldsmith SJ. (1990) Total-hip arthroplasty: Periprosthetic indium-111-labelled leukocyte activity and complementary technetium-99-m sulfur colloid imaging in suspected infection. *J Nucl Med* **31**: 1950–1955.

69. Love C, Marwin SE, Tomas MB, *et al.* (2004) Diagnosing infection in the failed joint replacement: A comparison of coincidence detection 18F-FDG and 111In-labeled leukocyte/99mTc-sulfur colloid marrow imaging. *J Nucl Med* **45**: 1864–1871.

Chapter 13

Lymphoscintigraphy and Nuclear Venography

E. Edmund Kim and Franklin Wong

Lymphatic drainage can be identified by the subcutaneous injection of small colloidal particles of size between 10 and 1,000 nm. This procedure is often utilized to locate the obstruction site of lymphatic drainage in patients with lymphedema. A series of static images up to 3 h of arm or leg are obtained after subcutaneous injection of 1 mCi of Tc-99m filtered sulfur colloid or nanocolloid in the web spaces between fingers or toes (Figs. 13.1–13.4).

More recently lymphoscintigraphy has been used for the identification of the first regional draining node from a metastasizing tumor (sentinel lymph node) (Fig. 13.1). This has made a dramatic effect on the management of patients with breast cancer and melanoma since it has become a valuable alternative to complete axillary lymph node dissection in patients with multifocal breast cancer.[1] Once identified and excised, the node may then be examined histologically for the presence of tumor cells. Positive identification of tumor within the sentinel node indicates a metastasis.

The technique usually involves peritumoral, sub-areolar, or peri- areolar interstitial injection of 0.5 mCi (on the day of surgery) or 2.5 mCi (in case of surgery on next day) of Tc-99m filtered sulfur colloid or nanocolloid in 2 ml (peri or subareolar injection, case of breast implant, injection around localizing needle tip) or 5 ml (peritumoral injection) saline. The draining node may be identified by dynamic imaging or by a series of static images for 3 h following injection. A body outline by transmission imaging using Tc-99m or Co-57 flood source is helpful to demonstrate the direction of lymphatic drainage. However, sing;e-photon emission computed tomography

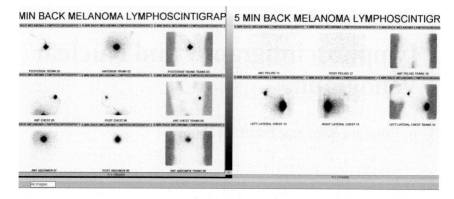

Fig. 13.1. Intradermal injection of 0.5 mCi Tc-99m sulfur colloid around the melanoma in the mid-back shows lymphatic vessel as well as focal activity drained into left inferior (level I) axillary lymph node.

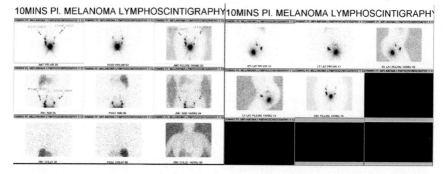

Fig. 13.2. Subcutaneous injection of 0.5 mCi Tc-99m sulfur colloid around the vulvar carcinoma shows activities drained into bilateral external iliac lymph nodes.

(SPECT)/CT is needed to localize the sentinel lymphnode precisely. Inferior (level I) axillary node is lateral to pectoralis minor muscle, mid (level II) is posterior or between pectoralis minor muscle, and superior (level III) is medial to pectoralis minor muscle. Inguinal node is below inferior epigastric vessel, and external iliac node is above inferior epigastric vessel (Fig. 13.3).

Surgical removal of sentinel node may be aided by use of an intraoperative sterile surgical probe (Geiger counter). During surgery, the surgeon can use the probe to localize the increased count rate from accumulation of the tracer in the node, which will point the site for surgical excision.

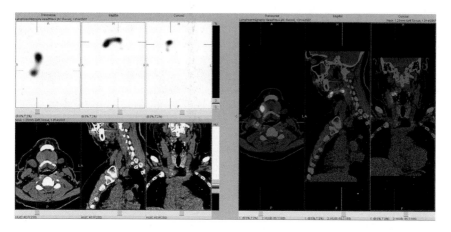

Fig. 13.3. SPECT/CT of the neck after intradermal injection of 0.5 mCi Tc-99m sulfur colloid around the melanoma in right cheek shows activities drained into right sublingual and right upper jugular lymph nodes.

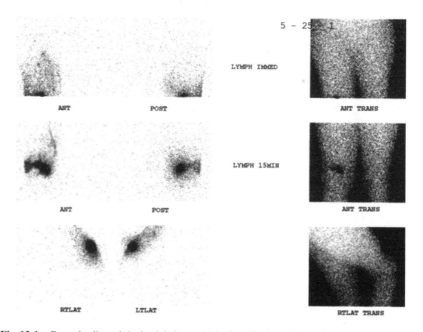

Fig. 13.4. Dermal collaterals in the right lower thigh after injection of 0.5 mCi Tc-99m sulfur colloid, suggesting lymphatic obstruction.

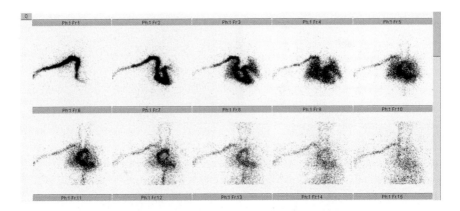

Fig. 13.5. Normal venogram of right upper extremity with Tc-99m DTPA injection.

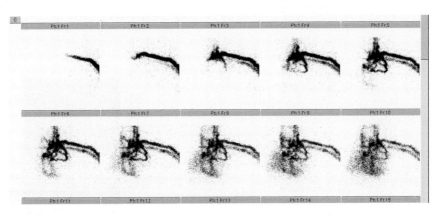

Fig. 13.6. Complete obstruction of left subclavian vein with collaterals. There is no visualization of left innominate vein.

Radionuclide venography (Figs. 13.5–13.7) has been used to evaluate a venous thrombosis, and its correlation with contrast venography ranges from 84% to 99%. Multiple factors for the discrepancy between two studies include variable age and size of the thrombus, presence of varicose vein, and large venous valve. The basic technique of the radionuclide leg venography involves the injection of 2–2.5 mCi Tc-99m MAA particles into the each dorsal foot vein with the tourniquet applied at the ankle to facilitate the deep venous system. After the tourniquets are removed, the superficial venous systems are evaluated by the sequential imaging of lower leg, thigh,

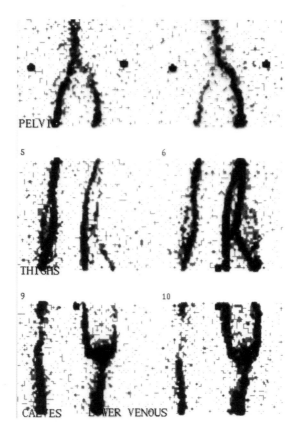

Fig. 13.7. Complete obstruction of left calf and popliteal veins with superficial saphenous vein. No femoral vein is noted.

and pelvis (Fig. 13.7). Delayed static images are obtained to search for local retention of the activity to suggest a blood clot. Both mechanical trapping and electrostatic forces are responsible for the adherence of the particles to the clot. This study is technically easier to perform, and a baseline lung scan is also provided without additional agent or radiation exposure. Duplex ultrasound has replaced conventional contrast venography. However, ultrasound has limited sensitivity for asymptomatic thrombosis and may be positive in as few as one-third of cases where pulmonary emboli have been confirmed. Radionuclide venography of upper extremity is performed by injecting 2 mCi Tc-99m DTPA or sulfur colloid into each antecubital vein (first on the side of suspected thrombosis). Sequential dynamic images show

331

a significant stasis or collateral channel with venous obstruction (Fig. 13.6). Additional injection of 1 mCi Tc-99m MAA or sulfur colloid is often used to evaluate the patency of central venous catheter.

The specific detection of thrombosis is the measurement of radiolabled fibrinogen incorporated into forming thrombi. Another method uses ^{111}In-labeled autologous platelets. Organized thrombi do not sequester circulating platelets. However, those agents are not easily available for clinical practice.

Reference

1. Goyal A, Newcombe RG, Mansel RE, *et al.* (2004) ALMANIC trials group. *Euro J Surg Oncol* **30**: 475–479.

Chapter 14
Infection and Inflammation Imaging

So-Won Oh, Ukihide Tateishi, Yu-Kyeong Kim,
Jin-Chul Paeng and E. Edmund Kim

14.1. Introduction

Nuclear medicine imaging provides physiological information on infection and inflammation which may be sometimes missed by conventional anatomical imaging modalities such as ultrasonography, computed tomography, or magnetic resonance imaging. In this regard, nuclear medicine imaging could be useful in the diagnosis of infection and inflammation, assessment of inflammation activity, evaluation of treatment response, etc. Especially in the diagnosis of fever of unknown origin (FUO), the utilization of whole-body image in nuclear medicine is advantageous to find a fever focus.

According to the purpose of imaging and patient's condition, sophisticated considerations are needed to choose radiopharmaceuticals for infection and inflammation imaging. For example, radiopharmaceuticals accumulating in various fever foci, including inflammation as well as tumor, are recommended for diagnosis of FUO. To diagnose infectious osteomyelitis or abscess, it is better to choose radiopharmaceuticals specific to bacterial infection rather than non-specific radiopharmaceuticals. In addition, it is very important that radiopharmaceuticals are taken up in proportion to the activity of infection or inflammation.

The development of new imaging instruments has brought about new possibilities in medicine. Conventional radiopharmaceuticals such as ^{111}In, ^{99m}Tc-labeled leukocytes, and ^{67}Ga have been used in infection and inflammation imaging. As positron emission tomography (PET) or PET in combination with computed tomography (CT) has widely been used in a variety of institutions, FDG emerged as a new radiopharmaceutical for the infection and inflammation imaging. Recently, the introduction of single-photon emission computed tomography (SPECT)/CT is expected to increase diagnostic credibility by adding precise anatomical information to the conventional gamma camera imaging and to promote the development of new radiopharmaceuticals based on the pathophysiology of infection and inflammation.

14.2. Pathophysiology of Infection and Inflammation

Inflammation, a biological response to various harmful stimuli such as microorganism infection or tissue injuries, is a very complicated systematic reaction, including vascular response, migration, and activation of leukocytes. Inflammation can be classified as either acute or chronic according to the underlying pathophysiological mechanisms and time course. Vascular reactions and cellular reactions are two major factors playing a key role in inflammation.

Vascular reaction of inflammation in consequence brings circulating serum proteins and leukocytes to inflammatory sites. First, vascular dilation mediated mainly by histamine and nitrous oxide occurs, and increase in microvascular permeability follows. As a result, serum proteins and water escape into the extravascular space, which leads to increase in blood viscosity and stasis of blood flow. These series of reaction allow leukocytes aggregate and adhere to the vascular endothelial cells, and then permit migration of leukocytes into the interstitial space.

Cellular reaction of inflammation consists of leukocyte migration, accumulation, and activation. Migrated leukocytes are rolling through interaction with the vascular endothelial cell surface. After binding to the endothelium, leukocytes are able to migrate across the endothelium and are then recruited to the inflammatory sites via chemotaxis.

14.3. Targeting Strategies for Infection and Inflammation Imaging

14.3.1. *Increase in vascular permeability*

Vascular permeability increases in the early phase of inflammation, which is a major target for the infection and inflammation imaging. This process is generally targeted by non-specific radiopharmaceuticals but it is also a basic mechanism used by specific radiopharmaceuticals accumulating in the inflammatory sites. Radiolabeled human immunoglobulin (HIG), a non-specific antibody, accumulates in the inflammatory sites mainly by increasing vascular permeability but also partly by binding with bacteria or inflammatory cells.

14.3.2. *Endothelial activation*

Matrix proteins are presented on the vascular endothelial cells to bind with leukocytes during inflammation, which could be used as a target for the infection and inflammation imaging. E-selectin, which is presented during the rolling process or binding matrix such as ICAM-1 that makes stable binding to integrins, are representative proteins as the target for the infection and inflammation imaging. F(ab')$_2$ antibodies to anti-E-selectin or anti-IACAM-1 labeled with ^{111}In or ^{99m}Tc have been reported to show high diagnostic results.

14.3.3. *Leukocyte accumulation*

Many radiopharmaceuticals accumulate in inflammatory sites by means of leukocyte activation. Autologous leukocytes labeled with ^{99m}Tc or ^{111}In are recruited to the inflammatory sites via chemotaxis without any difference to other non-radiolabeled leukocytes. ^{67}Ga moves to the inflammatory sites after binding with serum transferrin, and then binds with transferrin receptor (CD71) of leukocytes or lactoferrin secreted from the leukocytes. FDG uptake in the inflammatory sites increases through accumulation of leukocytes as well as increase in glycolytic activity of activated leukocytes. On the other hand, FDG-labeled leukocytes have also been reported to be useful in the infection and inflammation imaging.

14.3.4. *Microorganisms*

In infectious inflammation sites, microorganisms or its metabolites could be a target for the imaging. ^{99m}Tc-cyprofloxacin, a representative radiopharmaceutical directly targeted at microorganisms, is expected to be specific to bacterial infection because ciprofloxacin is a quinolone antibiotic inhibiting bacterial proliferation by binding with bacterial DNA gyrase. Microorganism activity also plays a role in ^{67}Ga scan; ^{67}Ga binds to siderophores of bacteria.

14.4. Radiopharmaceuticals

14.4.1. *Radiolabeled leukocytes*

In radiolabeled leukocyte imaging, ^{111}In and ^{99m}Tc-HMPAO are generally used. ^{111}In-leukocyte images are obtained at 30 min, 4 h, 18 ~ 24 h, respectively, after intravenous administration of 18.5~37 MBq. Among these images, images acquired at 18 ~ 24 h are mostly important and highly sensitive. ^{111}In labeling is advantageous to make a highly specific image due to irreversible binding of ^{111}In with leukocytes, but it could be disadvantageous in terms of radiation exposure and imaging quality considering a long half-life (2.8 days) and high energy photon peaks (172, 247 keV). In addition, ^{111}In-leukocyte scan should be scheduled at least a few days before the imaging because of production schedule of ^{111}In at a medical cyclotron.

^{99m}Tc-HMPAO leukocytes have similar *in vivo* pharmacokinetics and radiolabeling mechanism as that of ^{111}In-leukocytes. ^{99m}Tc-HMPAO leukocyte images are obtained at 4 h after intravenous administration of 740 MBq due to its short half-life (6 h). The use of ^{99m}Tc-HMPAO is much more convenient than ^{111}In in clinical practice since ^{99m}Tc is easily produced by a generator. In spite of this convenience, ^{99m}Tc-HMPAO leukocyte scan has several disadvantages stemming from its physiology. The free form of ^{99m}Tc-HMPAO is often secreted into the bile and urine, which causes non-specific uptake in the gallbladder, urinary system, and intestines. Thus, ^{111}In-leukocyte scan is favored in the diagnosis of intestinal abscess, inflammatory colitis, and renal or transplanted kidney infection.

Radiolabeled leukocyte images should be interpreted in consideration of *in vivo* pharmacokinetics of the radiolabeled leukocytes. Lung capillary

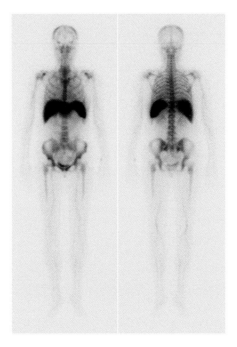

Fig. 14.1.   Anterior and posterior images of the whole body at 4 h after intravenous injection of ^{99m}Tc-HMPAO–labeled leukocytes. ^{99m}Tc-HMPAO leukocytes are normally distributed in the blood pool and reticuloendothelial system including liver, spleen, and bone marrow.

system, reticuloendothelial systems of the liver and spleen, and vascular system are well visualized in the early phase (Fig. 14.1). A few hours later, radioactivity in the lung and blood pool decreases and that in the reticuloendothelial systems increase. After sufficient time elapse, radioactivity other than that in the liver, spleen, and bone marrow are considered abnormal.

14.4.2. ^{67}Ga

After intravenously administered as ^{67}Ga-citrate, ^{67}Ga forms ^{67}Ga-transferrin complex in the blood circulation and is transported to inflammatory sites by means of increase in blood flow and vascular permeability. At the inflammatory sites, ^{67}Ga binds to transferrin receptor on leukocytes or lactoferrin secreted from leukocytes or siderophore of bacteria. In acidic pH, ^{67}Ga has a higher affinity for lactoferrin than transferrin.

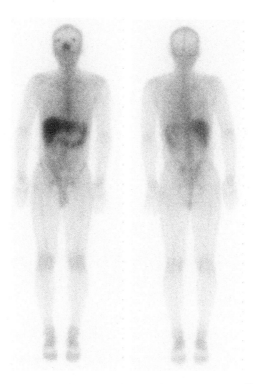

Fig. 14.2. Normal whole body images at 24 h after intravenous injection of ^{67}Ga. The distribution of ^{67}Ga is observed in the lacrymal glands, salivary glands, liver, and bone marrow. In addition, non-specific uptake is seen in the gastrointestinal system.

The distribution of ^{67}Ga differs by its pharmacokinetics and physiology. Normally, ^{67}Ga uptake is observed in the liver, spleen, and bone (Fig. 14.2). Genitourinary and gastrointestinal systems are also observed due to ^{67}Ga excretion. Accordingly, kidneys are well visualized 24 hours after administration of ^{67}Ga. ^{67}Ga uptake in tissues elaborating lactoferrin such as the salivary and lacrimal glands, is considered normal. ^{67}Ga uptake in these organs, however, could be abnormally increased due to production of lactoferrin in certain circumstances, i.e., inflammation. In addition, breast uptake increases in pregnancy and menarche, and thymus uptake is often observed in children.

^{67}Ga images are obtained using a medium or high energy collimator at 24, 48, and 72 h after intravenous administration of 185 MBq. ^{67}Ga is not an optimal radiopharmaceutical due to a long half-life of 3.76 days, high-energy gamma rays ranging from 100–400 keV, and slow clearance from the body.

14.4.3. *FDG*

FDG uptake increases in activated leukocyte as inflammation stimulates GLUT-1 and GLUT-3 expression on the leukocytes. In either infectious or non-infectious inflammatory disease, non-specific FDG uptake could be observed. It has been continuously reported that the diagnostic efficiencies of FDG-PET are comparable or even superior to those of radiolabeled leukocytes or ^{67}Ga scan in both infectious and non-infectious inflammatory diseases.

Recently, FDG-labeled leukocyte PET has been suggested for infection and inflammation imaging. However, the clinical usefulness of FDG-labeled leukocyte PET seems limited because FDG labeling of leukocytes is unstable; approximately 30% of FDG is excreted out of the leukocytes, and sufficient time is not allowed for the leukocyte accumulation due to short half-life of FDG.

14.4.4. *Radiolabeled antibody*

Various radiolabeled antibodies, including non-specific HIG or monoclonal antibodies to leukocytes, have been developed for infection and inflammation imaging. HIG radiolabeled with ^{111}In or ^{99m}Tc accumulates in the inflammatory sites by means of increase in vascular permeability, and it has been reported to be useful in diagnosis of FUO or immunodeficiency patients. NCA-95 (non-specific cross-reacting antigen-95) presented on the granulocyte surface is a commonly used target for monoclonal antibodies. Radiolabeled anti-NCA-95 or Fab' segment of anti-NCA-95 were already commercialized for the infection and inflammation imaging.

14.4.5. *[99m]Tc-ciprofloxacin*

[99m]Tc-ciprofloxacin (Infecton®), a quinolone antibiotic inhibiting bacterial DNA gyrase, was developed as a radiopharmaceutical specific to bacterial infection. ^{99m}Tc-ciprofloxacin is primarily eliminated by renal excretion,

thus the uptake is very low in the liver, gastrointestinal system, and bone marrow. It has been reported to be useful in diagnosis of osteomyelitis and abdominal infection.

14.5. Clinical Applications

14.5.1. *Fever of unknown origin*

Fever of unknown origin (FUO) is determined as fever higher than 38.3°C developing every day or intermittently persists at least 3 weeks, but the cause of fever has not been identified despite a one-week investigation in hospital. Recently, criteria on the hospital administration were changed to include out-patient setting; three out-patient visits or three days in hospital without elucidation of a cause or one week of intelligent and invasive ambulatory investigation.

The most common cause of FUO is infection, accounting for ~30%–40%, but more than half of FUO is caused by autoimmune diseases, connective tissue diseases, and neoplasms. In this regard, nuclear medicine could efficiently reveal the cause of FUO in terms of both time and spatially because it is able to visualize the whole body and detect pathophysiological changes prior to anatomical changes. Particularly, nuclear medicine imaging is very sensitive for both tumorous and non-tumorous fever focus.

In diagnosis of FUO, ^{67}Ga scan is more useful than radiolabeled leukocyte scan. ^{67}Ga scan could detect both tumorous and inflammatory lesions, whereas radiolabeled leukocyte scan hardly detects chronic inflammatory lesions. In particular, ^{67}Ga scan is helpful to diagnose various pulmonary disease such as pneumonia, tuberculosis, and sarcoidosis (Fig. 14.3). On the other hand, radiolabeled leukocyte scan shows superior diagnostic results than those of ^{67}Ga scan in infectious disease, especially in the abdominal lesions.

FDG-PET has also widely been used in diagnosis of FUO because FDG uptake could be increased in either tumorous or non-tumorous condition. Indeed, FDG-PET has proven useful for inflammation and infection through many clinical investigations as PET (or PET/CT) became more accessible in a variety of institutions.

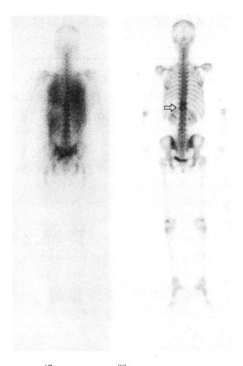

Fig. 14.3. Posterior images of ^{67}Ga scan (a) and ^{99m}Tc-MDP scan (b) in a patient who complained of fever and lower back pain. Diffuse ^{67}Ga uptake in the lungs, and increased ^{99m}Tc-MDP uptake in the 11th and 12th thoracic vertebrae (arrow) are observed. In ^{67}Ga scan, however, no abnormal finding is seen in the thoracic vertebrae. This patient was diagnosed with military tuberculosis and Pott's disease.

14.5.2. *Immunodeficiency patient*

Chest radiographs and laboratory tests are generally diagnostics of choice in diagnosis of immunodeficiency syndrome (AIDS)-related pulmonary infections, but nuclear medicine imaging could be helpful when radiographic findings are ambiguous, especially in patients without specific symptoms or signs. In particular, nuclear medicine imaging is useful for differential diagnosis of Kaposi sarcoma from pneumonia.

Pulmonary Kaposi sarcoma presents similar radiological features to those of lymphoma or pneumonia on chest radiographs, which often makes differential diagnosis difficult. In such cases, ^{67}Ga scan could provide a diagnostic clue as Kaposi sarcoma itself does not show ^{67}Ga uptake while pneumonia or concurrent infection with Kaposi sarcoma present ^{67}Ga uptake.

^{201}Tl scan could be added for more specific diagnosis since Kaposi sarcoma generally takes up ^{201}Tl.

^{111}In-leukocyte scan is more sensitive than ^{67}Ga scan in bacterial pneumonia, but not in pneumocystis pneumonia (PCP). Infectious lesion is usually seen as a focal uptake on the leukocyte scan, but this is non-specific for PCP. On the other hands, PCP presents diffuse intense uptake on ^{67}Ga scan.

14.5.3. *Inflammatory bowel disease*

Inflammatory bowel disease (IBD) generally refers to two distinct diseases among various inflammatory diseases that could involve in the intestines; ulcerative colitis (UC) and Crohn's disease (CD). Nuclear medicine imaging defines extent of inflammation in the intestines and diagnoses complications such as bowel obstruction in patients who are suspected for IBD. In particular, nuclear medicine imaging is useful to detect recurrent diseases and evaluate disease activity in patients who are already diagnosed with IBD.

In IBD, radiolabeled leukocyte scan is favored since ^{67}Ga scan is disadvantageous in evaluation of abdominal lesions due to normal excretion of ^{67}Ga into the intestines. Moreover, radiolabeled leukocyte scan shows a high sensitivity and specificity both greater than 90% in diagnosis of IBD, and it could differentiate CD and UC based on localizing characteristics. CD can involve literally any part of the gastrointestinal tract, so it may affect the small intestine but it frequently spares the rectum. In addition, a skip area might exist in CD. On the contrary, UC is usually limited to the colon including the rectum as the name suggests (Fig. 14.4).

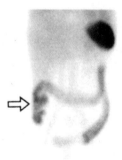

Fig. 14.4. Anterior image of the abdomen in a patient with ulcerative colitis 1 h after intravenous injection of ^{99m}Tc-HMPAO leukocyte. Diffuse increased uptake is seen in the whole colon (arrow).

14.5.4. *Prosthesis infection*

It is often difficult to differentiate aseptic loosening from prosthetic joint infection because these two major complications share very similar clinical symptoms and signs. Bone scan, however, has a relatively high sensitivity and a low specificity in diagnosis of bone and joint infection. Indeed, both aseptic loosening and prosthetic infection are observed as diffuse uptake around the prosthesis on bone scan. Besides, the addition of three-phase scan does not enhance diagnostic results in prosthetic infection, unlikely in osteomyelitis.

Nuclear medicine imaging could be useful in the diagnosis of prosthetic joint infection. Addition of ^{67}Ga scan to bone scan was reported to increase the diagnostic accuracy up to approximately 80%. In cases in which no focal uptake is seen on ^{67}Ga scan, the possibility of prosthetic infection could be excluded in consideration of its high specificity. Radiolabeled leukocyte scan is theoretically more specific to prosthetic infection than ^{67}Ga scan, but the sensitivity of the leukocyte is somewhat lower than expected because prosthetic infections are mostly chronic (Fig. 14.5). Lastly, FDG-PET shows a high sensitivity and a low specificity in prosthetic infection because FDG is non-specifically taken up in both prosthetic infection and aseptic loosening.

14.5.5. *Respiratory disease*

Pulmonary sarcoidosis is usually seen as a hot uptake on ^{67}Ga scan, but this finding is non-specific because ^{67}Ga could be taken up in various inflammatory and benign pulmonary diseases. Unique patterns such as symmetric uptake in the bilateral lacrimal glands and salivary glands (panda sign) and in the bilateral hilar nodes and right main bronchus (lambda sign) may increase a diagnostic specificity. ^{67}Ga scan could be used in evaluation of treatment response to corticosteroids. The degree of ^{67}Ga uptake in pulmonary sarcoidosis decreases after the steroid therapy, which is well correlated with clinical improvements. Likely in pulmonary sarcoidosis, ^{67}Ga uptake could be used for the assessment of disease activity in various parenchymal lung diseases such as idiopathic pulmonary fibrosis, pneumoconiosis, and tuberculosis.

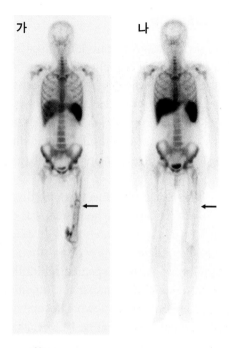

Fig. 14.5. Anterior images of ^{99m}Tc-HMPAO leukocyte scan in a patient who had intramedullary nailing in the left femur. Diffuse increased uptake around the nailing that was well visualized immediately after surgery (a) almost disappeared 2 months after treatment for osteomyelitis (b).

14.5.6. *Cardiovascular system*

Infective endocarditis (IE) mainly involves the cardiac valves and often forms vegetations on the valvular surface, and the detection of vegetations by echocardiography is one of the major criteria for diagnosis of IE. However, echocardiography may fail to properly diagnose a current infection in patients with structural abnormalities in the cardiac valves such as previous scarring, or without forming vegetations. ^{99m}Tc-labeled leukocyte scan could be helpful when echocardiographical diagnosis is limited, but clinical evidence is not sufficient to recommend a routine use of ^{99m}Tc-labeled leukocyte scan in such a case.

14.5.7. *Other applications*

Three-phase bone scan is very useful in diagnosis of osteomyelitis, but the diagnosis is made based on non-specific findings such as increase in blood

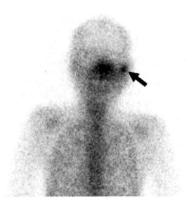

Fig. 14.6. Anterior image of ^{67}Ga scan in a patient with malignant otitis media. Focal ^{67}Ga uptake in the skull base area suggests that the infection constituted skull base osteomyelitis (arrow).

flow or bone metabolism. Accordingly, it is often difficult to distinguish osteomyelitis from fractures or tumors. In such a case, the infection and inflammation imaging, including radiolabeled leukocyte scan or ^{67}Ga scan, could be helpful for the differential diagnosis. ^{67}Ga scan is recommended in chronic osteomyelitis or infection of the axial bones because radiolabeled leukocyte scan shows a low diagnostic accuracy in chronic inflammation (Fig. 14.6). In diagnosis of acute osteomyelitis or peripheral bone infection such as diabetic foot, radiolabeled leukocyte scan shows better diagnostic results than those of ^{67}Ga scan. On the other hand, the infection and inflammation imaging is also used in the evaluation of disease activity of the autoimmune disease such as rheumatoid arthritis.

14.6. PET/CT of Inflammation

14.6.1. *Introduction*

Positron emission tomography/computed tomography (PET/CT) may play an important role in the assessment of a multitude of inflammatory processes. Functional imaging is a part of the non-invasive diagnostic procedure for assessment of inflammation and should be correlated with the referring anatomic modalities such as X-ray, CT, magnetic resonance imaging (MRI), or ultrasound. A number of radiotracers such as gallium-67 (^{67}Ga) and white blood cells labeled with either technetium-99m (^{99m}Tc) or indium-111 (^{111}In) have served to detect inflammation. With the increasing use of fluorine-18-fluorodeoxyglucose (^{18}F-FDG), uptake of tracer in inflammatory processes has been described before.

Accumulation of increased FDG uptake in inflammatory processes was initially described as a cause for false-positive results. Thus, diagnosis and monitoring of inflammatory processes may represent an additional important indication for ^{18}F-FDG-PET/CT.

14.6.2. *Mechanism of uptake in inflammatory processes*

Inflammatory cells such as activated lymphocytes, neutrophils, and macrophages are mostly present in inflammatory processes. These cells exhibit overexpression of hexokinase and glucose transporter proteins with a high affinity for ^{18}F-FDG.[1]

Inflammatory cells have a high capacity for accumulating FDG by stimulation of cytokines. PET/CT study can also detect unexpected inflammatory processes at cancer screening setting. In a study of cancer screening trial, a total of 62 subjects (1.4%) had unexpected abnormal finding.[2] Of these, typical benign lesions consisted of dystrophic calcification with inflammation, non-specific inflammation, and reactive lymphadenopathies in the soft tissue. Normal physiological or inflammatory pathologic ^{18}F-FDG uptake can be confused with malignancy.[3-6] Interpretive pitfalls are often encountered on PET/CT images mistaken for malignancy. Physiological uptakes of bone and soft tissue regions include skeletal muscle and bone marrow.

PET/CT may be used in the clinical setting for imaging and evaluation of infection and inflammation in humans. Most papers describing the use of PET/CT for detection of inflammatory processes were under the situation of nodal staging in malignancies. The generalized inflammatory response of lymph nodes is a common cause of ^{18}FDG uptake, but reactive lymph nodes are also found in cases with malignant tumors. Glycolytic metabolism is elevated in the infiltration associated with inflammatory processes, absorption of necrotic debris, focal hematoma, lymphatic obstruction, or thrombus. The precise reasons for ^{18}F-FDG uptake in these lesions are unclear. However, such lesions are often associated with abundant inflammatory cells or hemorrhagic process which can explain ^{18}F-FDG uptake within the lesion.

The use of PET/CT in the evaluation of inflammatory processes, similar to their implementation for cancer imaging, has decreased the overall uncertainty and the number of equivocal readings. In order to improve the differential diagnosis between malignant and inflammatory processes, the use of threshold standardized uptake value (SUV) has also been performed in many studies. Pathologic confirmation of various inflammatory processes is not usually obtained in all patients. However, disease activity in inflammatory processes may have caused the slight increase in the serum CRP or ESR level noted in clinical setting.

14.6.3. *Disease activity and accumulation*

A number of practical advantages make PET/CT one of the procedures for assessment of inflammation. ^{18}F-FDG has favorable tracer kinetics with rapid accumulation in inflammatory processes. The short physical half-life may result in lower radiation doses delivered to patients who undergo other imaging procedures using ionizing radiation. The fact that the physical characteristics of the agent require the procedure to be performed within an approximate time of 2 h represents an advantage of clinical results within a short time span. ^{18}F-FDG is taken up by macrophages and immature granulation tissue in experimental animal models. In addition, some cytokines such as tumor necrosis factor-α(TNF-α), which plays a major role in synovitis in patients with rheumatoid arthritis, regulates glucose transport and metabolism (Fig. 14.7). The degree of ^{18}F-FDG uptake significantly correlated with the results of physical examination and laboratory tests for evaluating disease activity in patients with inflammatory diseases.[7,8] A number of inflammatory diseases may cause significant uptake of ^{18}F-FDG that may simulate malignant lesion (Table 14.1). In the chest, active tuberculosis, non-tuberculous mycobacterium infection, sarcoidosis, organizing pneumonia, and histoplasmosis have been reported as showing increased ^{18}F-FDG uptake.[9] The degree of accumulation may correlate well with disease activity in inflammatory processes (Fig. 14.8).

Although ^{18}F-FDG-PET/CT may be a simple non-invasive method to estimate disease activity of inflammation except for its employment of radiation, clinical importance of this modality has not been evaluated in most inflammatory diseases. ^{18}F-FDG-PET may assist in identifying active

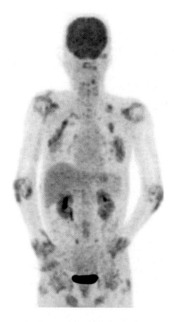

Fig. 14.7. A man aged 60 years with RA. Coronal PET maximum intensity projection image shows multiple involvements of major joints as well as bilateral metacarpophalamgeal and metatarsopharangeal joints. The SUV_{max} of the involved joints ranged from 1.5 (left elbow) to 3.5 (right shoulder). Physical examination reveals the presence of swelling in the wrist, knee, ankle, and MCP bilaterally.

inflammation and quantitative measure of ^{18}F-FDG accumulation would correlate with serum markers of inflammation in patients with inflammatory disease.

14.6.4. *Limitations*

Limitations of ^{18}F-FDG-PET/CT of inflammation are related to the normal tracer biodistribution of ^{18}F-FDG. Lesions of ^{18}F-FDG-avid foci located in organs in close vicinity to areas of high physiologic tracer uptake may be misinterpreted as false-positive as well as false-negative findings.

^{18}F-FDG imaging may have a lower sensitivity in the presence of hyperglycemia. A decrease in ^{18}F-FDG uptake in experimental inflammatory processes has been found in hyperglycemia due to a decreased expression of glucose transporters as well as direct competition with unlabeled glucose for ^{18}F-FDG uptake. Findings relating active inflammation evaluated by ^{18}F-FDG PET/CT in patients with inflammatory diseases may suggest

Table 14.1.

PET/CT Detectable Major Inflammatory Processes

Brain	Cerebritis, Meningitis
Head and neck	Pharyngitis, Laryngitis, Tonsillits, Chronic thyroiditis, Periodontitis, Sinusitis, Mastoiditis
Chest	Tuberculosis, NTM infection, Mycotic infection, Pneumonia, Sarcoidosis, Mediastinal fibrosis, Esophagitis, Angitis
Breast	Mastitis
Large vessel	Aortitis, Graft infection
GI tract	Gastritis, Ulcer, Duodenitis, Inflammatory bowel disease (Crohn disease, Ulcerative colitis), Diverticulitis, Colitis
Bile duct	Cholecystitis, Cholangitis
Pancreas	Autoimmune pancreatitis, Acute and chronic pancreatitis
Skelton	Arthritis, Rheumatoid arthiritis, Myelitis, Bone marrow hyperstimulation, Radiation induced osteomyelitis, Osteomyelitis
Soft tissue	Keroid, Dermatitis, Myositis, Retroperitoneal fibrosis

that the degree of ^{18}F-FDG uptake may be a useful tool to monitor active inflammation. A practical issue that has not yet received sufficient evaluation is the potential influence of prior therapy on ^{18}F-FDG uptake.

14.6.5. *Tracers*

Compared with ^{18}F-FDG for imaging inflammation, ^{18}F-FDG-labeled leukocytes is a more specific agent for detection of inflammation with the high spatial resolution and improved sensitivity. *In vitro* study of ^{18}F-FDG–labeled human granulocytes shows a significant uptake in all sterile and septic inflammation models. The normal biodistribution of ^{18}F-FDG–labeled leukocytes reveals secretion of only small amounts of tracers in gastrointestinal and urinary tracts. This may serve as a possible tracer for suspected inflammatory processes in these organs.

In a clinical study of ^{18}F-FDG–labeled leukocytes to detect suspected or documented infectious processes revealed accuracy of 90%.[10] Another clinical study in patients with suspected musculoskeletal infections revealed

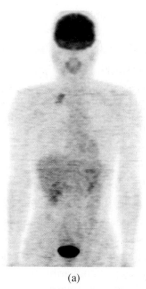

(a)

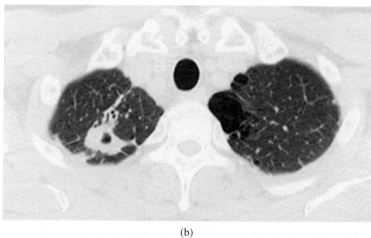

(b)

Fig. 14.8. (a) and (b) A man aged 50 years with non-tuberculous mycobacteria infection. Coronal PET maximum intensity projection image shows abnormal uptake in the apex of the right lung (a). Axial CT image shows cavitary lesion with thickened wall (b).

sensitivity of 87%, specificity of 82%, and accuracy of 84%, respectively.[11] Other possible tracers for inflammatory processes include the use of [68Ga] stand-alone or [68Ga]-labeled peptides. However, further study is needed to clarify the diagnostic performance in the clinical setting.

14.7. Conclusion

^{18}F-FDG-PET/CT has become an exciting modality for diagnostic imaging of inflammation in many settings. It appears to have an incremental value over anatomic imaging methods in the assessment of both acute and chronic inflammatory diseases. Due to the non-specific uptake mechanism of ^{18}F-FDG, most studies assessing ^{18}F-FDG PET/CT in inflammatory processes include only a small number of patients.

Further studies need to be performed in order to provide the clinical decision-making and cost-effectiveness calculations.

References

1. Kumar V, Abbas AK, Fauto N. (2004) *Pathologic Basis of Disease*. 7th edn, p. 47–86, Elsevier Saunders, Philadelphia.
2. Bleek-Rovers CP, Boerman OC, Rennen HJJM, Corstens FHM, Oyen WJG. (2004) Radiolabeled compounds in diagnosis of infectious and inflammatory disease. *Curr Pharm Des* **10**: 2935–2950.
3. Danpure HJ, Osman S. (1988) A review of methods of separating and radiolabeling human leukocytes. *Nucl Med Commun* **9**: 681–685.
4. *Harrison's Principles of Internal Medicine*, 16th edn. The McGraw-Hill Companies, ISBN 0-07-140235-7.
5. Dumarey N, Egrise D, Blocklet D, Stallenberg B, Remmelink M, del Marmol V, *et al.* (2006) Imaging infection with ^{18}F-FDG-labeled leukocyte PET/CT: Initial experience in 21 patients. *J Nucl Med* **47**: 625–632.
6. Bar-Shalom R, Yefremov N, Guralnik L, Keider Z, Engel A, Nitecki S, *et al.* (2006) SPECT/CT using ^{67}Ga and ^{111}In-labeled leukocyte scintigraphy for diagnosis of infection. *J Nucl Med* **47**: 587–594.
7. Fischman AJ, Rubin RH, Khaw BA, Callahan RJ, Wilkinson R, Keech F, *et al.* (1998) Detection of acute inflammation with ^{111}In-labeled nonspecific polyclonal IgG. *SeminNucl Med* **18**: 335–344.
8. Becker W, Bair J, Behr T, Repp R, Strechenbach H, Beck H, *et al.* (1994) Detection of soft-tissue infection and osteomyelitis using a technetium-99m-labeled anti-granulocyte monoclonal antibody fragment. *J Nucl Med* **35**: 1436–1443.
9. Sarda L, Cremieux AC, Lebellec Y, Meylemans A, Lebtahi R, Hayem G, *et al.* (2003) Inability of ^{99m}Tc-ciprofloxacin scintigraphy to discriminate between septic and sterile osteoarticular diseases. *J Nucl Med* **44**: 920–926.
10. Becker W, Meller J. (2001) The role of nuclear medicine in infection and inflammation. *Lancet Infect Dis* **1**: 326–333.
11. Knockaert DG, Mortelmans LA, De Roo MC, Bobbaers HJ. (1994) Clinical value of gallium-67 scintigraphy in evaluation of fever of unknown origin. *Clin Infect Dis* **18**: 601–605.

12. Meller J, Sahlmann CO, Scheel AK. (2007) ^{18}F-FDG PET and PET/CT in fever of unknown origin. *J Nucl Med* **48**: 35–45.

13. Kjaer A, Lebech AM, Eigtved A, Hojgaard L. (2004) Fever of unknown origin: Prospective comparison of diagnostic value of ^{18}F-FDG PET and ^{111}In-granulocyte scintigraphy. *Eur J Nucl Med Mol Imaging* **31**: 622–626.

14. Kerry JE, Marshall C, Griffiths PA, James MW, Scott BB. (2005) Comparison between Tc-HMPAO labeled white cells and TcLeukoScan in the investigation of inflammatory bowel disease. *Nucl Med Commun* **26**: 245–251.

15. Stumper KD, Romero J, Ziegler O, Kamel EM, von Schulthess, Strobel K, *et al.* (2006) The value of FDG-PET in patients with painful total knee arthroplasty. *Eur J Nucl Med Mol Imaging* **33**: 1218–1225.

16. Kuhl U, Lauer B, Souvatzoglu M, Vosberg H, Schultheisis HP. (1998) Antimyosin-scintigraphy and immunohistologic analysis of endomyocardial biopsy in patients with clinically suspected myocarditis-evidence of myocardial cell damage and inflammation in the absence of histologic signs of myocarditis. *J Am Coll Cardiol* **32**: 1371–1376.

17. Weisdorf DJ, Craddock PR, Jacob HS. (1982) Glycogenolysis versus glucose transport in human granulocytes: Differential activation in phagocytesis and chemo taxis. *Blood* **60**: 888–893.

18. Maeda T, Tateishi U, Terauchi T, Hamashima C, Moriyama N, Arai Y, Kim EE, Sugimura K. (2007) Unsuspected bone and soft tissue lesions identified at cancer screening using positron emission tomography. *Jpn J Clin Oncol* **37**: 207–215.

19. Brigid GA, Flanagan FL, Dehdashti F. (1997) Whole-body positron emission tomography: Normal variations, pitfalls, and technical considerations. *AJR* **169**: 1675–1680.

20. Cook GJ, Fogelman I, Maisey MN. (1996) Normal physiological and benign pathological variants of 18-fluoro-2-deoxyglucose positron-emission tomography scanning: Potential for error in interpretation. *Semin Nucl Med* **26**: 308–314.

21. Engel H, Steinert H, Buck A, Berthold T, Huch Boni RA, von Schulthess GK. (1996) Whole-body PET: Physiological and artifactual fluorodeoxyglucose accumulations. *J Nucl Med* **37**: 441–446.

22. Zhuang H, Alavi A. (2002) 18-fluorodeoxyglucose positron emission tomographic imaging in the detection and monitoring of infection and inflammation. *Semin Nucl Med* **32**: 47–59.

23. Wipke BT, Wang Z, Kim J, McCarthy TJ, Allen PM. (2002) Dynamic visualization of joint specific autoimmune response through positron emission tomography. *Nat Immunol* **3**: 366–372.

24. Fonseca A, Wagner J, Yamaga LI, Osawa A, da Cunha ML, Scheinberg M. (2008) (18) F-FDG PET imaging of rheumatoid articular and extraarticular synovitis. *J Clin Rheumatol* **14**: 307.

25. Tateishi U, Hasegawa T, Seki K, Terauchi T, Moriyama N, Arai Y. (2006) Disease activity and 18F-FDG uptake in organizing pneumonia: Semi-quantitative evaluation using computed tomography and positron emission tomography. *Eur J Nucl Med Mol Imaging* **33**: 906–912.

Chapter 15
Tumor Imaging

Ukihide Tateishi and E. Edmund Kim

15.1. Introduction

Positron emission tomography (PET) helps reduce many of the limitations of anatomic imaging. When PET combines with anatomic images in fusion images, especially those generated with dedicated PET in combination with computed tomography (PET/CT) systems, it provides both anatomic precision and functional information in a single data set. The use of PET/CT in tumor management has shown remarkable growth in the past few years as a wide range of papers have been published representing the broad applicability with fluorodeoxyglucose (FDG).

The molecular etiologies of tumors have been increasingly understood. There are many hallmarks of tumor, which include the following characteristics: self sufficiency in growth signals; apoptosis; insensitivity to anti-growth signals; tissue invasion and metastasis; replicative potential; and angiogenesis. On the other hand, there are general characteristics: the increased rate of proliferation, over- or under-expression of receptors/tumor antigens, presence of hypoxia and/or necrosis, increased metabolism of glucose, amino acids, membrane precursors, and other substrates such as glutamine, DNA precursors, and accelerated rate of apoptosis. Each of these phenotypic features represents a possible target for tumor imaging with PET, and many of these processes have been targeted with PET tracers.

15.2. Glucose Metabolism

FDG is currently the most commonly used and versatile tracer for tumor imaging. Increased glucose metabolism is not specific for tumor. The

353

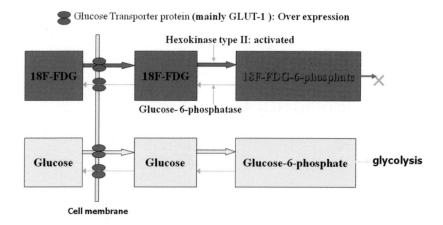

Fig. 15.1.

dominant tracer used in clinical PET to date, FDG had been developed as a tracer to evaluate the initial steps of glucose metabolism in the brain. FDG is transported into target cells, such as those in the brain or tumors. Transported FDG is phosphorylated by hexokinase II subtype. Glucose 6-phosphate is metabolized further; however, the FDG tracer is not substantially further metabolized after conversion to FDG 6-phosphate. FDG 6-phosphate is retained as the polar molecule and can be imaged by PET/CT (Fig. 15.1).

15.3. Glucose Transporter

The glucose transfer mediated by glucose transporter protein 1 (GLUT1) plays a pivotal role in the development and malignant behavior of cancer cells.[1] GLUT-1 belongs to the sugar transporter family and is the dominant protein expressed in cancer cells. The pioneering study was designed to quantify GLUT-1 expression by human rhabdomyosarcoma cells, and the authors demonstrated that GLUT-1 accounted for a major part of the basal and insulin-stimulated glucose transport *in vitro*.

Overexpression of facilitative glucose transporters on the cell surface is common, with the GLUT1 and GLUT3 transporters. GLUT is overexpressed in many tumors.[2-6] Glucose transporters are the molecular species that facilitate FDG transit into the cell. Some of the hexokinase enzymes, especially in hexokinase II, can be overexpressed in tumor. These are important proteins in the early phases of glucose metabolism.

The number of viable tumor cells expressing GLUT1 on the cell membrane appears to correlate well with the extent of FDG uptake in a given type of tumor. This association between GLUT1 protein levels and tumor FDG uptake is generally the case, but not invariably present. Strong relationships between GLUT1 membrane expression and FDG uptake have been shown in various histologic subtypes of tumors. The relationships between number of tumor cells, glucose transporters, flow, hexokinase levels, serum insulin levels, oxygen tension, cell cycle status, adenosine triphosphate levels, and receptor status seen at PET/CT are complicated.

15.4. Uptake by Tumor Cells

A major decline in FDG uptake may be attributed to successful therapeutic effect of tumor cells. However, the precise duration required following chemotherapy to optimally assess for treatment efficacy is not yet fully resolved. Receptor stimulation by agonists can increase tracer uptake. As in the acute cellular response to irradiation or chemotherapy, tumor cell uses glucose at an increased level in response to treatment in the early phases after treatment. In the presence of certain chemotherapies, FDG uptake in tumors can decline to a greater extent than the number of viable tumor cells.

15.5. Blood Flow and Uptake

Blood flow is measured by $H_2[^{15}O]$ (^{15}O-water) and, compared with FDG uptake, they correlate reasonably.[7,8] This evidence suggests that tumor uptake and blood flow are reasonably well linked. Using kinetic modeling approaches, some studies in humans have shown that tumors with higher standard uptake values (SUVs) actually had lower κ_3 values than a group of tumors with high κ_3 values. This supports the importance of delivery and transport of the tracer to the net FDG accumulation in tumors.

Schematic Compartmental Model of Contrast Medium Flow-Through Pattern

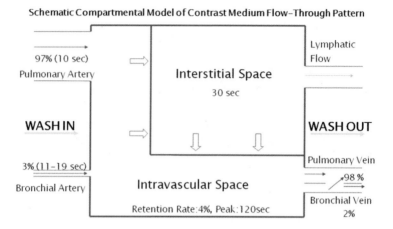

NORMAL LUNG

Fig. 15.2.

The quantification of blood flow within tumor is also currently performed using dynamic contrast-enhanced magn etic resonance imaging (DCE-MRI) for monitoring effects of chemotherapy.[9–12] DCE-MRI allows measurements of kinetic parameters related to perfusion and permeability. Pharmacodynamic markers obtained by sequential DCE-MRI are sensitive to detect early response to chemotherapy in various cancer types and can reflect histopathologic response after chemotherapy.

For further understanding, schematic compartmental model of contrast medium flow-through pattern in the normal lung is demonstrated (Fig. 15.2). Analysis of the compartmental model of the lung is complicated compared to other organs of the trunk, because wash-in in the normal lung consists both of pulmonary artery and bronchial artery. Contrast medium passes two compartments of intravascular space and interstitial space within the peak of 120 sec. On the other hand, wash-out in the normal lung is mainly pulmonary vain and the factor of the presence of bronchial vein is limited. When the other organ of the trunk is considered, wash-in of the target organ is usually branches of aorta. DCE-MRI parameters, including transfer constant (K_{trans}), the rate constant (κ_{ep}), and the area under curve (AUC), are potent predictor of outcome (Fig. 15.3). Although both sequential PET and DCE-MRI allow more precise visualization of

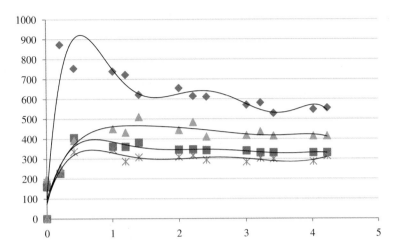

Fig. 15.3. The scatter plots of time-intensity curve of DCE-MRI. The *x*-axis represents time after administration of contrast medium (second) and the *y*-axis shows signal intensity of target lesion. The SI of tumor is 500 in maximum (green) compared to aortic peak of over 900 (blue). The SI of the tumor decreases after second cycle (brown) and sixth cycle (light blue).

tumor response to chemotherapy as biomarkers, the relationship between sequential PET and DCE-MRI for assessment of chemotherapy in cancer is not fully clarified.

15.6. Specific Pitfalls of PET/CT

Lesions less than 5 mm in size, either in the thorax or elsewhere in the body are not detected on PET/CT due to spatial resolution and count limitations. The positive scan results are much more useful and reliable than negative scan results when the lesions are small.

Early days after surgery are insufficient for evaluation with PET/CT because there is normal uptake in immature granulation tissue of surgical wounds and scars. If a wound is infected, the determination is quite difficult because PET/CT results are often positive in infections. Again, discussion with the referring physician may result in a postponement of the PET study for several months or until the infection has resolved.

Claustrophobic patients, patients with severe movement disorders, patients who are morbidly obese, patients who cannot lie on their backs or side, and poorly controlled diabetics are excluded as candidates for PET/CT.

15.7. PET/CT of Hematologic Malignancies

15.7.1. *Introduction*

Many reports have shown the use and value of PET, PET/CT imaging of malignant lymphomas for pretherapeutic staging, therapy control, interim response assessment of various combinations of radio-, chemo-, immuno- and radioimmunotherapy, and evaluation of prognosis.[13,14]

Malignant lymphoma most often involves lymph nodes and axial lymphatic pathways at the initial staging. Nodal involvement within the axial lymphatic pathways results from disparate disease status. Tumor stage in malignant lymphoma is assessed initially by conventional imaging modalities such as, PET, PET/CT, CT, MRI, and [67]Gallium scintigraphy, which can play an important role in the initial determination of the stage because they provide morphologic information on the extent of disease. FDG-PET or PET/CT is a valuable tool for staging of patients with malignant lymphoma, therapeutic effect, and prediction of prognosis in most histologic subtypes.[15–21] The anatomic location and specific features of fluorine-18-FDG (^{18}F-FDG) accumulation often provide insights into disease activity and can sometimes explain occult disease progression. This review summarizes outlines of clinical utility in PET or PET/CT for management of malignant lymphoma.

15.7.2. *Staging*

All studies comparing FDG-PET or PET/CT to CT reported a 10% to 20% higher accuracy of FDG-PET or PET/CT for staging of malignant lymphoma and resulted in treatment changes of 10% to 20% in patients. Many of the lesions detected with PET or PET/CT are in lymph nodes of sub-centimeter in size, which are considered normal nodes on CT (Fig. 15.4).

Limitations of FDG-PET or PET/CT for staging are diffuse bone marrow involvement with less than 60% accuracy in NHL, with a reduced sensitivity in some indolent (low-grade) lymphomas. The sensitivity of FDG-PET or PET/CT is excellent (approximately 95%) in follicular lymphoma, moderate (74%) in mantle cell lymphoma, and limited (approximately 50%) in small lymphocytic lymphoma and mucosa-associated lymphoid tissue lymphoma.

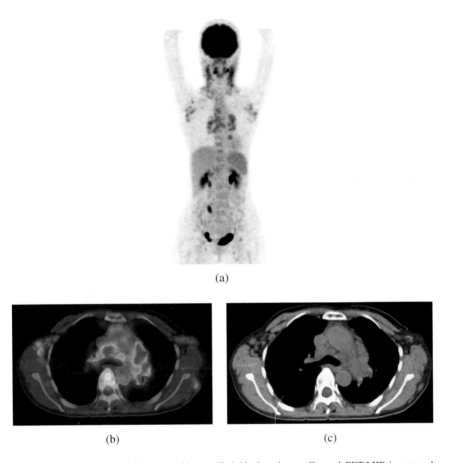

(a)

(b)   (c)

Fig. 15.4. A woman aged 60 years with non-Hodgkin lymphoma. Coronal PET-MIP image and axial PET/CT image shows abnormal uptake in axillary nodes and hilar nodes bilaterally as well as multiple mediastinal nodes and subcutaneous nodes (Fig. 15.4[a] and [b]). Corresponded axial CT image demonstrates enlarged and normal-sized nodes (Fig. 15.4[c]). Figure 15.4(c) shows abdominal level of axial PET/CT before (Fig. 15.4[d]) and after treatment (Fig. 14[d] and [e]) in this patient. Accumulation of FDG appears significant in the liver and spleen before therapy. However, a decrease of uptake is found after therapy. Corresponding axial CT images demonstrate a decrease in size of spleen (Fig. 15.4[f] and [g]).

Another application of PET/CT for staging of malignant lymphoma is contrast-enhanced PET/CT.[22-25] The lymphatic chains of the trunk are complicated and numerous. However, precise localization of lymph nodes in these regions is sometimes difficult only by non-contrasted images except for a bulky lesion. Contrast-enhanced PET/CT can reduce the number of

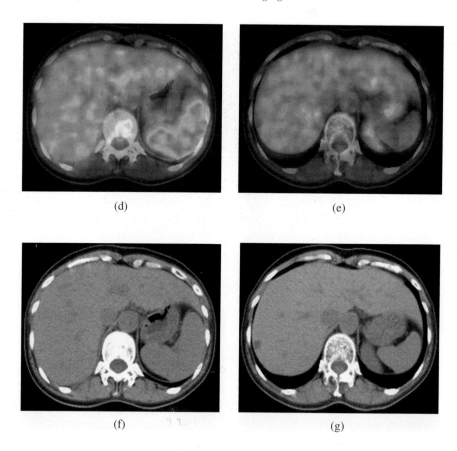

(d)   (e)

(f)   (g)

Fig. 15.4. *(Continued)*

overstaged patients compared with non-contrasted PET/CT. In contrast, clinical stage will change from stage I or II to stage IV in patients who have a single focus along the lymphatic pathways. In addition, contrast-enhanced PET/CT depicts intravascular extension of tumor that cannot be diagnosed with non-contrasted PET/CT.

15.7.3. *Response monitoring*

Criteria for response assessment and response categories have been established for lymphoma and are commonly known as the International

Workshop Classification (IWC). The IWC predominantly relies on anatomical imaging modalities such as CT.

Criteria for response assessment have been recently revised, and PET or PET/CT has been implemented.[26] The reason for revision was that it had been long recognized that lymphoma masses, when bulky on presentation, may not disappear completely if the disease has been eradicated completely. The introduction of functional metabolic imaging using FDG PET or PET/CT has proven to be helpful in accurate assessment of remission post-treatment and in characterizing residual masses.

PET after completion of chemotherapy should be performed at least 3 weeks after chemotherapy, and 8 to 12 weeks after irradiation or chemoradiation. Mediastinal blood pool activity is recommended as the reference. Visual assessment of potential lymphoma manifestations is regarded as adequate. Mild and diffusely increased uptake in residual masses 2 cm or greater in diameter with intensity less than or equal to mediastinal blood pool should be considered negative. Residual hepatic or splenic lesions greater than 1.5 cm on CT and FDG uptake greater than or equal to that of liver or spleen should be considered positive. The accuracy of PET is high enough to be used as a standard reference for assessment of remission and results in replacement of CT in avid lymphomas.

Complete clinical responses in malignant lymphoma are seen frequently compared to solid tumors. However, shorter end points are needed in phase II trials conducted in relapsed patients and those with refractory disease. The lack of response using FDG-PET criteria correlated with progression-free survival and overall survival in both Hodgkin's and non-Hodgkin's lymphoma (NHL). These data suggest an opportunity to qualify FDG-PET as an accurate early measure of response and to refine current standards for assessment of tumor response in patients with malignant lymphoma.

The ability to get an early and accurate assessment of response is an important tool in the management of a patient with malignant lymphoma since prognosis is usually poor in non-responding and relapsed patients. The early and intensive treatment including high-dose chemotherapy with autologous stem cell transplant may be of benefit to selected patients.

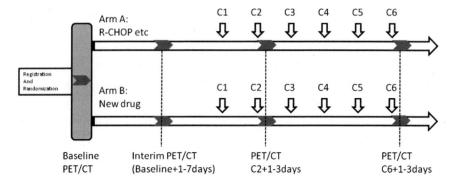

Fig. 15.5. A protocol of possible randomized control study using sequential PET/CT. Sequential PET/CT will be performed during cycles after baseline scan (red arrow). The results of interim PET/CT and C2 PET/CT may affect a choice of drug for non-responder.

15.7.4. *Evaluation of prognosis*

Achieving a complete remission is a major objective in patients with Hodgkin's lymphoma or NHL because it is usually associated with a longer progression-free survival than a partial remission.

About 40% of patients with aggressive NHL fail to achieve complete remission (CR) with initial standard chemotherapy, which is a prerequisite for cure. Overall, long-term cure is achieved only in 60% of the patients. This means that a substantial portion of patients may not respond to their initial treatment. PET has been investigated to potentially improve the accuracy of early response assessment (Figure 15.5). CR is evident on a repeated PET or PET/CT after one to three cycles of chemotherapy much earlier than size reduction of lymphoma masses seen on CT. Such an early CR on PET, presumably reflecting high chemosensitivity, correlates with better prognosis. Early PET is a more accurate predictor of outcome than post-treatment PET. The early interim PET is an accurate and independent predictor of progression free survival and overall survival.

15.7.5. *Proliferative activity in malignant lymphoma*

Proliferative activity of lymphomas is linked to biologic aggressiveness. Imaging of proliferative activity in individual lymphoma manifestations may improve early detection of the development of aggressive transformation of low-grade lymphoma.

Fluorothymidine (FLT) is the radiopharmaceutical that is most widely used at present for imaging proliferative activity. FLT is taken up by the cell through passive diffusion and facilitated sodium-positive-dependent, nucleoside transporter–mediated inward transport. Within the cell, FLT is phosphorylated by TK1 to FLT monophosphate and to a limited degree also to the di- and triphosphate. Only minor amounts of FLT are incorporated into DNA and result in DNA chain terminations. TK1 is virtually absent in quiescent cells but is upregulated several folds in proliferating cells during the late Gl and S phase of the cell cycle. The use of FLT might obviate quantitative tracer kinetic methods that are potentially required when other radiotracers such as FDG are used for grading NHL. However, FLT does have the challenge of high-level uptake in the liver and bone marrow, making it likely that lesion detection will be more difficult in these tissues than with FDG.

Table 15.1. Recommended timing of PET (PET/CT) scans in lymphoma clinical trials.

Histology	Pretreatment	Mid-Treatment	Response Assessment	Post-Treatment Surveillance
Routinely FDG avid				
DLBCL	Yes*	Clinical trial	Yes	No
HL	Yes*	Clinical trial	Yes	No
Follicular NHL	No[†]	Clinical trial	No[†]	No
MCL	No[†]	Clinical trial	No[†]	No
Variably FDG avid				
Other aggressive NHLs	No[†]	Clinical trial	No[†,‡]	No
Other indolent NHLs	No[†]	Clinical trial	No[†‡]	No

Abbreviations: DLBCL, diffuse large B-cell lymphoma; HL, Hodgkin's lymphoma; MCL, mantle-cell lymphoma; ORR, overall response rate.

*Recommended but not required pretreatment.
[†]Recommended only if ORR/CR is a primary study end point.
[‡]Recommended only if PET is positive pre-treatment.
Source: Chung JK, Lee YJ, Kim SK, Jeong JM, Lee DS, Lee MC. Comparison of [18F]fluorode-oxyglucose uptake with glucose transporter-1 expression and proliferation rate in human glioma and non-small-cell lung cancer. *Nucl Med Commun* 2004; **25**(1): 11–17.

Table 15.2.   Response definitions for clinical trials.

Response	Definition	Nodal Masses	Spleen, Liver	Bone Marrow
CR	Disappearance of all evidence of disease	(a) FDG-avid or PET positive prior to therapy; mass of any size permitted if PET negative (b) Variably FDG-avid or PET negative; regression to normal size on CT	Not palpable, nodules disappeared	Infiltrate cleared on repeat biopsy; if indeterminate by morphology, immunohistochemistry should be negative
PR	Regression of measurable disease and no new sites	$\geq$50% decrease in SPD of up to 6 largest dominant masses; no increase in size of other nodes (a) FDG-avid or PET positive prior to therapy; one or more PET positive at previously involved site (b) Variably FDG-avid or PET negative; regression on CT	$\geq$50% decrease in SPD of nodules (for single nodule in greatest transverse diameter); no increase in size of liver or spleen	Irrelevant if positive prior to therapy; cell type should be specified
SD	Failure to attain CR/PR or PD	(a) FDG-avid or PET positive prior to therapy; PET positive at prior sites of disease and no new sites of disease on CT or PET		

(Continued)

Table 15.2. (*Continued*)

Response	Definition	Nodal Masses	Spleen, Liver	Bone Marrow
		(b) Variably FDG-avid or PET negative; no change in size of previous lesions on CT		
Relapsed disease or PD	Any new lesion or increase by ≥50% of previously involved sites from nadir	Appearance of a new lesion(s) > 1.5 cm in any axis, ≥50% increase in SPD of more than one node, or ≥50% increase in longest diameter of a previously identified node > 1 cm in short axis Lesions PET positive if FDG-avid lymphoma or PET positive prior to therapy	> 50% increase from nadir in the SPD of any previous lesions	New or recurrent involvement

Abbreviations: PR, partial remission; SPD, sum of the product of the diameters; SD, stable disease; PD, progressive disease.

Source: Chung JK, Lee YJ, Kim SK, Jeong JM, Lee DS, Lee MC. Comparison of [18F]fluorodeoxyglucose uptake with glucose transporter-1 expression and proliferation rate in human glioma and non-small-cell lung cancer. *Nucl Med Commun* 2004; **25**(1): 11–17.

15.8. Conclusion

In malignant lymphoma, the definition of a clinical response by anatomic imaging should be refined with a confirmatory FDG-PET scan to detect residual disease in those patients with normal-sized nodes or to rule out disease in those with enlarged nodes. The ability to get more early and accurate assessment of response is an important tool in the management of a patient with lymphoma since prognosis is usually poor in non-responding and relapsed patients, and early intensive treatment may be of benefit to selected patients.

References

1. Ito S, Nemoto T, Satoh S, Sekihara H, Seyama Y, Kubota S. (2000) Human rhabdomyosarcoma cells retain insulin-regulated glucose transport activity through glucose transporter 1. *Arch Biochem Biophys* 373: 72–82.
2. Chung JK, Lee YJ, Kim SK, Jeong JM, Lee DS, Lee MC. (2004) Comparison of [18F]fluorodeoxyglucose uptake with glucose transporter-1 expression and proliferation rate in human glioma and non-small-cell lung cancer. *Nucl Med Commun*; 25(1): 11–17.
3. Mamede M, Higashi T, Kitaichi M, Ishizu K, Ishimori T, Nakamoto Y, Yanagihara K, Li M, Tanaka F, Wada H, Manabe T, Saga T. (2005) [18F]FDG uptake and PCNA, Glut-1, and hexokinase-II expressions in cancers and inflammatory lesions of the lung. *Neoplasia*; 7: 369–379.
4. Brown RS, Leung JY, Fisher SJ, Frey KA, Ethier SP, Wahl RL. (1996) Intratumoral distribution of tritiated-FDG in breast carcinoma: Correlation between Glut-1 expression and FDG uptake. *J Nucl Med*; 37(6): 1042–1047.
5. Reske SN, Grillenberger KG, Glatting G, Port M, Hildebrandt M, Gansauge F, *et al.* (1997) Overexpression of glucose transporter 1 and increased FDG uptake in pancreatic carcinoma. *J Nucl Med*; 38: 1344–1348.
6. Higashi T, Tamaki N, Honda T, Torizuka T, Kimura T, Inokuma T, *et al.* (1997) Expression of glucose transporters in human pancreatic tumors compared with increased FDG accumulation in PET study. *J Nucl Med*; 38: 1337–1344.
7. Mankoff DA, Dunnwald LK, Gralow JR, *et al.* (2002) Blood flow and metabolism in locally advanced breast cancer: Relationship to response to therapy. *J Nucl Med*; 43: 500–509.
8. Dunnwald LK, Gralow JR, Ellis GK, Livingston RB, Linden HM, Specht JM, *et al.* (2008) Tumor metabolism and blood flow changes by positron emission tomography: Relation to survival in patients treated with neoadjuvant chemotherapy for locally advanced breast cancer. *J Clin Oncol*; 26: 4449–4457.

9. Tofts PS, Brix G, Buckley DL, *et al.* (1999) Estimating kinetic parameters from dynamic contrast-enhanced T1-weighted MRI of a diffusable tracer: Standardized quantities and symbols. *J Magn Reson Imaging*; **10**: 223–232.

10. Brix G, Henze M, Knopp MV, *et al.* (2001) Comparison of pharmacokinetic MRI and [18F] fluorodeoxyglucose PET in the diagnosis of breast cancer: initial experience. *Eur Radiol*; **11**: 2058–2070.

11. Knopp MV, von Tengg-Kobligk H, Choyke PL. (2003) Functional magnetic resonance imaging in oncology for diagnosis and therapy monitoring. *Mol Cancer Ther*; **2**: 419–426.

12. Hayes C, Padhani AR, Leach MO. (2002) Assessing changes in tumour vascular function using dynamic contrast-enhanced magnetic resonance imaging. *NMR in Biomed*; **15**: 154–163.

13. Ito S, Nemoto T, Satoh S, Sekihara H, Seyama Y, Kubota S. (2000) Human rhabdomyosarcoma cells retain insulin-regulated glucose transport activity through glucose transporter 1. *Arch Biochem Biophys*; **373**: 72–82.

14. Chung JK, Lee YJ, Kim SK, Jeong JM, Lee DS, Lee MC. (2004) Comparison of [18F]fluorodeoxyglucose uptake with glucose transporter-1 expression and proliferation rate in human glioma and non-small-cell lung cancer. *Nucl Med Commun*; **25**(1): 11–17.

15. Mamede M, Higashi T, Kitaichi M, Ishizu K, Ishimori T, Nakamoto Y, Yanagihara K, Li M, Tanaka F, Wada H, Manabe T, Saga T. (2005) [18F]FDG uptake and PCNA, Glut-1, and hexokinase-II expressions in cancers and inflammatory lesions of the lung. *Neoplasia*; **7**: 369–379.

16. Brown RS, Leung JY, Fisher SJ, Frey KA, Ethier SP, Wahl RL. (1996) Intratumoral distribution of tritiated-FDG in breast carcinoma: Correlation between Glut-1 expression and FDG uptake. *J Nucl Med*; **37**(6): 1042–1047.

17. Reske SN, Grillenberger KG, Glatting G, Port M, Hildebrandt M, Gansauge F, *et al.* (1997) Overexpression of glucose transporter 1 and increased FDG uptake in pancreatic carcinoma. *J Nucl Med*; **38**: 1344–1348.

18. Higashi T, Tamaki N, Honda T, Torizuka T, Kimura T, Inokuma T, *et al.* (1997) Expression of glucose transporters in human pancreatic tumors compared with increased FDG accumulation in PET study. *J Nucl Med*; **38**: 1337–1344.

19. Mankoff DA, Dunnwald LK, Gralow JR, *et al.* (2002) Blood flow and metabolism in locally advanced breast cancer: Relationship to response to therapy. *J Nucl Med*; **43**: 500–509.

20. Dunnwald LK, Gralow JR, Ellis GK, Livingston RB, Linden HM, Specht JM, *et al.* (2008) Tumor metabolism and blood flow changes by positron emission tomography: Relation to survival in patients treated with neoadjuvant chemotherapy for locally advanced breast cancer. *J Clin Oncol*; **26**: 4449–4457.

21. Tofts PS, Brix G, Buckley DL, *et al.* (1999) Estimating kinetic parameters from dynamic contrast-enhanced T1-weighted MRI of a diffusable tracer: Standardized quantities and symbols. *J Magn Reson Imaging*; **10**: 223–232.

22. Brix G, Henze M, Knopp MV, *et al.* (2001) Comparison of pharmacokinetic MRI and [18F] fluorodeoxyglucose PET in the diagnosis of breast cancer: Initial experience. *Eur Radiol*; **11**: 2058–2070.

23. Knopp MV, von Tengg-Kobligk H, Choyke PL. (2003) Functional magnetic resonance imaging in oncology for diagnosis and therapy monitoring. *Mol Cancer Ther*; **2**: 419–426.
24. Hayes C, Padhani AR, Leach MO. (2002) Assessing changes in tumour vascular function using dynamic contrast-enhanced magnetic resonance imaging. *NMR in Biomed*; **15**: 154–163.

Chapter 16
Receptor-Binding Peptide Imaging

E. Edmund Kim and Richard Baum

During the past two decades, radiolabeled receptor-binding peptides have emerged as an important class of radiopharmaceuticals that promise to dramatically change the field of nuclear medicine with new methods of synthesizing longer peptides in large quantities and purifying, characterizing, and optimizing them.[1] Peptides, are a small chain of amino acids coupled by peptide bond CONH and usually comprise less than 50 amino acids. At 100 amino acids or more, the string of amino acids is considered a protein (Fig. 16.1). The maximum molecular weight of a peptide is approximately 5,500 Da, since the average amino acid residue weight is about 110 Da. In contrast to antibody, this low-molecular-weight renders peptides rapid clearance and tissue penetration and low in antigenicity.[1] There are more than 900 well-characterized endogenous peptides that offer the possibility of wide applications in clinical medicine. Endogenous peptides have physiologic effects that may cause side effects, and thus it is preferable to use high-specific-activity compounds or antagonists that would exert high receptor specificity without physiologic effects. Receptor imaging is a localization of a radiolabeled compound that binds to cellular sites (receptors) with a high degree of affinity and specificity. Receptor binding is the first step in pharmacologic and hormonal signaling, and it is followed by a cascade of biochemical effects after receptor interaction. Approximately 80% of the hormonal messenges are peptides in mammals.[1]

Most peptides have a very short biologic half-life because of rapid proteolysis by circulating enzymes which usually have very defined specificities. Judicious use of D-amino acids and the end-capping process can induce resistance to *in vivo* enzymatic degradation. Hydrophilic peptides may be

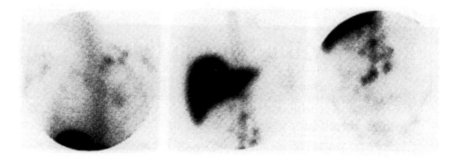

Fig. 16.1. Anterior static images of chest and abdomen at 72 hours after injection of [111]In (ProstaScint) show metastatic prostate cancers in retroperitoneal, left hilar, and left supraclavicular lymph nodes with prostatic membrane antigen.

removed rapidly by the kidneys, and lipophilic peptides can be sequestered by the liver and may be eliminated by hepatobiliary excretion. Peptides should be radiolabeled at a certain position that will not interfere with their binding to their biologic target. A chelate is frequently covalently coupled to the peptide. This process can adversely influence the biologic activity or receptor specificity of a peptide. Binding to the receptor on the target surface generally triggers the signal transduction mechanism of the target cell for the transmission of the biological effect to the target tissue. The specific receptor-binding property of the ligand can be exploited by labeling the ligand as a radiopharmaceutical to image and/or treat tissues expressing particular receptors. Such ligands, e.g., hormones and neurotransmitters, can act as chemical messengers.

Virtually every tumor type has shown an antibody prepared to some component of the tumor cell, and tumor-derived antigens are usually one of several types. They are epitopes that are uniquely expressed on tumors. Any of the known cell or tumor regulator receptor may be used as antigens. The clinical utility of radiolabeled monoclonal antibodies has been limited to date, probably due to poor contrast between the target and background and thus often repeat and delayed imaging. Multiple factors influence the clinical utility of scintigraphic agents and they represent characteristics of the agents, characteristics of the lesion, nature of interaction between the agent and the lesion, as well as the background. It is not surprising to observe that greater the percentage of injected dose taken up by the tumor, smaller the lesion detected.

16.1. Receptor Targeting in Oncology

Tumors may overexpress various receptor types. Somatostatin (SST) receptors (SSTRs) are expressed in the majority of neuroendocrine tumors (Figs. 16.2–16.4), neuroblastomas, some pheochromocytomas, medullary thyroid carcinomas, small cell lung cancers (SCLCs), and prostate cancers. Vasoactive intestinal peptide (VIP) receptors are expressed in neuroendocrine tumors, astrocytomas, meningiomas, and lymphomas.

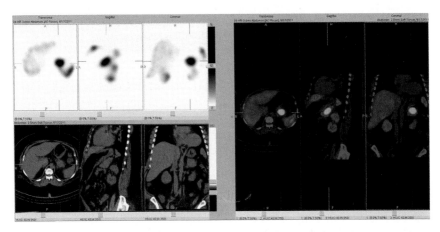

Fig. 16.2. Markedly increased uptake of ^{111}In octreotide in the neuroendocrine tumor in the pancreatic tail with SSTR 2 and/or 5.

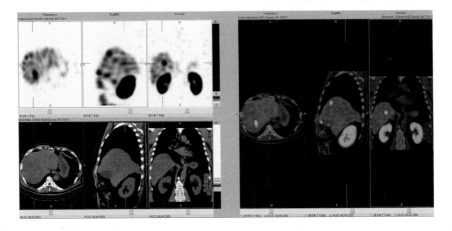

Fig. 16.3. [111]In octreotide scan shows metastatic hepatic lesions of neuroendocrine tumor.

371

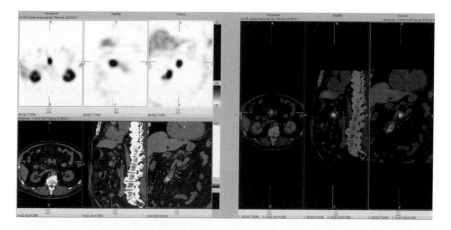

Fig. 16.4. Uptake of ^{111}In octreotide in the mesenteric metastatic lesion of neuroendocrine tumor.

Gastrin-releasing peptide (GRP) receptors have shown to be expressed in prostate carcinomars, and cholecystokinin (CCK)-B/gastrin receptors are expressed in almost all medullary thyroid carcinomas, SCLCs, some ovarian cancers, and astrocytomas. Neurotensin (NT) receptors are expressed in Ewing's sarcomas, meningiomas, astrocytomas and ductal pancreatic adenocarcinomas. The majority of breast cancers express calcitonin receptors.[2] Radiolabeled peptides binding each of these receptors (Fig. 16.5) have been

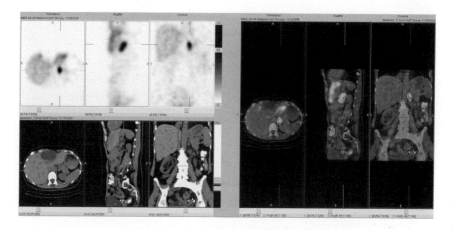

Fig. 16.5. Uptake of I-123 MIBG in left pheochromcytoma with chromaffin granules.

tested as a vehicle to target cancer lesions for the diagnostic peptide–receptor radionuclide imaging (PRRI) using gamma emitters and also peptide–receptor radionuclide therapy (PRRT) using beta emitters.

16.2. Somatostatin

Somatostatin (SST) is a peptide hormone produced by degradation of a precursor protein and inhibits the secretion of various hormones such as gastrin, insulin, and growth hormone. It also acts as a neurotransmitter in the brain and as a therapeutic agent for endocrine-active tumors. SST is a 14-amino-acid polypeptide with one disulfide bridge between two cysteine residues. The wild-type SST is very susceptible to enzymatic degradation, and thus an 8-amino-acid analogue of this tetradecapeptide, designated as octreotide, has been developed. Octreotide binds with high affinity to SSTR2 and SSTR5, to lesser extent to SSTR3, but it does not bind to SSTR1 or SSTR4. The third amino acid, phenylalanine, has been replaced by a tyrosine (Tyr) residue to allow radioiodination of the octreotide. Octreotide has been substituted N-terminally with DTPA to allow efficient labeling with ^{111}In, and ^{111}In DTPA-octreotide showed less hepatobiliary clearance than the ^{123}I labeled one.[2] ^{111}In emits not only gamma rays but also short-range Auger electrons that can be cytotoxic after internalization of the radiolabeled peptides.

Besides octreotide, a series of other SSTR-binding peptides has been developed. It has been suggested that lanreotide, unlike octreotide, has a high affinity for SSTR3 and SSTR4.[3] A new SST analog, 1,4,7,10-tetraaza-cyclododecane-N, N', N", N"'-tetraacetic acid (DOTA)-Tyr3-octreotide has been developed, and DOTA-Tyr3-octreotide showed a higher binding affinity for SSTR2 than DTPA-octreotide.

Interest and research in ^{68}Ge and ^{68}Ga (having half-lives of 9 months and 68 minutes, respectively) have been recently revived since a major advantage of ^{68}Ge/^{68}Ga generator is its continuous source of ^{68}Ga, independently from an on-site cyclotron. ^{68}Ga DOTA-NOC has been found to be superior to ^{68}Ga DOTA-TATE and used for routine receptor positron emission tomography/computed tomography (PET/CT) of neuroendocrine tumors.[4] DOTANOC has very high affinity for receptor subtypes 2, 3, and 5.[5]

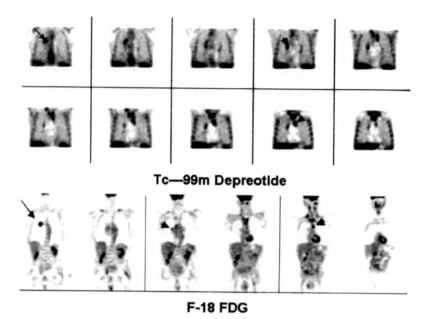

Tc—99m Depreotide

F-18 FDG

Fig. 16.6. Uptakes of Tc-99m depreotide (P829) and ^{18}F-FDG in lung cancer in the posterior right upper lung and metastatic bilateral paratracheal lymph nodes with SSTR 2, 3 and/or 5.

A cyclic somatostatin analogue lacking a disulfide bridge that can be labeled with Tc-99m was developed. Tc-99m depreotide (NeoTect; P829) binds with high affinity to SSTR2,SSTR3, and SSTR5.[2] Tc-99m P829 scintigraphy correctly identified or excluded in 27 of 30 patients with solitary pulmonary nodules (Fig. 16.6). It also revealed visualization of breast cancer lesions in 7 of 8 patients and in 6 of 6 patients with melanomas.[1] A peptide designated as vapreotide (RC160) was labeled with ^{123}I, ^{111}In, ^{99m}Tc, or [188]Re. In contrast to octreotide, vapreotide has been reported to pass the blood brain barrier and thus may be used to image brain tumors.[2]

16.3. Vasoactive Intestinal Peptide

Vasoactive Intestinal Peptide (VIP) is a 28-amino-acid peptide with a wide range of biological activites and an affinity for the SSTR3 receptor that is bound by p829 and lanreotide. VIP receptors are widely distributed throughout the gastrointestinal tract and also expressed on adenocarcinomas, melanomas, neuroblastomas, and breast and pancreatic carcinomas.[2] VIP promotes both the growth and proliferation of normal and malignant cells. [123]I VIP would not be a cost-effective competitor for ^{111}In octreotide in detecting neuroendocrine tumors. [123]I VIP was superior to ^{111}In octreotide for identifiying the lesions of colorectal carcinomas.[1] [123]I VIP could fill a diagnostic gap in detecting pancreatic cancer.

16.4. Bombesin, Calcitonin, and Cholecystokinin

Bombeisin is a 14-amino-acid neuropeptide which has a high affinity for gastrin-releasing peptide (GRP) receptor. GRP is overexpressed in a variety of cancers, and their activation stimulates both cell growth and proliferation. Despite similar receptor affinity, the agonist (In-111 DTPA-Pro 1,Tyr4-bombeisin) was internalized by bombesin receptor-positive cells, whereas the antagonist (In-111 DTPA-Tyr5, Phe6-bombesin) was not. The agonist showed much higher tumor uptake.[2]

Calcitonin receptors are overexpressed in the majority of breast cancer cell lines, and P1410 is a calcitonin receptor–binding peptide, which has a 4-amino-acid chelating sequence. The peptide can be labeled with Tc-99m or Re-188. Cholecystokinin (CCK) and gastrin are peptides in the brain and the intestines. They are frequently overexpressed in medullary thyroid cancer, small cell lung cancer, astrocytoma, and stromal ovarian cancer. Receptor-specific uptake of ^{111}In DOTA CCK was demonstrated in the stomach and in tumor metastases.[2]

16.5. Epidermal Growth Factor and Vitronectin Receptor

Epidermal growth factor (EGF) is a large peptide involved in cell growth. Its upregulation is inversely correlated with estrogen receptor expression and directly correlated with poor response to hormonal therapy. Labeling with Tc-99m or In-111 did not reduce the receptor affinity.[2] Integrins are heterodimeric transmembrane glycoproteins consisting of alpha and beta subunits. They are receptors involved in cell adhesion processes and highly expressed in sprouting endothelium. The tripeptic sequence Arg-Gly-Asp

(RGD) is the primary site of recognition by vitronectin receptor, which is highly expressed on osteosarcomas, neuroblastomas, melanomas, and lung, breast, prostate, and bladder cancers. A decapeptide, containing two RGD sequences and cystein residue to facilitate labeling with Tc-99m was synthesized and characterized.

16.6. Infectious and Inflammatory Imaging Peptides

Infection is a condition caused by microorganisms that may lead to an inflammatory response. Inflammation is the response of tissues to injury to serum molecules and cells of the immune system to the affected site. The inflammatory response is characterized by locally increased blood flow, increased vascular permeability, enhanced transudation of plasma proteins, and enhanced influx of leukocytes. The ideal radiopharmaceutical for infection imaging should accumulate rapidly in infectious and inflammatory foci and rapidly clear from non-inflamed tissues. Peptides with high affinity for receptors as expressed preferentially on infiltrating leukocytes could meet such criteria.

483-H contains a heparin-binding sequence from the C-terminus of platelet factor-4 that facilitates cell binding to Tc-99m and binds to circulating and inflammation-activated leukocytes. RP-128 is a small peptide directed to the tuftsin receptor. Tuftsin, a leukokinin-derived tetrapeptide, stimulates chemotaxis and phagocytosis of polymorphonuclear (PMN) leukocytes, monocytes, and macrophages. RP-128 consists of a 5-amino-acid receptor antagonist linked by a Gly to a N_3S amino acid Tc-99m binder.

The most extensively studied chemotactic peptides have been derivatives of N-formyl-Met-Leu-Phe, which is an analogue of peptides secreted by bacteria that promote the migration of both PMN and monocytes to the site of bacterial invasion. More work has been directed to increasing the stability of the Tc-99m complex and chemically modifying the peptide to improve antagonist formyl peptide receptor binding.

Radiolabeled antimicrobial peptides have been synthesized in PMN and stored in granules. These peptides possibly differentiate an infectious from non-infectious inflammation. Elastase is an enzyme secreted by activated

PMN in response to inflammatory stimuli, and a high-affinity inhibitor is present in tissues. Peptide analogues of this inhibitor have been developed with the use of phage display technology.

Interleukin (IL)-1 binds receptors expressed mainly on granulocytes, monocytes, and lymphocytes with high affinity. The naturally occurring IL-1 receptor antagonist was labeled with ^{123}I to evaluate a rheumatoid arthritis. Chronic inflammation was targeted with ^{123}I or Tc-99m by means of specific binding to IL-2 receptors, expressed on activated T lymphocytes. It seems a suitable agent for targeting mononuclear cell infiltration in autoimmune disorders such as Hashimoto thyroiditis and Crohn's disease.[1,2]

16.7. Thrombus Imaging Peptides

The detection of thrombi and emboli by hot spot imaging has been a goal in radiopharmaceutical development. The homeostasis process maintains a precarious balance between the thrombogenic substances and antithrombotics. Most clotting factors are enzymes that become proteases when activated. When blood vessel ruptures and the sub-endothelium is exposed, a platelet plug is formed. Platelets release stored adenosine diphosphate and thromboxane A_2, which stimulates the platelets to aggregate. This activation exposes the glycoprotein (GP) IIb/IIIa receptor on the platelet 's surface. Fibrinogen present in the blood adheres to this receptor and forms a bridge between platelets, promoting further clumping. [125]I fibrinogen is no longer commercially available. Most of the antiplatelet antibodies were directed against the GP IIb/IIIa receptor.

AcuTect (P280) is a dimer which contains an RGD mimetic sequence, S-aminoprophyl-L-cystein (apc)-GD. The sensitivity, specificity, and agreement rates of nuclear venogram using Tc-99m AcuTect were 91%, 84% and 87%, respectively, when the clinical information was taken into consideration (Fig. 16.7). DMP-444 (HYNICtide) consists of a rigid RGD analogue, 6-aminocaproic acid (Aca), attached to amynobenzyl benzoic acid, and a hydrazinonicotyl (HYNIC) group for Tc-99m binding. Bitistatin, called disintegrin, binds to GP IIb/IIIa platelet receptor with high affinity. This large peptide has been labeled with [123]I. The fibrin-binding domain (FBD) peptide consists of 5 repeated sequences which contain 20 cysteine residues. [111]In or

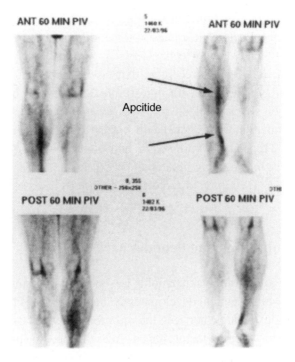

Fig. 16.7. Delayed static images at 60 minutes after injection of Tc-99m apcitide (P820) show new DVT in right calf vein.

Tc-99m labeled FBD has been tested in animals. TP 850 is a peptide from N-terminal of the alpha chain of fibrin that binds to the C-terminal gamma chain. This agent depends on fibrin binding and not on the accumulation of activated platelet, and thus has the potential to detect both acute and aged clots.[1,2]

References

1. Weiner RE, Thakur M. (2001) Radiolabeled peptides in diagnosis and therapy. *Semin Nucl Med* **4**: 296–311.
2. Boerman OC, Oyen WJG, Corstens FHM. (2000) Radio-labeled receptor-binding peptides: A new class of radiopharmaceuticals. *Semin Nucl Med* **30**: 195–208.
3. Smith-Jones PM, Bischof C, Leimer M, *et al.* (1999) DOTA-lanreotide: A novel somatostatin analog for tumor diagnosis and therapy. *Endocrinology* **140**: 5136–5148.

4. Breeman WAP, de Blois E, Chan HS *et al.* (2011) Ga-68 labeled DOTA-peptides and radiopharmaceuticals for PET: Current status of research, clinical applications, and future perspectives. *Semin Nucl Med* **41**: 314–321.
5. Prasad V, Ambrosini V, Hommann M, *et al.* (2010) Detection of unknown primary neuroendocrine tumors (CUP-NET) using Ga-68 DOTA-NOC receptor PET/CT. *Eur J Nucl Med Mol Imaging* **37**: 67–77.

Chapter 17
In vivo Molecular Imaging

Keon Wook Kang

Molecular imaging is a technology visualizing molecular targets or processes of cells, tissues, and body through imaging. It is a conversion technology combining two major disciplines: molecular biology and *in vivo* imaging. Molecular imaging has two components: molecular probes to targeting specific biomarkers in, on, and around cells, and sensors to detect the signals from those probes. Various signals from the molecular probes can be used, such as gamma-ray, light, magnetic resonance, and ultrasound. Matching sensing technologies are used for detecting signals such as positron emission tomography (PET), single-photon emission computed tomography (SPECT), optical imaging system, magnetic resonance imaging (MRI), and ultrasonography. We can detect the amount or activities of transporters, receptors, peptides, enzymes, and gene expressions using small molecules, peptides, antibodies, and synthetic nanoparticles. Recently, the scope of molecular imaging has been enlarging, scaling down to cellular, sub-cellular, or single molecular level using live cell fluorescent microscopy, multi-photon microscopy, atomic force microscopy, and *in vivo* confocal microscopy.

Applications of molecular imaging include medical utilizations in hospitals, biological research in science, and drug development in pharmaceutical industry. Medical applications include early diagnosis, companion diagnostics for tailored medicine, therapeutic monitoring, and predicting prognosis of diseases such as cancer, neurological, and cardiovascular diseases. Biomedical applications include research on signal transduction pathways, molecular interactions, gene expressions, RNAi, cell trafficking, and stem cell differentiation. Industrial applications include drug development, lead optimization, and prediction of effects or adverse effects using *in vivo* imaging of biodistribution, pharmacokinetics, pharmacodynamics, non-invasive measuring targeting efficiency, and duration of efficacy of small molecule drugs, peptides, genes, cells, and nanodrug delivery systems in preclinical and clinical settings.

17.1. Molecular Imaging and Nuclear Medicine

Nuclear medicine leads molecular imaging using radiopharmaceuticals as high-sensitive molecular probes. Traditional radioiodine imaging is one of the good examples of molecular imaging and theragnosis (Fig. 17.1). Radioiodine therapy and gamma ray imaging, which began from the late 1930s, is still an effective treatment and monitoring method of patients

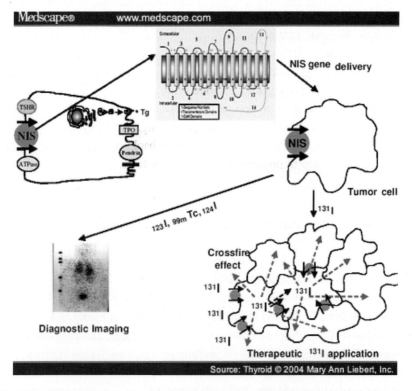

Fig. 17.1. Molecular mechanism of radioiodine imaging and therapy (Thyroid 2004, Mary Ann Liebert, Inc).

with thyroid cancer in clinics. Radioiodine ^{131}I accumulates in thyroid or differentiated thyroid cancer cells through sodium/iodide symporter (NIS), and the whole-body gamma camera imaging reveals molecular activity of NIS from patients.

The major advantages of nuclear medicine technique are ultra-high sensitivity and high penetration property in the body. Nanomolar or picomolar level of molecular probes can be detected, which is 1000 times more sensitive than MRI. In these levels of concentration, even toxic materials can be injected into humans without any harmful or pharmacological effects. High tissue penetration property of gamma ray renders tomography imaging of body and quantification of molecular probes *in vivo*, which is not possible in optical imaging.

However, the nuclear medicine technique also has limitations. Spatial resolution is limited to the millimeter range, whereas optical imaging can be scaled down to microscopic level. Another limitation is that nuclear medicine imaging cannot discriminate metabolites from its mother molecules because radioactivity does not alter by changing of chemical structures. Recently, optical imaging by switchable optical probes increases signal-to-noise ratio using fluorescence resonance energy transfer (FRET) technology. This probe can be designed to turn on only when the desired molecular event occurs. However, radioactive signals are always turned on since it cannot be switched on and off. So the background activity reduces signal-to-noise ratio in nuclear medicine technology.

17.2. Molecular Imaging and Positron Emission Tomography

Positron emission tomography (PET) is a valuable tool for molecular imaging. It has higher sensitivity and better spatial resolution than gamma camera imaging or SPECT. Absolute quantification of molecular probes is possible due to attenuation, scatter, and random correction. One of the major advantages is that various radioisotopes are available from cyclotrons and generators. Positron-emitting radioisotopes such as ^{11}C, ^{15}O, ^{13}N, and ^{18}F are components of molecules consisting of peptides, nucleotides, and drugs. Therefore, labeling with these radioisotopes does not alter

Table 17.1. Molecular mechanism of PET radiopharmaceuticals.

Mode of Action	Radiopharmaceuticals
Substrate metabolism	^{18}F-FDG, O-15 O2, C-11 acetate, C-11 choline
Protein synthesis	C-11 methionine, C-11 tyrosine
DNA synthesis	C-11 thymidine, ^{18}F-FLT, ^{18}F-FMAU
Hypoxia or Angiogenesis	^{18}F-FMISO, Cu-64 ATSM, Ga-68 RGD peptide
Drugs	C-11 cocaine, N-13 cisplatin, ^{18}F-fluorouracil
Receptor affinity	C-11 raclopride, C-11 carfentanil, ^{18}F-FP-Gluc-TOCA
Neurotransmitter biochemistry	^{18}F-fluorodopa, ^{18}F-FESP, C-11 ephedrine
Amyloid plaque	C-11 PIB, ^{18}F-AV-1
Gene expression	^{18}F-FHBG, I-124 FIAU
Antibodies	I-124 anti-CEA minibody, Cu-64 anti-Her2 minibody

the chemical structures of molecules which we want to look at *in vivo*. Theoretically, any molecules can be radiolabeled, and these probes can trace and reveal its molecular behavior *in vivo* according to their mode of actions (Table 17.1). The most common example of molecular tracer is F-18-2-fluoro-2-deoxyglucose (^{18}F-FDG). FDG-PET reflects the activity of glucose metabolism *in vivo* as ^{18}F-FDG trapped in cells by glucose transporter and hexokinase. Due to the increased glucose metabolism of cancer, FDG became the most common PET agent for oncologic diagnosis such as differential diagnosis, staging, monitoring therapy, and detecting recurrence of cancer in clinics. Other promising agents for PET are C-11 Pittsburgh compound B (PIB) and ^{18}F AV-1 targeting β-amyloid proteins in the brain for early diagnosis of Alzheimer's disease.

Radiolabeled antibodies, peptides, and aptamers can be used for PET imaging. For example, [124]I-labeled Herceptin could be used for evaluating Her2 status *in vivo* and RGD peptides for evaluating angiogenesis. Cyclic RGD (Arg-Gly-Asp) peptide is known to bind with $\alpha v \beta_3$ integrin expressed in the angiogenic endothelial cells. PET using Ga-68 RGD peptide, Arg-Gly-Asp-D-Tyr-Lys [c(RGDyK)] conjugated with NOTA (1,4,7-triazacyclononane-1,4,7-triacetic acid) and labeled with positron emitter Ga-68, showed angiogenic activities of tumors in patients. Angiogenesis PET could predict the response of malignant tumors to anti-angiogenic therapy such as bevacizumab and might help to select appropriate patients.

One of the limitations using PET is that it lacks detailed anatomical information. Even though spatial resolution of recent PET scanners improved to $1 \sim 2$ mm range, PET detects and reveals the only the location of molecular probes and not the anatomical structures. So multimodal imaging systems such as PET/CT or PET/MR will solve this limitation.

17.3. Reporter Gene Imaging

The name molecular imaging originated from "molecular-genetic imaging," which is imaging reporter genes. In the field of molecular biology, measuring certain gene expression levels have been determined by assaying reporter gene expression in cells from decades ago. A recombinant plasmid that expresses simultaneously a gene of interest and a reporter gene, such as luciferase, and green fluorescent protein is transfected into target cells. If the gene of interest is a therapeutic gene, reporter gene imaging enables the locations, durations, and magnitudes of therapeutic gene expressions *in vivo*.

For nuclear medicine technology, various imaging reporter genes matched with positron- and gamma-emitting probes have been developed. The Herpes simplex virus-1 thymidine kinase (HSV_1-tk) system has been used most commonly. The plasmid HSV_1-tk is transcribed to HSV_1-tk mRNA, which is then translated to HSV_1-TK protein enzyme. The expressed TK then phosphorylates its substrates, acyclovir, ganciclovir, or penciclovir, which are drugs to treat Herpes viral infection by killing infected cells. Thus HSV_1-tk has been tried for suicidal gene therapy for cancers. If we use radiolabeled penciclovir analogue, ^{18}F 9-(4-fluoro-3-hydroxymethylbutyl)-guanine (^{18}F-FHBG), which accumulate in transfected cells and it emits positrons that can be visualized by PET. Thus, PET can localize and measure the activity of HSV_1-tk reporter gene expression. ^{18}F-FHBG has been approved by the U.S. Food and Drug Administration (FDA) as an investigational drug.

To improve substrate uptake, several different reporter probes have been tested. FMAU and FIAU were once abandoned for anti-viral therapeutics due to their mitochondrial toxicities and lethal effects on neurons and liver in clinical studies. However, by taking advantage of the high sensitivities of PET and SPECT, it is possible to administer trace doses of these drugs labeled with radioisotopes (^{18}F-FMAU, ^{131}I FIAU) and probe *HSV*$_1$-*tk* expression *in vivo*. Because of its high sensitivity and selectivity, FEAU has been suggested to be a promising reporter probe for *HSV*$_1$-*tk*.

A number of investigators examine the use of gamma emitters for reporter gene imaging. The simplest and the most applicable one is NIS gene system. Iodine enters thyroid cells with sodium through NIS. The NIS gene was identified in 1996 by Carrasco in the rat, and its human equivalent (hNIS) was isolated and cloned using the complementary DNA sequence of rat NIS. NIS has many advantages as an imaging reporter gene because of the wide availability of its substrates, i.e., radioiodines and Tc-99m. Reporter gene imaging using NIS is easy to apply, because all nuclear medicine departments have access to gamma cameras, SPECT, radioiodines, and Tc-99m.

Optical imaging modalities such as fluorescence and bioluminescence imaging are simple, cheap, and convenient. Many molecular biologists already get used to luciferase assay or spectrometer measurement using firefly luciferase or green fluorescent reporter gene in cells. For the sake of *in vivo* optical imaging system equipped with high-sensitivity, low-noise, cooled CCD camera, imaging can be acquired *in vivo* using optical reporter genes. However, the attenuation effect of light photons in the tissues or organs limits its use only in small animals. Moreover, photon intensities may not reflect reporter gene expression proportionately, and quantification of gene expression is not possible.

Reporter gene imaging can be applied to the monitoring of cell therapy, such as immune or stem cells. After stem cells have been administered in the body systemically or locally, they may migrate, repopulate, and differentiate. Reporter gene imaging techniques can provide information on cell trafficking, cell viability, and cell numbers. After the stable transfection of cells with an imaging reporter gene, an imaging system matched with imaging probe can visualize the distribution and survival of stem cells longitudinally. Successful differentiation of stem cells into functional cells can be also visualized using reporter genes with tissue-specific promoters.

17.4. Multimodal Molecular Imaging

Fluorescent materials, radioisotopes, and MRI enhancers can be used for optical imaging, PET, or MRI. Since each modality has its own advantages and limitations, the single modal imaging method does not provide optimal solutions for solving the issues of sensitivity, resolution, and tissue penetration of signal. PET has high sensitivity but poor spatial resolution, and it provides poor anatomical information. MRI has high spatial resolution but poorer sensitivity than PET or optical imaging. Advances in clinical imaging are being made through combinations of different imaging modalities, such as PET/CT and PET/MRI. Fluorescent signal has poor tissue penetration but can be detected by a videoscope during medical or surgical procedures, or by a fluorescent microscope in subcellular level. Multimodal technique combining PET/MRI/optical imaging will overcome the limitations of each modality.

Combined PET/CT is widely used in clinics to overcome this issue. Recently, combining PET with MRI scanner was actively under investigation, and clinical PET/MRI scanner will be commercially available in the near future. Unlike CT scanner, MRI can detect signals from the nanoparticles as a molecular probe. Although MRI probes are much less sensitive than PET probes, it can be monitored longer than PET probes because it is not affected by the physical half-life of radioisotopes.

PET/MRI/fluorescent triple modality imaging using multifunctional nanoparticles can guide surgical operation especially minimal invasive procedures such as endoscopic, laparoscopic or robotic surgery (Fig. 17.2). When PEGylated magnetic silica nanoparticles containing near-infrared fluorescent dye, NIR-797 isothiocyanate, and iron oxide core conjugated with ^{68}Ga NOTA was injected subcutaneously into foot-pad on the leg of mice, these nanoparticles localized sentinel lymph nodes by triple-modal imaging using an animal PET/CT scanner, animal MRI, and *in vivo* optical imaging system.

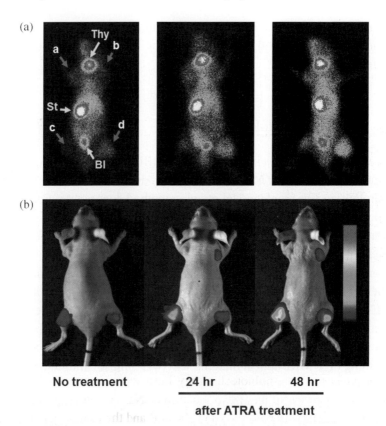

Fig. 17.2. Non-invasive and repetitive gamma camera imaging of Tc-99m by NIS (a) and bioluminescence imaging by luciferase (b) to the response of ATRA (all transretinoic acid) in nude mice bearing SK-HEP1 and SK-RARE/NL tumors. Xenograft tumors derived from SK-HEP1 (a, 1X10^7 wild-type)and SK-RARE/NL cells (b, 1×10^6; c, 1×10^7; d, 1×10^8) were grown in male nude mice (Thy = thyroid; St = stomach; Bl = bladder).

(*Source*: Tseng JR *et al.* (2008) Preclinical efficacy of the c-Met inhibitor CE-355621 in a U87 MG mouse xenograft model evaluated by 18F-FDG small-animal PET. *J Nucl Med* **49**(1): 129–134.)

If we use triple modality molecular probes targeting cancer in patients with malignant tumor, we can assess the locations of tumors and metastatic lymph nodes using whole body PET/MRI (Fig. 17.3). And then surgeon can locate the tumors, tumor margin, and lymph nodes by fluorescent signal using a videoscope during the operation. The pathologist then can assess tumor margin and lymph nodes using fluorescent microscope. Finally, post-operative MRI can confirm all the lesions are removed.

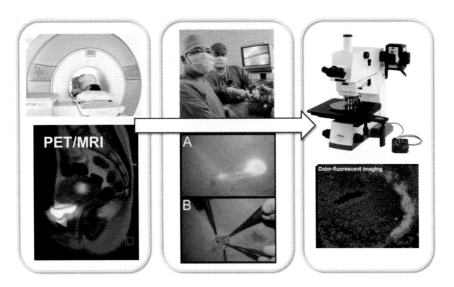

Fig. 17.3. Surgical guidance using PET/MRI/fluorescent imaging after injecting multimodal nanoparticles.

17.5. Molecular Imaging Using Nanoparticles

Recent advances in nanobiotechnology have identified many candidates of molecular probes for medical applications. Nanotechnology can control the size of materials in nanoscale (1–100 nm) and the unique chemical and physical properties of them. Nanoparticles are able to carry fluorescent dye, radioisotope, drugs, genes, and targeting biomarkers on their surface and inside. Some nanoparticles, such as quantum dots, exhibit fluorescence itself with different colors according to their size. Nanoparticle can carry fluorescent dyes inside or on their surface. Nanoparticles containing iron oxide can emit magnetic resonance signal under high magnetic field. If nanoparticles labeled with radioisotopes, they can be detected by gamma cameras or PET scanners. Nanoparticles can handle multiple chemical properties and has a potential for multifunctional and multimodal properties. These multifunction nanoparticles as multimodal molecular probes can be used for diagnostics both *in vitro* and *in vivo*, as well as therapeutic purposes.

One of the applications is molecular imaging targeting biomarkers. For example, quantum dot–conjugated Herceptin could be used for evaluating Her2 status in tissues and *in vivo* as a companion diagnostics to select appropriate patients who will be treated using Herceptin. Fluorescent nanoparticles, such as quantum dots and nanosilica containing fluorescent dye are emerging imaging materials for biology and medicine. In comparison with organic fluorescent dyes, fluorescent nanoparticles have unique optical properties such as superior signal brightness, resistance to photobleaching, and multiple fluorescence colors. These properties are most promising for improving the sensitivity and multiplexing capabilities of molecular imaging both *in vitro* and *in vivo*.

We can add targeting function to the nanoparticles by conjugating three-dimensional (3D) scaffold such as antibodies, peptides, and aptamers. As a result, the particles can trace targets and reveal the lesions after systemic administration. If we combine nanotechnology and high-throughput proteomics searching for individual biomarkers, personalized targeting therapy can be possible after validating the targeting efficiency using multimodal multiplexing *in vivo* imaging.

17.6. Translational Research Using Molecular Imaging

Small animal PET cameras have been developed to meet the need for translational research from bench to bedside (Fig. 17.4). Recently, commercialized animal PET scanner has a spatial resolution of 1 mm. In addition, high-resolution small animal SPECT systems with multi-pinhole collimators have also been developed to overcome poor sensitivity of gamma imaging. Molecular imaging in animals using nuclear medicine technology can be easily translated into human because the same modality is available in clinics. Furthermore, advances in imaging technology have now resulted in the development of fused imaging modalities, such as PET/CT, SPECT/CT, and PET/MRI. These fusion modalities allow us to obtain biological information in combination with precise anatomical localization in a single imaging session.

One of the common applications of non-invasive *in vivo* molecular imaging such as FDG PET and luciferase reporter gene optical imaging in animal is a visually monitoring of tumor burden at primary sites. It also offers a longitudinal monitoring method for cancer progression, metastasis, and therapy in whole body of animals without sacrificing them.

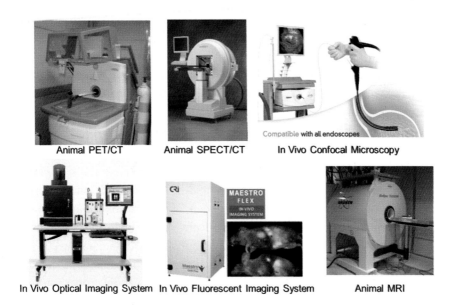

Animal PET/CT   Animal SPECT/CT   In Vivo Confocal Microscopy

In Vivo Optical Imaging System   In Vivo Fluorescent Imaging System   Animal MRI

Fig. 17.4. *In vivo* animal imaging equipments for translational research.

Another application is a pre-clinical testing for drug development. Radiolabeled new drugs can be measured and located effectively and quantitatively in animals by either animal PET or SPECT scanner after injecting drugs into animals. These can evaluate biodistribution, pharmacodynamics, pharmacokinetics, excretion pathways, and possibly toxicologic aspects of investigational new drugs, which would lead to more efficient and rational candidate drug screening protocols, and considerable cost and time reductions.

Transgenic mice expressing a specific reporter gene can be produced by injecting a gene fragment of interest into fertilized eggs. The major advantage of reporter animals is that they provide measurable endpoints for evaluating drug efficacy in all tissues. They provide us an opportunity to better understand physiological and pathological mechanisms and allow the effects of therapies in models of specific diseases. The differentiation of stem cells to mature functional cells in the target tissues is critical for successful stem cell therapy. A transgenic mouse model with alpha-myosin heavy chain (MHC) promoter and NIS as a reporter gene was developed to image differentiation of cardiomyocyte. Nuclear medicine images obtained using I-131 and I-124 in transgenic mice showed radioiodine uptake only in the myocardium. By injecting bone marrow–derived stem cells obtained from these transgenic animals into other animals with myocardial infarct, radioiodine scintigraphy or PET could be used to confirm the differentiation of stem cells into mature cardiomyocytes.

Continued improvements in instrumentation, the identification of novel targets and genes, and the availability of improved imaging probes indicate that molecular imaging is likely to play an important role in clinic as well as basic research. Furthermore, dual- or triple-reporter constructs for optical and nuclear medicine imaging provide opportunities for multi-modal imaging, and should ease the transition between laboratory studies and clinical application. The collaborative efforts of physicists, molecular biologists, radiochemists, bioengineers, computer scientists, and clinicians have led to substantial recent advances in detection devices, imaging analysis software, tissue- or disease-specific reporter genes, and target-specific probes. Molecular imaging is expected to play a major role in the personalized healthcare and therapy in the near future.

References

1. Lee HY, Chung JK, Lee JJ, Oh SW, Kang KW, Park DJ, Cho BY, Lee MC. (2010) Radioiodine treatment of differentiated thyroid carcinoma: The experience at Seoul National University Hospital. *Current Medical Imaging Reviews* **6**: 2–7.
2. Lee HY, Kang KW, Kim TY, Lee YS, Jeong JM, Han SW, Paeng JC, Chung JK, Lee MC, Lee DS. (2010) Angiogenesis imaging using 68Ga-RGD PET: Preliminary report from Seoul National University Hospital. *Current Medical Imaging Reviews* **6**(1): 56–59.
3. Jeon YH, Kim YH, Choi K, Piao JY, Quan B, Lee YS, Jeong JM, Chung JK, Lee DS, Lee MC, Lee J, Chung DS, Kang KW. (2010) *In vivo* imaging of sentinel nodes using fluorescent silica nanoparticles in living mice. *Mol Imaging Biol* **12**(2): 155–162.
4. Tseng JR, Kang KW, Dandekar M, Yaghoubi S, Lee JH, Christensen JG, Muir S, Vincent PW, Michaud NR, Gambhir SS. (2008) Preclinical efficacy of the c-Met inhibitor CE-355621 in a U87 MG mouse xenograft model evaluated by 18F-FDG small-animal PET. *J Nucl Med* **49**(1): 129–134.
5. Kang KW, Jeong JM, Beer AJ. (2010) Angiogenesis PET using radiolabeled RGD peptides. Chapter 12 In: Fanti S, Farsad M, Mansi L, eds. *PET-CT Beyond FDG*, pp. 195–211, Springer, Berlin.
6. Kang JH, Chung JK. (2008) Molecular-genetic imaging based on reporter gene expression. *J Nucl Med* **49**(Suppl 2): 164S–79S.

7. Willmann JK, van Bruggen N, Dinkelborg LM, Gambhir SS. (2008) Molecular imaging in drug development. *Nat Rev Drug Discov* **7**(7): 591–607.
8. Gambhir SS. (2002) Molecular imaging of cancer with positron emission tomography. *Nat Rev Cancer* **2**(9): 683–693.
9. Tjuvajev JG, Finn R, Watanabe K, Joshi R, Oku T, Kennedy J, Beattie B, Koutcher J, Larson S, Blasberg RG. (1996) Noninvasive imaging of herpes virus thymidine kinase gene transfer and expression: a potential method for monitoring clinical gene therapy. *Cancer Res* **56**(18): 4087–4095.
10. Kang KW, Min JJ, Chen X, Gambhir SS. Comparison of [(14)C]FMAU, [(3)H]FEAU, [(14)C]FIAU, and [(3)H]PCV for monitoring reporter gene expression of wild type and mutant herpes simplex virus type 1 thymidine kinase in cell culture. *Mol Imaging Biol* **7**: 296–303.
11. Kang JH, Lee DS, Paeng JC, Lee JS, Kim YH, Lee YJ, Hwang DW, Jeong JM, Lim SM, Chung JK, Lee MC. (2005) Development of a sodium/iodide symporter (NIS)-transgenic mouse for imaging of cardiomyocyte-specific reporter gene expression. *J Nucl Med* **46**(3): 479–483.

Chapter 18
In Vitro Nuclear Medicine Tests

E. Edmund Kim

18.1. Carbon-14 Urea Breath Test

The causal relationship between *Helicobacter pylori* (HP) and chronic gastritis is well known, and only small fraction of HP-positive patients develop peptic ulcer disease (PUD). However, almost all patients with duodenal ulcer and most patients with other than non-steroidal anti-inflammatory drug-induced gastric ulcer are infected with HP. It has been known that HP infection is associated with adenocarcinoma and lymphoma in the stomach.[1]

The symptoms of gastric ulcer can include abdominal pain just below the ribcage, indigestion, nausea, vomiting, loss of appetite, weight loss, and anemia. The presence of active HP infection can be diagnosed non-invasively with the carbon-14 (^{14}C) urea breath test (UBT), which is based on the detection of urease produced by HP. The presence of urease can be equated with HP infection since it is not present in normal tissues and other urease-producing bacteria do not colonize the stomach. Orally administered ^{14}C urea will be hydrolyzed into ammonia and ^{14}C carbon dioxide; ^{14}C carbon dioxide is absorbed into the circulation and exhaled by the lungs, and thus the presence of a significant amount of ^{14}C carbon dioxide indicates active HP infection.

Indications

(a) To document HP eradication following anti-HP therapy for duodenal ulcer patients.
(b) For initial diagnosis as well as follow-up of gastric ulcer patients.

Procedure

1. Patient preparation: Patients should be off antibiotics and bismuth compounds such as Pepto Bismol for 30 days as well as Sucralfate and proton-pump inhibitors such as Prilosec and Prevacid for 2 weeks before the test. Patients should fast for more than 6 hours.
2. Precaution: None
3. Radiopharmaceutical: ^{14}C urea in capsule form containing 1 mg urea labeled with 1 uCi (37 kBq) ^{14}C, which is a pure beta emitter with a physical half-life of 3,730 years and maximum energy of 160 keV.
4. Procedure:
    4.1. Breath sample collection: Test begins with the patient swallowing the capsule containing 1 uCi ^{14}C urea with 20 ml warm water. The patient drinks another 20 ml of water at 3 min after dose. At 10 min postdose the patient is asked to take a deep breath, hold it for 5–10 sec, and then exhale through a straw into a mylar balloon. Another optional breath sample can be obtained at 15 min postdose.
    4.2. Breath sample analysis: 2.5 ml trapping solution is pipetted into a scintillation vial for each balloon. The trapping solution contains 1 mmol hyamine, methanol, and thymolphthalein. The air from the balloons is transferred into the scintillation vials using air pump and plastic tubing. The color change from blue to colorless of the collection fluid indicates the endpoint of transfer. At this point, 1 mmol CO_2 has been trapped. To each vial, 10 ml of suitable scintillation fluid is added and mixed thoroughly. A blank background sample and also a standard are counted for 5–20 min in a liquid scintillation counter using ^{14}C window.
5. Calculations: Raw sample counts per minute (cpm) should be background corrected and can be converted into disintegrations per minute (dpm) using the following equations:

$$dpm = \frac{(\text{sample cpm} - \text{blank cpm})}{\text{efficiency}} \qquad efficiency = \frac{(\text{standard cpm} - \text{blank cpm})}{\text{standard dpm}}$$

^{14}C standard should be prepared by adding a known volume (50 ul) of calibrated ^{14}C reference standard breath sample. The same volume of scintillation fluid as used for the patient samples is added. The sample should be counted with every set of patient samples. The efficiency of the counter for this test and scintillation cocktail can be determined.

6. Interpretation and Report

   Less than 50 dpm at 10 min = negative for HP; 50–199 dpm at 10 min = indeterminate for HP; more than 200 dpm at 10 min = positive for HP. Aside from patient's demographics, the report should include indication, procedure, result, interpretation, normal values, and limitations.

7. Source of errors

   False-negative results: antibiotics, Bismuth, Sucralfate, Prilosec, Prevacid, non-fasting, and gastric surgery

   False-positive results: achlorhydria, gastric surgery with bacterial overgrowth, and chemiluminescence

18.2. Schilling Test

Pernicious anemia is a form of megaloblastic anemia caused by inadequate secretion of gastric intrinsic factor (IF) and diagnosed easily with pancytopenia and megaloblastic bone marrow. Megaloblastic anemia mostly proves to be a nutritional defect caused by deficiency of vitamin B12, folic acid, or both. Vitamin B12 (cyanocobalamin) is freed from ingested animal protein by acid digestion in the stomach and bound by IF secreted by gastric parietal cells. B12 IF complex passes into the ileum where it attaches to specific receptors and absorbed. It is delivered to the liver with B12 delivery protein, transcobalamin II which binds nearly 30% of total serum cobalamin. Total vitamin B12 in the body is 5 mg, and pernicious anemia occurs when the vitamin B12 pool has been reduced to 10% of normal. Vitamin B12 deficiency may lead to glossitis, belching, indigestion, anorexia, and diarrhea.

Vitamin B12 absorption test introduced by Schilling in 1953 requires oral ingestion of 0.5 ug of ^{57}Co-labeled vitamin B12 and 0.5 ug of ^{58}Co-labeled vitamin B12 plus IF. Within 2 hours, an injection of 1 mg of unlabeled vitamin B12 is given intramuscularly to saturate vitamin B12 receptors in tissue and plasma. Much of the radiolabeled vitamin B12 is excreted in the urine, and the urine excretion of the activity is calculated as a percentage of the dose ingested. Normal excretion is 10%–45%, and normal IF-bound to free ratio is 0.7–1.3. Pernicious anemia shows greater than 1.7 bound to free ratio while malabsorption revelas 0.7–1.3 ratio.[2]

18.3. Blood Volume

The volume of fluid in a closed compartment can be measured with the use of radioactive material if it is distributed uniformly. By determining the extent to which the tracer becomes diluted when mixed uniformly in the fluid, the volume of the liquid can be calculated on the basis of the dilution technique:

$$V2 = C1 \times V1/C2,$$

where $C1$ and $V1$ are the concentration and volume before the dilution, respectively. Volume of diluents (ml) = Tracer quantity (cpm)/Tracer concentration in diluents (cpm/ml.

Total blood volume (BV) is measured by summing red cell volume (RCV) and plasma volume (PV) on the assumption that RCV is virtually the same as that of total circulating blood cells.

$$BV = RCV/0.9\ Ht \quad or \quad PV/(1 - 0.9Ht),$$

where 0.9 represents a mean of the ratio of whole body hematocrit (Ht) to venous Ht. In the RCV measurement, red cells from 15-ml whole blood are labeled with ^{51}Cr sodium chromate (28 days $T_{1/2}$ and 320 keV of ^{51}Cr), and the known amount of labeled red cell suspension is injected. Approximately 10–15 min later, a blood sample is taken from the vein other than that used for the injection.

$$RCV = S \times D \times V \times H/B,$$

where S = cpm/ml in diluted standard; D = final volume/RBC volume put into it; V = labeled RBC injected; and B = cpm/ml of blood sample after mixing. Normal values of RCV are 25–35 ml/kg in adult males and 20–30 ml/kg in females.

^{125}I (60 days $T_{1/2}$ and 30 keV) is used for estimation of PV. Since albumin diffuses rapidly into the extravascular spaces, it is better to take multiple timed (10, 20 and 30 min) blood samples.

$$PV = S \times D \times V/P$$

where S = cpm/ml standard, D = diluted standard, V = labeled albumin volume injected, and P = cpm/ml sample corrected to time 0 on semilog paper. Normal value of PV is about 40 ml/kg in both men and women.[3]

Polycythemia is a sustained abnormal increase of RCV, and increased hemoglobin level is accompanied by increased erythrocytes. Relative plocythemia is caused by fluid loss, extravascular shift of fluid, or Gaisbock's syndrome. Primary absolute polycythemia (erythemia, polycythemia vera) is a chronic myeloproliferative disorder with overproduction of erythrocytes and abnormalities of granulocytic as well as thrombocytic elements. Symptoms are due to increased blood viscosity, and dusky redness is noticeable on lips and fingernails. The lab findings include erythrocytosis, leukocytosis, thrombocytosis, and increased leukocyte alkaline phosphatase. Therapy using 2–3 mCi P-32 (13.5 days $T_{1/2}$ and 695 keV beta) is effective to suppress excessive hematopoiesis. Secondary absolute polycythemia (erythrocytosis) is associated with increased erythropoietic production. Erythropoietin is produced mostly in the kidney and less in liver. Renal or hepatic disorder, hypoxia due to cardiac or pulmonary disease, obesity, ascites, or abnormal hemoglobin level causes an erythrocytosis. Renal cell carcinoma, hemangioblastoma in the posterior fossa, pheochromocytoma, as well as lung, breast, and rectal cancers have been associated with polycythemia.

18.4. Cell Survival and Sequestration

To perform a red cell survival study, autologous red blood cells are incubated with 0.25–0.3 mCi ^{51}Cr sodium chromate, and 0.05–0.1 mCi labeled cells are injected. Serial blood samples are obtained starting 30 min after tracer injection and then for 3–5 days. The activity per milliliter of whole blood is determined, and the results are plotted on semilog paper. The rate of disappearance reflects not only the removal of senescent red cells from the circulation (about one percent per day) but also a variable degree of Cr-51 elution from the labeled cells (about one percent per day). Normally $T_{1/2}$ of Cr-51 labeled red blood cells is about 28 days, with a range of 24 to 38 days.

Shortened survival of ^{51}Cr-labeled red blood cells may be in hemolytic anemias, sickle cell disease, iron deficiency anemia, spehrocytosis, malaria, bleeding ulcer, and blood transfusion during the survival study.

Platelets can be labeled with ^{111}In oxine (2.3 days $T_{1/2}$, 175 and 225 keV) or ^{51}Cr sodium chromate to measure platelet turnover in patients with theombocytopenic diseases. Mean platelet survival determined from the blood radioactivity disappearance curve is approximately 10 days.[4]

Along with the survival time measurement, external organ counting over the heart, liver, and spleen is performed to locate the sites of red cell or platelet sequestration and destruction. The organ counting is affected by the concentration of the activity in the organ and also size of the organ. Normally, the spleen to hepatic count density ratio ranges from 0.5 to 1.5. The ratio progressively rises in patients with splenic sequestration of red cells or platelets. Splenic sequestration is seen in patients with hypersplenism, spherocytosis, and sickle cell anemia. In adults with sickle cell anemia, the liver is a predominant site of red cell sequestration. In patients with idiopathic thrombocytopenic purpura, a high splenic to hepatic count density ratio indicates that splenectomy will induce a remission.

References

1. Balon H, Gold CA, Dworkin HJ, McCormick VA, Freeitas JE. (1998) Procedure guideline for carbon-14 urea breath test. *J Nucl Med* **39**: 2012–2015
2. Zuckier LS, Chervu LR. (1984) Schilling evaluation of pernicious anemia: Current status. *J Nucl Med* **25**: 1032–1039.
3. International Committee for Standardization in Hematology. (1980) Recommended methods for measurement of red-cell and plasma volume. *J Nucl Med* **21**: 793–800.
4. Vollertsen RS, Fuster V, Conn DL, *et al.* (1982) *In vivo* platelet survival in rheumatoid arthritis. *Mayo Clin Proc* **57**: 620–624.

Chapter 19

Therapeutic Applications of Radiopharmaceuticals

Franklin C. Wong and E. Edmund Kim

19.1. Introduction to Radionuclide Therapy

The use of radiopharmaceuticals in treating human diseases depends on the irreversible destruction to ablate abnormal tissues. Radiopharmaceuticals are mostly used in cancer therapy, although they are also used to treat non-malignant diseases such as Graves disease, by systemic administration, and arthropathy in hemophiliacs, by locoregional injection into bursas of knee joints. Radiopharmaceuticals follow the same metabolic pathways as their non-radioactive counterparts because of similar biologic activities which depend on biochemical properties of the molecule. With exceptions of radioactive atoms such as iodides and lanthanides, biochemical properties often reside in the non-radioactive moiety, which can be designed to direct the attached radionuclide to delivery radiation.

Non-radioactive pharmaceuticals mostly act through reversible biochemical mechanisms such as receptor binding and enzyme inhibition or activation. On the other hand, upon arrival to the target tissue, therapeutic radiopharmaceuticals deposit ionizing radiations from alpha, beta, and/or gamma emissions. These emissions cause free radical showers that irreversibly alter the surrounding tissues. In contrast to dehydrating or cauterizing agents, such as acids, alkaline, or talc, that immediately cause tissue alternations, radiopharmaceuticals deposit their radiation over their residence times or several effective half-lives (i.e., hours to days). Longer duration to deposit the radiation results in lesser tendency to induce violent inflammatory reactions in host tissues and render a smoother clinical course during treatment and recovery. While

401

non-radioactive drugs are limited by their diffusion across biologic barriers to reach target tissues, radiopharmacueticals do not respect barriers and can ablate tissues beyond several millimeters in depth. The cross-fire effects will destroy target tissues even though radionuclides are not in direct contact.

While the measure of radioactivity for diagnostic use is usually in units of mCi or MBq, the therapeutic use of radiopharmaceuticals involves additional concepts, e.g., radiation-absorbed doses such as Gy or Sv. Theoretically, the use of absorbed dose provides a better correlation with outcomes. In practice, the estimation of absorbed doses is limited by low accuracy because of lack of verification methodology. It also suffers from low precision, with the coefficient of variation often greater than 25%. The measure of success of treatment varies and depends on the disease being treated and is subject to interpretation by the patient and referring physician. For Graves disease, it is the control of hyperthyroidism. For thyroid cancer and lymphoma, it is the time to recurrence. For control of painful osseous metastasis, it is the decrease in the use of pain medication. Often, the outcome measure is by default the gestalt impression of the referring physicians who consider all available clinically relevant information, including biomarkers, imaging findings, and patient performance status.

This chapter reviews radiopharmaceuticals for therapy and the systemic and locoregional treatment routes and highlights the scientific and practical aspects. Certainly, important issues of regulatory control and patient informed consent need to be strictly complied.

19.2. Radiopharmaceuticals for Therapy

19.2.1. *Therapeutic radionuclides*

The requirement for the successful deposition of therapeutic radionuclide is its specific accumulation into target tissues and low retention of radioactivity from non-target sites. In our armamentarium are small organic molecules, inorganic moieties, as well as antibodies, peptides, minibodies, nucleotides, and ligands, with specific receptor affinity. The following 12 radionuclides have been used for cancer therapy in routine clinical care as well as in clinical trials: ^{32}P, ^{89}Sr, ^{90}Y, ^{111}In, ^{117m}Sn, ^{131}I, ^{166}Ho, ^{153}Sm, ^{177}Lu, ^{186}Re, ^{188}Re, and ^{223}Ra.

Although residence time is the ultimate determinant of radiation-absorbed dose, desirable physical half-life should be from few hours and several days; the emitted particles of radiation should have a range of several millimeters in tissues. They should be produced with high radionuclide purity, radiochemical purity, and specific activity to allow subsequent processing to produce radiopharmaceuticals. The ratio of non-penetrating to penetrating radiation should be high. The daughter should be short-lived or stable.

19.2.2. *The ranges of emitted particle radiation in the tissue*

Alpha α-particles have the shortest range of about $100\,\mu$m in water or soft tissues and can have therapeutic effects if they reach the cell membrane, such as binding to a cell-surface receptor. Beta emissions, including Auger electrons, have a range of 1–$10\,\mu$m and can have therapeutic effect if they overcome the cell membrane to reach the nucleus to ablate the DNA. Low-energy, high-intensity electrons, emitted following electron capture (EC) and isomeric transition (IT), have variable ranges and may result in significant amounts of secondary radiation. While high-energy gamma radiations may generate secondary radiation by scattering, low-energy gamma rays are better absorbed by tissues and may serve as basis for locoregional radiation in the case of GlialSite using high activities of ^{125}I and reach up to $60\,$Gy in 1cm depth.[1]

19.2.3. *Biodistribution of radiopharmaceuticals determines residence time of radionuclides in the target tissue and non-target tissues*

Irrespective of the route of administration, the distribution of radionuclides is determined by tissue physiology such as blood flow and fluid dynamics as well as tissue biochemistry such as receptor binding and enzymatic processes. The radiation-absorbed doses results from contribution of all radionuclides retained in all organs and tissues in the body. The measure of tissue retention of radionuclides is the residence time, which would be 1.44 times the effective half-life if the uptake is instantaneous and the washout follows a mono-exponential decay scheme. In less than ideal situations, such as that usually encountered during routine clinical care of patients, the estimation of radiation dosimetry is a difficult task in which there are few concrete variables and low precision in their estimation.

19.2.4. *Dosimetry of radiopharmaceuticals*

The accuracy in radiation dosimetry depends on the accurate estimation of residence time and specific radiation-absorbed doses (or S value) of the radionuclide reaching the target. A formula has been established by the MIRD Committee, which published a table of S values, to translate cumulated activity in different organs to radiation absorbed dose. An ideal method to calculate radiation dosimetry is to perform simulation such as Monte Carlo methods to estimate the radiation-deposited dose from all radiation sources in the body of all shapes to all organs for each patient. It is tedious and lengthy beyond the current computing capabilities to be clinically useful for each patient. With refinement on geometric assumptions from earlier efforts of MIRDOSE3, organ-specific and whole-body age-specific models have been developed and are included in an FDA-approved software OLINDA[2] and subsequently OLINDA2 to apply fixed geometry models to derive absorbed dose calculation. Fixed geometry models have the disadvantage, however, of not matching the actual patient body habitus. Various versions of patient-specific dosimetry software are under development. One example is a deterministic approach that allows post-estimation refinement for repeated approximation for better accuracy.[3,4]

19.2.5. *Radionuclides of therapeutic interest*

While the biodistribution of radiopharmaceuticals is determined by the biochemical characteristics of the entire molecule consisting of the biologically active moiety and the radionuclide, the choice of the radionuclide determines the physical half-life and range of radiation to accomplish therapy.

Phosphorus-32
About 85% of total body phosphate is deposited in the skeleton, and 15% in muscle, liver, and spleen. It has a physical life of 14.3 days and emits

a β-particle with a maximum energy of 1.71 MeV and an average mean energy of 0.70 MeV. The mean and the maximum particle range in soft tissue are 3 and 8 mm, respectively.

Phosphorus-32 (^{32}P) has been used in the form of sodium orthophosphate (Na_2HPO_4), polymetaphosphate ($Na_6O_{18}P_6$), pyrophosphate (P_2O_7), and hydroxyethylidene diphosphonate (HEDP), which is approximately 20 times more concentrated in the bone mineral than ^{32}P. Its uptake depends on osteoblastic activity of the tissue. Following systemic administration, about 5%–10% of the administrated activity is excreted within 24 hours. ^{32}P was the first radionuclide introduced for the palliation of pain from bone metastases, polycythemia vera, and leukemia.

Strontium-89

Strontium-89 (^{89}Sr) is a pure beta emitter. It is a calcium analogue and has a physical life of 50.5 days and maximum β-particle energy of 1.46 MeV. The maximum and the average range in soft tissue are 7 mm and 2 mm, respectively. Inspite of its Bremsstrahlung radiations, current clinical gamma cameras cannot convey images with sufficient spatial resolution for localization. After intravenous injection, 50% of ^{89}Sr localize to bone, mostly in those areas with high osteoblastic activities. The deposited densities are 2 to 25 times greater in metastasis than in normal bone. The rest of the injected ^{89}Sr is excreted by the renal (80%) and gastrointestinal system (20%).

Yttrium-90

Yttrium-90 (^{90}Y) is a pure β-emitter with a physical half-life of 64.1 h (2.67 days) and it decays to stable Zirconium-90 (^{90}Zr). The β-rays that are emitted by its decay have an average value of 0.9367 MeV while their maximum energy reaches 2.284 MeV. Its average range in tissue is 2.5 mm and its maximum is 11 mm. Inspite of its Bremsstrahlung emissions, current clinical gamma cameras cannot produce images with sufficient spatial resolution for localization. The unique low-yield pair-production properties of ^{90}Y have been recently explored to be measured by positron emission tomography (PET) during locoregional cancer treatment[5] and therefore may allow radiation dosimetric estimation.

Indium-111

Indium-111 (^{111}In) has a physical half-life of 2.8 days and emits gamma rays at 171 and 245 keV as well as Auger electrons and 3 and 19 keV, which would be effective in ablating microorganelles within 10 m. Once this radionuclide is inside a cancer cell, Auger electrons that are emitted from ^{111}In can damage the DNA of the cancer cell.

Tin-117m

Tin-117m ([117m]Sn) has a half-life of 13.6 days and emits electrons at 160 KeV and photons at 159 KeV which allows scintigraphic imaging. It is a radionuclide used to treat primary or metastatic bone malignancies and is used in pain palliation.[6]

Iodine-131

Iodine-131 (^{131}I) has a physical half-life of 13.6 days and emits electrons with an average energy of 200 KeV (max 600 KeV) and gamma photons at 364 keV, which allow scintigraphic imaging. Its tissue range is 0.4 mm (max 2.4 mm). [131]I has been used in both its native form of iodide ([131]I$^-$ in sodium iodide) and organified forms such as ^{131}I-MIBG and labeled antibodies for treating Graves disease and cancers.

Samarium-153

Samarium-153 ([153]Sm) has a half-life of 1.95 days and emits electrons with an average energy of 230 KeV (max 810 KeV) and photons at 103 KeV, which allows scintigraphic imging. Its tissue range is 0.53 mm (max 3 mm). It is often used in the form of conjugate as [153]Sm-EDTMP to relief bone pain from osseous metastases.

Holmium-166

Holmium-166 ([166]Ho) is a β-emitter with two β-emissions, at 1.85 MeV and at 1.77 MeV, attributing to a mean range of 4 mm and a maximum of 8.7 mm in soft tissues. [145, 146]. It also emits γ-photons with energies of 1.38 MeV and 80.6 keV (6.6%), the latter of which can be imaged scintigraphically. The physical half-life of [166]Ho is 26.8 h.

Lutetium-177

Lutetium-177 (^{177}Lu) decays to stable Hafnium-177 with a half-life of 6.71 days. It emits beta radiation with a maximum energy of 498 keV and gamma rays with maximum energy of 208 and 113 keV, respectively, which allow scintigraphic imaging and dosimetry.[7] Its abilities for therapy and scintigraphy been demonstrated by the recent clinical trials of ^{177}Lu DOTA-TOC in the treatment of neuroendocrine tumors.

Rhenium-186

Rhenium-186 (^{186}Re) is a mainly a beta-emitter with a physical half-life of 89.3 hours, with beta-emissions of maximum energies of 1.077 MeV and 939 keV, respectively. Its gamma-emission of 137 keV (9%) enables scintigraphic imaging during therapy and biodistribution studies for patient-specific dosimetry.

Rhenium-188

Rhenium-188 (^{188}Re) decays with a half-life of 17 hours and emission of an energetic beta-particle with a maximum energy of 2.12 MeV and gamma-photons at 155 keV. ^{188}Re is a good radionuclide candidate for therapy because of its energetic emissions, shorter half-life, and convenient production from a ^{188}W/^{188}Re generator in contrast to ^{186}Re production, which requires neutron bombardment.

Radium-223

Radium-223 (^{223}Ra) is an alpha-emitter produced by a generator system using ^{227}Ac as parent nuclide. ^{223}Ra has a half-life of 11.43 days, while emitting alpha-particles at 5.65 MeV.[8] The cation of ^{223}Ra behaves similar to calcium and is incorporated into the bone matrix, especially to active osseous metastases.

19.3. Systemic Radionuclide Therapies in Practice

19.3.1. *Polycythemia vera using* ^{32}P

While blood-letting and chemotherapeutic agents such as hydroxurea, pipo-broman, and busulfan are alternatives to treat polycythemia vera, ^{32}P in the form of sodium orthophosphate ($Na_2H^{32}PO_4$) is a viable option when other methods fail. Blood-letting should be performed to achieve hematocrit level of 42%–47%. An initial dose of 2–3 mCi/m^2 is injected intravenously, with a total dose less than 5 mCi in order to avoid a bone marrow dose more than 1 Gy. The blood count should be monitored every three to four weeks. If a hematocrit level of 47% is reached and leukocyte and platelet counts are not reduced by 25% in 12 weeks, another blood-letting should be performed followed by another cycle of ^{32}P therapy, with a total dose 25% higher than the first dose. These cycles of blood-letting and ^{32}P therapy should be repeated with individual highest dose below 7 mCi.[9]

19.3.2. *Hyperthyroidism and Graves disease using* ^{131}I

Primary hyperthyroidism may be caused by Graves disease with elevated levels of thyroid-stimulating antibodies and toxic nodular goiter with autonomous thyroxine-producing nodules. Upon confirmation using serum thyroid-stimulating hormone (TSH) levels and imaging findings with ^{123}I NaI, endocrinologists may prefer some trial periods with anti-thyroidal medications in Graves disease before referring for ^{131}I NaI therapy. As part of the workup before radionuclide therapy, thyroid uptake of radioiodide is often obtained using small dose of ^{123}NaI (0.2–0.3 mCi) administered orally 4 hours before uptake and imaging. Additional uptake study at 24 hours is also obtained to exclude thyroiditis as a cause of hyperthyroidism.

Upon confirmation of elevated radioiodide uptake at 4 and 24 hours at ($>15\%$ and $>35\%$, respectively), radioiodide therapy using ^{131}I is conducted, typically in an out-patient setting for Graves disease. The goal is to deliver between 80 to 300 Gy to the thyroids.[10] For patients treated with 150 Gy and 300 Gy, long-term hypothyroidism can be achieved at 27% and 68%, respectively, and recurrent hyperthyroidism occurs at 27% and 8%, respectively.[10] The required radioactivity is proportional to the thyroid mass and inversely proportional to the 24-hour uptake.

Using a range of μCi/g desired from 50–80, the required ^{131}I activity is:

Required activity in μCi = (μCi/g desired)

$\times$ (thyroid mass in g)/24 h uptake

Using desired radiation-absorbed dose in cGy (5000 cGy–30000 cGy), required ^{131}I is:

Required activity in μCi = (cGy desired)

$\times$ (thyroid mass in g)/24 h uptake/93

This type of calculation requires an accurate estimation of thyroid mass and assumption of uniform distribution of radioiodide inside thyroids. An alternative method is a stepwise fixed-dose method which dictates iodide activities at 5, 10, 15, 20, and up to 30 mCi, depending upon the 24-hour thyroid uptake. Usually, the higher the uptake, the lower the prescribed dose level.

Toxic nodular goiters are more resistant to radioiodide therapy. However, with two to five times the activities typical for Graves disease, i.e., up to 150 mCi, there is a high chance of cure and rendering the patient hypothyroid. Potential side effects include thyroid storm upon initial release of stored thyroxine, especially with large thyroid gland mass. Patients can be protected from thyroid storm using beta-blockers. More typical is the eventual hypothyroidism which could be managed by supplemental thyroxin.

19.3.3. *Thyroid cancer remnants using* ^{131}I

The mainstay of thyroid cancer treatment is surgical resection of both thyroid lobes and suspicious lymph nodes. Often, in more than 90% of the cases, remnants of thyroid gland and/or thyroid cancers are visualized using the radioiodide scan. Initial preparation includes thyroxine withdrawal for four weeks followed by two weeks of cytomel and then two weeks without cytomel. An alternative to thyroxin withdrawal is the use of subcutaneous injection of Thyrogen (recombination TSH) over two days before radioiodide administration. Thyrogen is expensive but will allow the patient continue on thyroxin to avoid unpleasant effects of hypothyroidism.

Usually, a low iodide diet is prescribed for two to three weeks before the diagnostic test. Abstinence in the use of iodinated contrast for one to two months is required and high serum TSH level (>30 IU) is confirmed before small amounts (1–5 mCi) of ^{123}I NaI or ^{131}I NaI are orally administered. Delayed scintigraphic imaging is conducted to survey abnormal iodide uptake sides. Residual iodide-avid lesions can be visualized by whole-body scan, static images, or single-photon emission computed tomography (SPECT-CT). Therapeutic decisions will be made concerning radioactivity prescribed, and ^{131}I therapy will proceed according to a conventional guideline as stated in the following:

(a) For post-operative ablation of thyroid bed remnants, activity in the range of 2.75–5.50 GBq (75–150 mCi) is typically administered,
(b) With iodide-avid lesions in the neck or mediastinal lymph nodes, activity in the range of 5.55–7.40 GBq (150–200 mCi) used.

(c) For distant metastases, activity of >7.4 GBq (200 mCi) is often given. The radiation dose to the bone marrow, although rare, is typically the limiting factor.

Recent advances and reports from clinical trials have resulted in guidelines recommending more simplified algorithms for radioiodide therapy of thyroid cancer remnants, depending on the staging of disease, thyroglobulin levels, and extent of involvement as reported from surgery and determined by ultrasonography.[11–15] There is also a trend of using lower radioactivity (e.g., starting with 50 mCi) for uncomplicated post-surgical cases.

Post-therapy scans are often obtained and have been reported to yield more lesions than diagnostic scans, likely due to the higher administered activities of [131]I. Potential side effects include anemia because of known radiation effects above 400 mCi, swelling of post-surgical thyroid bed, nausea because of exposure to the entire dose of ^{131}I, and dry mouth of variable durations. As for the issue of fertility, the US Nuclear Regulatory Commission (NRC) has recommended a waiting period of six months for female patients before attempting to conceive while the American thyroid Association recommends one year of waiting so that reproductive cells recover from exposure to therapeutic dose of ^{131}I in cancer treatment.

The issue of patient release and hazard to the public has long been debated. The long-standing criteria of less than 30 mCi for out-patient treatment was relaxed to 33 mCi in 1997 in the US. It was further relaxed to allow out-patient treatment and release to the public if the treatment dose is below 220 mCi. Compliance to these rules is complicated by the differing rules.[16] In the US, patient-release criteria are governed by federal and state regulations and differ in states, especially among agreement and non-agreement states. In general, they can be summarized as from patient protection facility such as a dedicated room is as following:

(a) If the measured radiation exposure rate is below 7 mRem/Hr at 1 m, the patient can be discharged to home; if transfer to other in-patient facilities is intended, the radiation exposure rate should be below 2.5 mRem/Hr at 1 m.
(b) If there are reliable methods and documentation to assure the general public do not receive more than the NRC mandated thresholds (e.g., 5 mSv for non-pregnant adults). Multiple schemes have been devised

for these methods to estimate the risk and exposure to the general public based on estimation of 24-hour thyroid bed uptake, clearance time, and serial measurement of radiation exposure rates, as well as assumption of the behavior and habits of the public and people in the patients surroundings.

Out-patient schemes of accelerated release of patients treated with ^{131}I for thyroid cancer remnants have gained popularity in the recent years and may be further justified by savings from reduced in-patient stay. A recent backlash is the public dissent in the media concerning unknown exposure. The US NRC has advised physicians to advice all patients concerning radiation protection and not encourage patients to stay in public places such as hotels immediately after accelerated release from ^{131}I treatment of thyroid cancer remnants. It is important to observe all local rules and state and federal laws in the design of local out-patient treatment plans.

19.3.4. Refractory lymphomas using ^{90}Y- ibritumomab tiuxetan and ^{131}I

A good example of systemic therapeutic use of ^{90}Y is in the treatment of refractory non-Hodgkin's lymphomas in the form of ^{90}Y-ibritumomab-tiuxetan (Zevalin).[17–23] ^{90}Y is directed toward the tumor cells by the antibodies against CD20 on the surface of lymphoma cells. The binding attaches ^{90}Y to those lymphoma cells with CD20 on the surface and subjects the rest of the tumor to cross-fire effect. In order to decrease non-specific binding of radiolabeled ibritumomab tiuxetan to other organs, up to 650 mg of non-radioactive anti-CD20 antibody Rituximab is injected to saturate the binding sites a few hours before the administration of labeled antibodies. Care should be taken during such infusion to observe allergic reactions and fluid overloading.

Since ^{90}Y cannot be imaged by conventional means, an imaging surrogate is required to confirm its appropriate biodistribution and the lack of loculation after injection. Typically, after initial infusion of non-radioactive rituximab, 5 mCi of ^{111}I-ibritumomab tiuxetan is injected followed by delayed whole-body scintigraphy in 2–4 days. Upon scintigraphic confirmation of satisfactory biodistribution, the patient receives another infusion of rituxanmab followed by injection of ^{90}Y-ibritumomab-tiuxetan at a dose of

0.3 mCi/kg when platelet are low (100–150 k/ul) or 0.4 mCi/kg when there is normal bone-marrow function as indicated by platelets above 150 k/ul. The total prescribed dose should be below 32 mCi. This treatment regimen is typically reserved for refractory lymphoma and approved by the FDA as such. However, there are exciting data from recent clinical trials to suggest favorable results if it is used as a first-line regimen. The recent successful imaging studies of the pair-production of ^{90}Y using PET-CT has enabled the visualization of concentrated ^{90}Y[5] and brought hope to directly visualize and accurately quantify ^{90}Y-ibritumomab tiuxetan during therapy for dosimetry.

^{131}I-Tositumomab (Bexxar) is another approved radiolabeled antibody against CD20 to treat refractory lymphomas.[24–26] The radionuclide ^{131}I allows imaging and dosimetry, but earlier studies did not confirm the correlation between dosimetry and outcome probably because of poor accuracy of the dosimetry methodology. Nevertheless, initial workup involves the infusion of non-radioactive antibodies followed by 5 mCi of ^{131}I-Tositumomab and serial whole-body imaging for 5 days to determine the whole-body exposure to radioiodide by measuring clearance of ^{131}I. An upper limit between 75 cGy and 100 cGy of the whole-body absorbed dose is applied to calculate the prescribed dose. The typical treatment involves infusion of non-radioactive antibodies followed by injections of radioactivities varying between 60 and 150 mCi of ^{131}I-Tositumomab, depending the measured clearance rate of ^{131}I. Because of the high-energy gamma photons and long half-life of (8 days) of ^{131}I, radiation protection is a more important issue than that in ^{90}Y-zevalin.

19.3.5. *Painful osseous metastases using ^{89}Sr chloride and ^{153}Sm-EDTMP*

Treatment of painful osseous metastasis started in the 1940s with ^{32}P, which is no longer employed for this purpose. Current approved practice involves only ^{89}Sr chloride and ^{153}Sm-EDTMP, while the use of ^{223}Ra, ^{117m}Sn DTPA, ^{166}Ho-DOTMP, ^{186}Re-HEDP, and ^{188}Re-HEDP is experimental in clinical trials only.

A study was conducted with patients with painful bone metastases who both received therapeutic doses of ^{89}Sr chloride (Metastron) at 60 μCi/kg with volumes of the metastases determined from the high-resolution CT images and the bone density calculated from the mean Hounsfield unit.[27] The International Commission on Radiological Protection (ICRP) dosimetric model for bone (ICRP 30) was used and revealed mean absorbed dose to metastases at 20 cGy/MBq (740 cGy/mCi) to 24 cGy/MBq (889 cGy/mCi). In normal bone, the biological half-life of ^{89}Sr is approximately 14 days compared with more than 50 days in bone metastasis. This would ensure persistent and preferential culmination in osseous metastases. With the physical half-life of 50.5 days, the long effective half-life/residence time will deliver a continuous irradiation on cancer cells going through the different stages of cell cycle. After initial studies of various activities, a 4-mCi (150 MBq) fixed dose has been adopted, with occasional adjustment according to body weight or body surface area but not exceeding 4 mCi.[28]

The initial workup involves confirmation of active osseous metastasis, typically from a 99mTc MDP bone scan within a month. Care should be taken to ensure the absence of pending spinal cord compression by the osseous metastasis because focal radionuclide in close contact with the spinal cord would further exacerbate myelopathy or radiculopathy in progress. Pre-treatment with steroid would be another option if ^{89}Sr treatment is indeed carried out. The ^{89}Sr chloride dose is typically injected intravenously and great caution should be made to ensure patent venous access to avoid interstitial locualtion at the injection site. This treatment is effective in alleviating bone pain in 80% of cancer patients with metastasis to the bone. Potential side effects would be hematotoxicity and transient flare of pain.

Samarium-153 ([153]Sm) lexidronam (chemical name Samarium-153-ethylene diamine tetramethylene phosphonate [[153]Sm-EDTMP], trade name Quadramet) is a complex of a lanthanide Samarium with the chelator EDTMP for palliative treatment of painful osseous metastases.[29–33] The typical administered activity of [153]Sm-EDTMP is 1 mCi/kg (37 MBq/kg). Pain begins to improve in the first week for most patients, and the effects can last several months. [153]Sm-EDTMP is also used in treating primary bone cancer such as osteosarcoma on clinical trials with up to 6 mCi/kg doses.[29,34,35] It is rapidly eliminated through the urinary system. The total uptake of metastatic lesions is about (65.5 ± 15.5)% of the administration dose. The main adverse effects are hematotoxicities, similar to those of ^{89}Sr; precautions are similar to those of [89]Sr. Additional contraindication includes rare allergies from prior injection. One main difference is the shorter half-life of 1.95 days which would allow deposition of half of the total radiation absorbed dose to the target tissues to provide prompt tumor control. However, a high dose rate may also elicit more acute inflammation and a flare phenomenon of increasing bone pain in shorter timeframe.

Because of concerns of hematotoxicities, these radiopharmaceuticals are typically not administered concurrently with chemotherapeutic agent to avoid potentiation of adverse effects. However, clinical trials aiming at the eradication of cancer cell reserves in skeleton using concurrent chemotherapy and ^{89}Sr chloride[36] and ^{153}Sm-EDTMP[37] have been conducted. They reported favorable phase-1 findings of tolerable added toxicities.

In a comparative study of alpha-emitter ^{223}Ra and the beta-emitter ^{89}Sr, it was shown that cationic ^{223}Ra and ^{89}Sr had almost the same bone uptake. Estimates of dose deposition in bone marrow suggested an advantage of alpha-particle emitters for sparing bone marrow.[38] The use of the ^{223}Ra was extended to solid tumors and soft tissue metastases. When cationic ^{223}Ra is used in treating bone metastasis, an ICRP-67 dosimetry estimate indicated that for a 50 kBq per kg of body weight dose, the bone surfaces would receive 13.05 Sv. The average bone surface to red bone marrow dose ratio was estimated to be 10.3.[39,40] Because of the high payload of ^{223}Ra from its high linear energy transfer, only very small activity is required (e.g., 1–2 μCi/kg).

Another promising agent for the relief of painful osseous metastasis is Sn-117m(4+)/diethylenetriaminepentaacetic acid (DTPA), which emits photons of lower energies but not electrons. It concentrates exclusively on the bones and does not follow the excretion route through urine, and there are reports of a good therapeutic outcome.[6] It presents a great advantage as higher activities can be administered to patients for further alleviation due to its very low toxicity and dose absorption in the bone marrow.

19.3.6. *Neuroendocrine tumor using* ^{111}*In-octreotide,* ^{90}*Y- DOTA-TOC and* ^{177}*Lu-DOTA-TOC*

Radionuclide therapy of neuroendocrine tumors is only at the clinical trial stage. Although there are many promising agents, there are no

FDA-approved radiopharmaceuticals for the treatment of neuroendocrine tumor.

The neuroendocrine tumors have abundant surface receptors that avidly bind somatostatin ligands of subtype 2 and 5. Earlier studies using high levels of activities of ^{111}In-octreotide up to 500 mCi caused renal damage because of the prominent uptake by kidneys. Efforts to decrease renal toxicities using intravenous infusion of branched-chain amino acids results in other undesirable effects such as nausea and vomiting. Dosimetry of ^{111}In-octreotide therapy can be performed with planar or scintigraphic images. One of the widely used products for target therapy with radionuclides is the ^{90}Y-DOTA-[D-Phe1-Tyr3]-octreotide, which is a somatostatin analogue with high affinity for somatostatin subtype receptors SSTR2 and SSTR5. Octreotide analogues are localized primarily in spleen, kidneys, and liver, which together with the urine bladder get the highest absorbed dose.[41–50]

^{177}Lu-labeled octreotide analogues[45,47,49] have been used for the experimental treatment of metastasized neuroendocrine gastro-entero-pancreatic (GEP) tumors. Both [^{177}Lu-DOTA-,Tyr^3]-octreotide, known as ^{177}Lu-DOTATOC, and [^{177}Lu-DOTA-,Tyr^3]-octreotate, known as ^{177}Lu-DOTATATE, have identical biodistribution patterns.[51] However, comparing ^{177}Lu-DOTATATE with ^{177}Lu-DOTATOC reveals the mean ratio of tumor residence time was 2.1. Similarly, the residence times in normal organs are significantly longer for ^{177}Lu-DOTATATE, with mean ratios of 1.5 for spleen and 1.4 for kidneys. They are associated with less renal toxicities than with ^{90}Y or ^{111}In-analogues, probably related to shorter range of emissions.

19.4. Locoregional Radionuclide Therapies

19.4.1. *Concerns specific to locoregional radionuclide therapies*

19.4.1.1. *High efficacy*

Locoregional radionuclide therapy achieves geometric proximity to the target tissues via intracavitary, intraarterial, or interstitial routes and may require interventional or surgical procedures.[52,53] Toxicities of locoregional radionuclide therapy are related to return of radionuclide to the general circulation from lymphatics and/or diffusion across biologic barrier from the target tissue.

Intraarterial injection of particulate radiopharmaceuticals with particle sizes greater than that of capillaries ensures that particles are loculated in the target/tumor capillary bed. Alternatively, intraarterial injection of soluble tumor-avid radiopharmaceuticals may gain greater exposure to higher radioactivity from concentrated injectates. For lipophilic radiopharmaceuticals with high first-pass extraction such as ^{131}I lipiodol, there is even higher fraction of retention.

Intracavitary injection often requires a catheter to establish reliable and repeatable access to the cavity. For instance, during intraventricular radionuclide therapy, an intraventricular catheter is connected to a reservoir over the scalp. The patency of the cerebrospinal fluid (CSF) flow is typically evaluated by injection of 0.5 mCi ^{111}In DTPA. The half-life of ^{111}In allows prolonged observation of possible obstruction or delayed return to the general circulation. Although ^{111}In DTPA is the only US FDA–approved intrathecal radiopharmaceutical, alternative tracers include Tc-99m DTPA, which is more widely available.

Intracavitary ^{90}Y DOTA-TOC has been applied to treat glioma in post-surgical cavities. The intracavitary injection of ^{111}In octreotide allowed visualization of CSF compartments and subsequent systemic return from both interstitial and intrathecal routes. Favorable responses to Y-90 DOTA-TOC reported[42] further supporting interstitial/intracavitary treatment of brain tumors using unsealed soluble radiopharmaceuticals. Intracavitary radionuclide therapies in pleural, pericardial, or peritoneal compartments or post-surgical tumor bed also require radiographic and/or scintigraphic confirmation of adequate distribution of injectate, typically using Tc-99m macro-aggregated albumin (MAA) or sulfur colloids.

Even small intratumoral activity of Tl-201(0.5 mCi) delivering 2–8 Gy was able to eradicated brain tumor implants in rats.[54] Interstitial injection of particulate radiopharmaceuticals into tumor bed is limited by loculation around the injection site. The concentration of radiation in very confined volume necessitates multiple injections to the tumor. In fact, after ^{90}Y-Y(OH)$_3$ particles were injected in human superficial tumors in multiple locations within a tumor, there was local control.[55] Less than 5% of particles less than 1 μm diameter were drained through lymphatics. On the other hand, locoregional application of soluble radiopharmaceuticals such as ^{90}Y- DOTA-TOC[42] in post-surgical cavity after glioma resection may diffuse to neighboring tissues before returning to the systemic circulation via capillary bed and manage to ablate tumor cells at greater distance from the initial deposition. The interstitial use of soluble radiopharmaceuticals with tumor affinity may thus enhance the retention of radionuclide, resulting in even higher payload.

19.4.1.2. *Toxicity and interaction with host*

Toxicity of radionuclide therapy is determined by radiation-absorbed doses to critical organs manifesting as toxicities. Pharmacokinetic advantages of locoregional radionuclide therapy result in wide therapeutic windows allowing higher radiation absorbed doses (e.g., $>100\,\mathrm{Gy}$) delivered to the tumor bed, as long as the diffusion to surrounding tissue is limited. When tumor cells are exposed to lethal doses of radiation (100–$200\,\mathrm{Gy}$), they become metabolically inactive without initial structural disintegration. Since protein inactivation requires higher doses ($>1{,}000\,\mathrm{Gy}$), tumor cells and surrounding tissues will initially retain structural integrity. However, metabolic ablation results in the suppression of tumor defenses such as autocrine formation to resist host immunologic surveillance and tumor stromal impedance. Tumor-specific antigens will be orderly and stably presented to host immune systems, leading to priming of immune cells and tumor destruction by macrophages and/or cytotoxic mechanism. Indeed, non-radioactive locoregional tumor therapeutic experiments such as photodynamic therapy[56,57] and radiofrequency ablation have reported enhanced specific immune responses toward tumors.[58] Locoregional radionuclide therapy may have an important role. The lack of immediate violent inflammation because of low dose rate allows stable exposure and recognition of tumor-specific antigens for triggering of immune cascade upon future recurrence of malignancies. In contrast, conventional chemotherapy may impede competent immune responses. The potential immunologic benefit could be shared by systemic radionuclide therapy and proton beam and stereotactic radiotherapy. However, wider therapeutic windows of locoregional radionuclide therapy allow higher radiation-absorbed doses to the tumor bed to achieve more complete metabolic ablation.

19.4.1.3. *Dosimetry modeling and limits*

Accurate estimation of radiation-absorbed doses to tumor, surrounding tissues, and critical organs is important, especially for the design and modification of dosing regimes. An FDA-approved radionuclide dosimetry software OLINDA[2] is available for systemically administered radiopharmaceuticals under a fixed anatomy model. On the other hand, locoregional administration requires custom-designed dosimetry schemes. Fixed anatomy from anthropomorphic models is often applied but rigidly limited to standardized patients.[59] Any modification of initial assumptions or regions of interests requires a repeated lengthy simulation computation. Recent development involves the use of deterministic approach using *a priori* criteria to perform simulation.[3,4] and allows prompt post-processing and iterative modification of estimation. It can estimate external beam radiotherapy doses within 1%–2% variability. The accuracy of deterministic approach in radionuclide therapy is not known. Since image-based radionuclide therapy dosimetry is subject to variability at 14%–25%,[60] the use of dosimetry in radionuclide therapy should be guarded. Other considerations such as accuracy in estimation of injectate volume, geometry of injectate, and microdosimetry to sub-cellular organelles need to be further studied.

19.4.2. *The practice of locoregional radionuclide cancer therapy*

19.4.2.1. *Intraarterial palliative treatment of liver cancers*

Selective internal radiotherapy (SIRT) uses ^{90}Y microspheres, which are point sources of radiation that preferentially localize in the intratumoral arterial vasculature.[61–67] SIRT therapy takes advantage of the dual blood supply of the liver because the majority of hepatic tumors derive 80%–100% of their blood supply from the hepatic artery. ^{90}Y-microspheres have been used in medicine since 1960. Initial studies assume that all the activity infused is delivered uniformly throughout the liver upon arterial injection via selected hepatic arteries. Current FDA-approved ^{90}Y- microspheres are TheraSphere (glass-based spheres of smaller size 20–30 μm but higher payload per particle, by Nordion Inc. of Canada[63,65]) for the treatment of hepatocellular cancers and SIR-Sphere (polymer-based spheres of larger and less uniform particle size at 20–60 μm of lower payload per particle manufactured by SIRtex Inc., Australia[62,64]) for hepatic metastases from colorectal cancers.

They provide palliation of symptoms to improve the quality of life. Earlier studies did not show survival benefits. However, results from recent trials have found favorable survival benefits in selected groups of patients.[68,69] Both radiopharmaceuticals require placement of arterial catheter under fluoroscopic guidance to reach the specific hepatic artery and scintigraphic confirmation studies using ^{99m}Tc MAA. The scintigrams are needed to confirm location of perfusion inside the liver or specific lobe of the liver and to exclude extrahepatic perfusion to the abdomen. Pulmonary shunting is frequently noted and a cut-off value of 13%–20% is adopted to establish the feasibility of conducting the treatment. For ^{90}Y-TheraSpheres, the prescribed dosing activity depends on the intended radiation absorbed dose to the tumor which is estimated by CT and the MAA scintigram. Because of the loculated distribution, higher amount of radioactivity (e.g., up to >100 mCi) may be derived while less capillary bed will be embolized with ^{90}Y-TheraSpheres which have smaller sizes and higher payload per particle.

SIR-Spheres are larger particles with broader range of size distribution and less payload per particle. They may cause backflow when there is significant embolization of the arteries, thus preventing completion of the entire dose. The prescribed radiation-absorbed dose is to the entire liver or one lobe of the liver, usually in the range of 100 Gy. Adverse effects such as nausea, vomiting, and abdominal pain are related to acute radiation effects.

Using ^{99m}Tc MAA as a surrogate to calculate tumor radiation dosimetry,[70] it was found that if the activity were to be distributed uniformly within the liver, the radiation-absorbed dose to the entire liver of the patient would be 110 Gy. However, only the 16% of the normal liver received dose higher than 110 Gy, with a mean dose of 58 Gy, whereas 83% of the tumour received more than 110 Gy, with a mean dose of 163 Gy. As far as the other organs are concerned, the maximum dose to right kidney was 25 Gy and to the stomach was 60 Gy, which correlate well with the immediate adverse effects. Post-treatment Bremsstrahlung imaging studies have been performed to evaluate distribution, but the quality of scintigram and SEPCT is sub-optimal and not sufficient for dosimetry. With the recent studies to explore PET imaging of low-yield pair production from ^{90}Y,[5] more accurate dosimetry and correlation with clinical outcome may be possible, especially using the mode of locoregional therapy involving higher levels of radioactivity loculated in smaller volumes.

19.4.2.2. *Intrathecal treatment of meningeal carcinomatosis*

Meningeal metastasis remains one of the most difficult to manage problems of lethal cancer complications. The incidence varies among different cancer types but may be as high as 10% in melanoma patients and 25% in leukemia. Treatment using external beam radiation is general limited to 30 Gy as palliative measures, because of high risk of toxicity to underlying brain and spinal cord surrounding the arachnoid tumor deposits.

Intrathecal radionuclides can deliver tumorcidal levels of local radiation-absorbed doses to the arachnoids to ablate tumors with short-range radiations that neither require diffusion nor reach nervous tissues a few millimeters from the CSF interface. Considerations of intrathecal radionuclide therapy include high locoregional dosimetry to the arachnoid, low neurotoxicity, and low systemic toxicity. Many known radionuclide therapeutics may fulfill these criteria and serve as good candidates as long as temporal and spatial profiles of their intrathecal pharmacokinetics are ascertained.

Intrathecal injection of radionuclide has been reported with ^{131}I- radioiodinated serum albumin (RISA), In-111 DTPA, Tc-99m DTPA, I-131 sodium iodide and Yb-192 DTPA for diagnostic purposes. With availability of Ommaya reservoirs to perform repeated CSF aspirations, many intrathecal injections are done via this reservoir. A cisternogram using 0.5-mCi In-111 DTPA is performed before therapy to assure CSF patency and avoid loculation. Therapeutic trials using radionuclide with no tumor affinity such as 3 mCi ^{32}P chromic phosphate[71,72] or 1.5–5 mCi of ^{198}Au colloid[73,74] have been reported with efficacy but suffered from cauda equina syndrome. Hematotoxicity is the dose-limiting factor for tumor-targeting ^{131}I-labeled monoclonal antibodies (MoAb)[75–79] and tumor basement matrix tenascin-targeting MoAb 81C6 dose-escalating to up to 80 mCi with 60 mg protein content. Efficacies have been reported along with limiting hematotoxicity from the circulating radioiodinated antibodies and metabolites.[80] Another interesting parallel example is to explore theoretical models comparing intrathecal dosimetry of ^{131}I and ^{67}Ga.[81] The findings suggest favorable dosimetry for intrathecal use of Ga-67 because of the abundant Auger electrons.

19.4.2.3. *Pleural and pericardial effusion*

Pleural fluid is produced by the parietal pleura covering the structure of the thoracic cavity and lined by high-pressure intercostal arteries. More than 80% pleural flow is reabsorbed through the visceral pleura covering the lungs and the rest by subserosal lymphatics. When there is irritation of pleural serosa, which produces more fluid and reabsorbs less, malignant pleural effusion develops. Malignant cytology is found in up to 50% of pleural effusion. While positive cytology is an indication for intrathoracic therapy, the status of exudates is another indication, as determined by pleural fluid LDH level >200 mg/dl, pleural/serum LDH ratio >0.6 or pleural/serum protein >0.5.

Intrathoracic therapy is typically performed by close-tube thoracostomy and may involve sclerosing agents to obliterate the peritoneal cavity through chemical inflammation. ^{198}Au colloid was able to achieve 50%–75% total or partial response in malignant pleural effusion but was subject to long-term radiation hazards because of long half-life and is no longer commercially available.[82–90] ^{32}P chromic phosphate suspension has been reported with 50% responses. Typically, a thoracentesis is performed, followed by 2–3 mCi Tc-99m sulfur colloid to confirm distribution of the injectate. Then 10–15 mCi of 32P- chromic phosphate suspension is injected and flushed by 50 ml of saline. The patient is to change position every 10 minutes for 2 hours to facilitate distribution within the pleural space. This is a palliative procedure and has no impact on survival. The rate of pleural fluid production or the frequency of thoracentesis required to relief symptoms is used as the response.[86,87,91–94] Advantages of ^{90}Y include shorter physical half-life of 61 hours and ready detoxification schemes using EDTA.[86,91] Radiolabeled tumor-targeting monoclonal antibodies (mouse I-131 HMFG1, HMFG2, and AUA1) were used in a trial and reported response in 9 of 11 patients and was also applied to treat malignant pericardial effusion.[95–98]

A small amount of fluid is normally found in the pericardial sac and is typically drained by lymphatics. The diagnosis of malignant pericardial effusion can be made by cytology through pericardiocentesis, which is typically done in the subxiphoid approach. Radionuclide therapy may be preferable when a patient develop pericardial effusion under chemotherapy. Typically, after pericardiocentesis using a peritoneal catheter under ultrasound guidance, 0.5 mCi Tc-99m DTPA in 25 ml is instilled to confirm pericardial distribution. Then, 5 mCi of 32P chromic phosphate in 30–50 ml saline is instilled, followed by immediate removal of the catheter. Hemopericardium is a potential complication.[99] High response rates with as much as 16 of 28 patients with little complications were reported.[100,101] Another study report responses in three out of three patients using mouse monoclonal antibodies HMFG1, HMFG2 and AUA1 labeled with [131]I [98] but the advantages of tumor targeting is still to be proven.

19.4.2.4. *Peritoneal carcinomatosis*

Malignant ascites occurs commonly in metastatic ovarian, renal, and gastrointestinal cancer, mesothelioma, or lymphoma. Intracavitary radionuclide therapy is indicated for palliation when systemic therapy and paracentesis fail to relief symptoms of abdominal distention, dyspnea, cough, or hiccoughs from diaphragmatic irritation. Typically, a fenestrated peritoneal dialysis catheter is inserted followed by injection of tracer dose of 1 mCi of Tc-99m sulfur colloid and flushing with 250 ml saline. Confirmation of distribution is needed before the instillation of 15 to 25 mCi of ^{32}P chromic phosphate in 500 ml of saline. Potential adverse effects are nausea, vomiting, diarrhea, and abdominal pain, related to radiation peritonitis. Peritoneal fluid production cessation for 3 months is considered excellent, and marked slowing fluid formation is good response. Favorable results have been reported with ^{198}Au colloids and ^{90}Y colloids but they are not as effective as ^{32}P colloids.

Radiolabeled colloids such as ^{32}P chromic phosphate do not specifically target the tumor implants and plate out on the surfaces of viscera and may lead to bowel toxicity.[102] Radiolabeled antibodies have been applied to target tumor surface markers including mucins (MUC16/CA125,

MUC1),[103,104] glycoproteins (TAG72, aFR/gp38 or folate receptors),[105−110] and oligosaccharides (Lewis Y).[111] The average uptake of radionuclide by the tumor nodules was greater than 100-fold of that by intravenous injection. Locoregional toxicities such as bowel obstruction are expected to be less frequent with radioimmunotherapy which, however, may suffer from allergic reaction to foreign proteins.[112−114] A large-scale phase-3 study using ^{90}Y-90 murine IgG HMFG1 was able to achieve complete remission of epithelia ovarian cancer (stage IC–IV) after surgical resection, but there were no survival benefits.[104,115] Strategies in improving locoregional radioimmunotherapy include a better choice of radionuclide (e.g., ^{177}Lu over ^{90}Y), use of systemic de-incorporation agents, pre-targeting, and combination with other therapeutic modalities.

19.4.2.5. *Intracavitary treatment of cystic brain tumors*

Locoregional radionuclide therapy may be via sealed catheter such as 400–600 mCi of ^{125}I Iotrex contained in a surgically implanted inflatable Glial-Site balloon-catheter to deliver 60 Gy at 1 cm from the cavity surface for over 100 hours.[1,116−118] Alternatively, it may involve direct instillation of unsealed radiopharmaceuticals such as ^{90}Y-DOTA-TOC via stereotaxic injection or an external catheter surgically connected to the cavity. Owing to the proximity to the tumors from locoregional applications, non-specific radiocolloids from ^{198}Au, ^{32}P, ^{186}Re, or ^{90}Y have been used with variable efficacy reported.[119−122]

The cavity cyst is accessed by an Ommaya reservoir catheter. Assuming homogenous distribution and planning doses of 200–250 Gy to the cyst wall, good response was reported with ^{32}P colloids.[121,123−132] A formula has been simplified to derive the required activity for injection in microcurie $= 27.47 \times V/f$, where V is the tumor volume in ml and f is a volume-dependent dosimetry factor varying between 0.420 and 0.485 for spherical volumes of 0.5–65.5 ml.

After injection of 0.2–7.8 mCi ^{90}Y colloids during diagnostic punctures of craniopharyngioma, follow-up study found shrinkage of the tumors in a majority of patients. Transient visual field defects and third nerve palsy, hypothalamic injury, as well as increased intracranial pressure were observed probably because of the longer range of ^{90}Y and the location of tumor closed to the optic chiasm.[133] In 5 of the 29 injections, radioactivity was detected in the lumbar CSF, indicating leakage to the CSF.[134]

While metastatic brain tumors occur much more often than primary brain tumors, there are ongoing clinical trials to treat brain tumor with similar locoregional nuclide therapy such as using [125]I Iotrex in GlialSite balloon catheters.[118] Survival benefits (8 months versus 56 months) have been reported with systemic 3-step retargeted adjuvant radioimmunother-apy (PARIT) using biotinylated anti-tenascin monoclonal antibodies (BC2 and BC4 epitopes), followed by ^{90}Y-labeled biotin.[135,136] The dose-limiting hematotoxicity was reached at 80 mCi. ^{131}I-labeled monoclonal antibodies can be used with cumulative radioactivity up to 550 mCi in 3–10 cycles by direct instillation into post-surgical cavities in patients with anaplas-tic astrocytoma (AA) or GBM; patient survival was reported to be 46 and 19 months respectively.[135–142] Using ^{90}Y-labeled mAb in 3–5 cycles up to 85 mCi, patient survival was 90 and 20 months, respectively.[137,143,144] In combination with locoregional injection of 4 mg mitoxantrone every 20 days, this approach of locoregional regional PARIT at 10-week cycles using up to 27 mCi of [90]Y- biotin prolonged survival of 42% patients at 18 months.[145]

While radioimmunotherapy involves biologic products and multiple agents, ^{90}Y DOTA-TOC instillation into post-surgical cavity from resected tumors with somatostatin receptors is a simpler approach. After con-firmation of somatostatin receptor with [68]Ga- DOTA-TOC using PET, three patients were treated with ^{90}Y DOTA-TOC and the responses were favorable.[42] This approach will also allow more ready diffusion of the small molecule radionuclide to cross biologic barriers surrounding the cavity to reach tumor cells.

19.4.2.6. *Interstitial radionuclide therapies*

Intratumoral injection of ^{90}Y-colloids formed by alkaline precipitation of Y-90 chloride[55] resulted in up to 10% [90]Y distributed to liver, kidney, spleen, and bone marrow. Up to 5% of ^{90}Y is excreted in urine and up to 80% is retained in the tumor. Injectates with strength between 0.1 mCi/0.1 ml and 0.4 mCi/0.1 ml activity resulted in spherical necrotic volume of 0.7–0.8 cm in diameter, irrespective of radioactivity injected. When this method was applied clinically to treat superficial tumors, multiple injections of 0.15 mCi ^{90}Y colloid placed 1 cm apart resulted in transient reduction in tumor volume.

On the other hand, soluble molecules of smaller size (<10,000 Da) are cleared from the interstitial by capillary return. After interstitial injection, they may be able to diffuse more freely to reach a larger volume of distribution and bind specifically with tumor markers on the tumor cells. In spite of advantages of more volume of distribution and potential gain of tumor targeting, direct injection of soluble radiopharmaceuticals for locoregional tumor therapy has not been fully explored. Optimism should remain as illustrated by the earlier example of intratumoral injection of 0.5 mCi ^{201}Tl chloride eradicating brain tumor implants in rats.[54]

19.5. Conclusion

There have been increasing applications of radionuclide in therapy via systemic routes and locoregional approaches. Significant therapeutic and palliative benefits to cancer patients have been realized. Obstacles remain, such as establishing access to the tumor, which is, however, less onerous compared to the lack of biologic, toxicological, and dosimetry parameters. Nevertheless, these parameters have been made possible by advances in radiochemistry, imaging technology, and dosimetry algorithms. The translation of basic medical sciences through imaging sciences has enabled radionuclide therapy to firmly assume ancillary roles for cancer therapy. Furthermore, with better understanding of molecular mechanisms, imaging of biodistribution and modeling dosimetry, radionuclide therapy has reached the prime time in cancer therapy, as demonstrated by radioiodide treatment of thyroid cancer, radiopeptide therapy of neuroendocrine tumors, and radioimmunotherpy of lymphomas.

References

1. Wernicke AG, *et al.* (2010) The role of dose escalation with intracavitary brachytherapy in the treatment of localized CNS malignancies: Outcomes and toxicities of a prospective study. *Brachytherapy* **9**(1): 91–99.

2. Stabin MG, Sparks RB, Crowe E. (2005) OLINDA/EXM: The second-generation personal computer software for internal dose assessment in nuclear medicine. *J Nucl Med* **46**(6): 1023–1027.

3. Vassiliev ON, *et al.* (2008) Feasibility of a multigroup deterministic solution method for three-dimensional radiotherapy dose calculations. *Int J Radiat Oncol Biol Phys* **72**(1): 220–227.

4. Gifford KA, *et al.* (2008) Optimization of deterministic transport parameters for the calculation of the dose distribution around a high dose-rate 192Ir brachytherapy source. *Med Phys* **35**(6): 2279–2285.

5. Gates VL, *et al.* (2011) Internal pair production of ^{90}Y permits hepatic localization of microspheres using routine PET: Proof of concept. *J Nucl Med* **52**(1): 72–76.

6. Bishayee A, *et al.* (2000) Marrow-sparing effects of 117mSn(4+) diethylenetriamine-pentaacetic acid for radionuclide therapy of bone cancer. *J Nucl Med* **41**(12): 2043–2050.

7. Dvorakova Z, *et al.* (2008) Production of 177Lu at the new research reactor FRM-II: Irradiation yield of 176Lu(n,gamma)177Lu. *Appl Radiat Isot* **66**(2): 147–151.

8. Imam SK. (2001) Advancements in cancer therapy with alpha-emitters: A review. *Int J Radiat Oncol Biol Phys* **51**(1): 271–278.

9. Najean Y, Rain JD. (1997) Treatment of polycythemia vera: use of ^{32}P alone or in combination with maintenance therapy using hydroxyurea in 461 patients greater than 65 years of age. The French Polycythemia Study Group. *Blood* **89**(7): 2319–2327.

10. Reinhardt MJ, *et al.* (2002) Radioiodine therapy in Graves' disease based on tissue-absorbed dose calculations: Effect of pre-treatment thyroid volume on clinical outcome. *Eur J Nucl Med Mol Imaging* **29**(9): 1118–1124.

11. Miller BS, Doherty GM. (2011) An examination of recently revised differentiated thyroid cancer guidelines. *Curr Opin Oncol* **23**(1): 1–6.

12. Sacks W, *et al.* (2010) The effectiveness of radioactive iodine for treatment of low-risk thyroid cancer: A systematic analysis of the peer-reviewed literature from 1966 to April 2008. *Thyroid* **20**(11): 1235–1245.

13. Mallick UK. (2010) The revised American Thyroid Association management guidelines 2009 for patients with differentiated thyroid cancer: An evidence-based risk-adapted approach. *Clin Oncol (R Coll Radiol)* **22**(6): 472–474.

14. Boelaert K. (2010) Thyroid gland: Revised guidelines for the management of thyroid cancer. *Nat Rev Endocrinol* **6**(4): 185–186.

15. Famakinwa OM, *et al.* (2010) ATA practice guidelines for the treatment of differentiated thyroid cancer: Were they followed in the United States? *Am J Surg* **199**(2): 189–198.

16. Siegel JA, Marcus CS, Stabin MG. (2007) Licensee over-reliance on conservatisms in NRC guidance regarding the release of patients treated with 131I. *Health Phys* **93**(6): 667–677.

17. Hoffmann M, *et al.* (2011) ^{90}Y-ibritumomab tiuxetan (Zevalin) in heavily pretreated patients with mucosa associated lymphoid tissue lymphoma. *Leuk Lymphoma* **52**(1): 42–45.

18. Otte A. (2008) Diagnostic imaging prior to ^{90}Y-ibritumomab tiuxetan (Zevalin) treatment in follicular non-Hodgkin's lymphoma. *Hell J Nucl Med* **11**(1): 12–15.

19. Tennvall J, *et al.* (2007) EANM procedure guideline for radio-immunotherapy for B-cell lymphoma with ^{90}Y-radiolabelled ibritumomab tiuxetan (Zevalin). *Eur J Nucl Med Mol Imaging* **34**(4): 616–622.

20. Wiseman GA, Witzig TE. (2005) Yttrium-90 (^{90}Y) ibritumomab tiuxetan (Zevalin) induces long-term durable responses in patients with relapsed or refractory B-Cell non-Hodgkin's lymphoma. *Cancer Biother Radiopharm* **20**(2): 185–188.

21. White CA. (2004) Radioimmunotherapy in non-Hodgkin's lymphoma: Focus on ^{90}Y-ibritumomab tiuxetan (Zevalin). *J Exp Ther Oncol* **4**(4): 305–316.

22. Witzig TE. (2003) Efficacy and safety of ^{90}Y ibritumomab tiuxetan (Zevalin) radioimmunotherapy for non-Hodgkin's lymphoma. *Semin Oncol* **30**(6 Suppl 17): 11–16.

23. Wiseman GA, *et al.* (2000) Phase I/II ^{90}Y-Zevalin (yttrium-90 ibritumomab tiuxetan, IDEC-Y2B8) radioimmunotherapy dosimetry results in relapsed or refractory non-Hodgkin's lymphoma. *Eur J Nucl Med* **27**(7): 766–777.

24. Iagaru A, *et al.* (2010) 131I-Tositumomab (Bexxar) vs. ^{90}Y-Ibritumomab (Zevalin) therapy of low-grade refractory/relapsed non-Hodgkin lymphoma. *Mol Imaging Biol* **12**(2): 198–203.

25. Friedberg JW, Fisher RI. (2004) Iodine-131 tositumomab (Bexxar): Radioimmuno-conjugate therapy for indolent and transformed B-cell non-Hodgkin's lymphoma. *Expert Rev Anticancer Ther* **4**(1): 18–26.

26. Rutar FJ, *et al.* (2001) Feasibility and safety of outpatient Bexxar therapy (tositumomab and iodine I 131 tositumomab) for non-Hodgkin's lymphoma based on radiation doses to family members. *Clin Lymphoma* **2**(3): 164–172.

27. Blake GM, *et al.* (1987) 89Sr radionuclide therapy: Dosimetry and haematological toxicity in two patients with metastasising prostatic carcinoma. *Eur J Nucl Med* **13**(1): 41–46.

28. Kan MK. (1995) Palliation of bone pain in patients with metastatic cancer using strontium-89 (Metastron). *Cancer Nurs* **18**(4): 286–291.

29. Etchebehere EC, *et al.* (2004) Treatment of bone pain secondary to metastases using samarium-153-EDTMP. *Sao Paulo Med J* **122**(5): 208–212.

30. Maini CL, *et al.* (2004) 153Sm-EDTMP for bone pain palliation in skeletal metastases. *Eur J Nucl Med Mol Imaging* **31**(Suppl 1): S171–S178.

31. Kendler D, *et al.* (2004) An individual dosimetric approach to 153Sm-EDTMP therapy for pain palliation in bone metastases in correlation with clinical results. *Nucl Med Commun* **25**(4): 367–373.

32. Bayouth JE, *et al.* (1994) Dosimetry and toxicity of samarium-153-EDTMP administered for bone pain due to skeletal metastases. *J Nucl Med* **35**(1): 63–69.

33. Farhanghi M, *et al.* (1992) Samarium-153-EDTMP: Pharmacokinetic, toxicity and pain response using an escalating dose schedule in treatment of metastatic bone cancer. *J Nucl Med* **33**(8): 1451–1458.

34. Aas M, *et al.* (1999) Internal radionuclide therapy of primary osteosarcoma in dogs, using 153Sm-ethylene-diamino-tetramethylene-phosphonate (EDTMP). *Clin Cancer Res* **5**(10 Suppl): 3148s–3152s.

35. Moe L, *et al.* (1996) Maxillectomy and targeted radionuclide therapy with 153Sm-EDTMP in a recurrent canine osteosarcoma. *J Small Anim Pract* **37**(5): 241–246.

36. Tu SM, *et al.* (2005) Therapy tolerance in selected patients with androgen-independent prostate cancer following strontium-89 combined with chemotherapy. *J Clin Oncol* **23**(31): 7904–7910.

37. Tu SM, *et al.* (2009) Phase I study of concurrent weekly docetaxel and repeated samarium-153 lexidronam in patients with castration-resistant metastatic prostate cancer. *J Clin Oncol* **27**(20): 3319–3324.

38. Henriksen G, *et al.* (2003) Targeting of osseous sites with alpha-emitting 223Ra: Comparison with the beta-emitter 89Sr in mice. *J Nucl Med* **44**(2): 252–259.

39. Bruland OS, *et al.* (2006) High-linear energy transfer irradiation targeted to skeletal metastases by the alpha-emitter 223Ra: Adjuvant or alternative to conventional modalities? *Clin Cancer Res* **12**(20 Pt 2): 6250s–6257s.

40. Nilsson S, *et al.* (2005) First clinical experience with alpha-emitting radium-223 in the treatment of skeletal metastases. *Clin Cancer Res* **11**(12): 4451–4459.

41. Imhof A, *et al.* (2011) Response, survival, and long-term toxicity after therapy with the radiolabeled somatostatin analogue [^{90}Y-DOTA]-TOC in metastasized neuroendocrine cancers. *J Clin Oncol* **29**(17): 2416–2423.

42. Heute D, *et al.* (2010) Response of recurrent high-grade glioma to treatment with (90)Y-DOTATOC. *J Nucl Med* **51**(3): 397–400.

43. Menda Y, *et al.* (2010) Phase I trial of ^{90}Y-DOTATOC therapy in children and young adults with refractory solid tumors that express somatostatin receptors. *J Nucl Med* **51**(10): 1524–1531.

44. Sierra ML, *et al.* (2009) Lymphocytic toxicity in patients after peptide-receptor radionuclide therapy (PRRT) with 177Lu-DOTATATE and ^{90}Y-DOTATOC. *Cancer Biother Radiopharm* **24**(6): 659–665.

45. Bodei L, *et al.* (2008) Long-term evaluation of renal toxicity after peptide receptor radionuclide therapy with ^{90}Y-DOTATOC and 177Lu-DOTATATE: The role of associated risk factors. *Eur J Nucl Med Mol Imaging* **35**(10): 1847–1856.

46. Davi MV, *et al.* (2008) Multidisciplinary approach including receptor radionuclide therapy with ^{90}Y-DOTATOC ([^{90}Y-DOTA0, Tyr3]-octreotide) and 177Lu-DOTATATE ([177Lu-DOTA0, Tyr3]-octreotate) in ectopic cushing syndrome from a metastatic gastrinoma: A promising proposal. *Endocr Pract* **14**(2): 213–218.

47. de Jong M, *et al.* (2005) Combination radionuclide therapy using 177Lu- and ^{90}Y-labeled somatostatin analogs. *J Nucl Med* **46**(Suppl 1): 13S-17S.

48. Bodei L, *et al.* (2004) Receptor radionuclide therapy with ^{90}Y-[DOTA]0-Tyr3-octreotide (^{90}Y-DOTATOC) in neuroendocrine tumours. *Eur J Nucl Med Mol Imaging* **31**(7): 1038–1046.

49. Capello A, *et al.* (2003) Tyr3-octreotide and Tyr3-octreotate radiolabeled with 177Lu or ^{90}Y: Peptide receptor radionuclide therapy results *in vitro*. *Cancer Biother Radiopharm* **18**(5): 761–768.

50. Paganelli G, *et al.* (2002) ^{90}Y-DOTA-D-Phe1-Try3-octreotide in therapy of neuroendocrine malignancies. *Biopolymers* **66**(6): 393–398.

51. Esser JP, *et al.* (2006) Comparison of [(177)Lu-DOTA(0),Tyr(3)]octreotate and [(177)Lu-DOTA(0),Tyr(3)]octreotide: Which peptide is preferable for PRRT? *Eur J Nucl Med Mol Imaging* **33**(11): 1346–1351.

52. McCready VR, Cornes P. (2001) The potential of intratumoural unsealed radioactive source therapy. *Eur J Nucl Med* **28**(5): 567–569.

53. McCready VR. (1995) A different approach to the use of unsealed radionuclides for cancer therapy. *Eur J Nucl Med* **22**(1): 1–3.

54. Ljunggren K, *et al.* (2004) Absorbed dose distribution in glioma tumors in rat brain after therapeutic intratumoral injection of 201Tl-chloride. *Cancer Biother Radiopharm* **19**(5): 562–569.

55. Asakura H. (1964) [Intratumoral Injection Therapy with Yttrium-90 Chloride Colloid.]. *Nippon Igaku Hoshasen Gakkai Zasshi* **23**: 1493–1509.

56. Garg AD, *et al.* (2010) Photodynamic therapy: Illuminating the road from cell death towards anti-tumour immunity. *Apoptosis.*

57. Korbelik M. (2010) Photodynamic therapy-generated cancer vaccines. *Methods Mol Biol* **635**: 147–153.

58. Saji H, *et al.* (2006) [A possibility of overcoming local tumor immune tolerance by radiofrequency ablation in combination with intratumoral injection of naive dendritic cell]. *Gan To Kagaku Ryoho* **33**(12): 1736–1738.

59. Sparks RB, *et al.* (2002) Radiation dose distributions in normal tissue adjacent to tumors containing (131)I or (90)Y: The potential for toxicity. *J Nucl Med* **43**(8): 1110–1114.

60. Flower MA, McCready VR. (1997) Radionuclide therapy dose calculations: What accuracy can be achieved? *Eur J Nucl Med* **24**(12): 1462–1464.

61. Knesaurek K, *et al.* (2010) Quantitative comparison of yttrium-90 (^{90}Y)-microspheres and technetium-99m (99mTc)-macroaggregated albumin SPECT images for planning ^{90}Y therapy of liver cancer. *Technol Cancer Res Treat* **9**(3): 253–262.

62. Schleipman AR, Gallagher PW, Gerbaudo VH. (2009) Optimizing safety of selective internal radiation therapy (SIRT) of hepatic tumors with ^{90}Y resin microspheres: A systematic approach to preparation and radiometric procedures. *Health Phys* **96**(2 Suppl): S16–S21.

63. Riaz A, *et al.* (2009) Yttrium-90 radioembolization using TheraSphere in the management of primary and secondary liver tumors. *Q J Nucl Med Mol Imaging* **53**(3): 311–316.

64. Stubbs RS, O'Brien I, Correia MM. (2006) Selective internal radiation therapy with ^{90}Y microspheres for colorectal liver metastases: Single-centre experience with 100 patients. *ANZ J Surg* **76**(8): 696–703.

65. Lewandowski RJ, *et al.* (2005) ^{90}Y microsphere (TheraSphere) treatment for unresectable colorectal cancer metastases of the liver: response to treatment at targeted doses of 135–150 Gy as measured by [18F]fluorodeoxyglucose positron emission tomography and computed tomographic imaging. *J Vasc Interv Radiol* **16**(12): 1641–1651.

66. Campbell AM, Bailey IH, Burton MA. (2000) Analysis of the distribution of intra-arterial microspheres in human liver following hepatic yttrium-90 microsphere therapy. *Phys Med Biol* **45**(4): 1023–1033.

67. Lau WY, *et al.* (1998) Selective internal radiation therapy for nonresectable hepatocellular carcinoma with intraarterial infusion of 90yttrium microspheres. *Int J Radiat Oncol Biol Phys* **40**(3): 583–592.

68. Uthappa MC, Ravikumar R, Gupta A. (2011) Selective internal radiation therapy: ^{90}Y (yttrium) labeled microspheres for liver malignancies (primary and metastatic). *Indian J Cancer* **48**(1): 18–23.

69. Saxena A, *et al.* (2010) Factors predicting response and survival after yttrium-90 radioembolization of unresectable neuroendocrine tumor liver metastases: A critical appraisal of 48 cases. *Ann Surg* **251**(5): 910–916.

70. Sarfaraz M, *et al.* (2004) Radiation absorbed dose distribution in a patient treated with yttrium-90 microspheres for hepatocellular carcinoma. *Med Phys* **31**(9): 2449–2253.

71. Altenbrunn HJ. (1978) [Radionuclide therapy of malignant tumors]. *Z Gesamte Inn Med* **33**(14): 475–484.

72. Muriel FS, *et al.* (1976) Remission maintenance therapy for meningeal leukaemia: Intrathecal methotrexate and dexamethasone versus intrathecal craniospinal irradiation with a radiocolloid. *Br J Haematol* **34**(1): 119–127.

73. Brunhober J, *et al.* (1981) [Intrathecal radiogold application for meningosis "prophylaxis" in children with leukemias and non-Hodgkin lymphomas. II. Results and problems from viewpoint of nuclear medicine]. *Radiobiol Radiother (Berl)* **22**(5): 570–578.

74. Doge H, Hliscs R. (1984) Intrathecal therapy with 198Au-colloid for meningosis prophylaxis. *Eur J Nucl Med* **9**(3): 125–128.

75. Moseley RP, *et al.* (1990) Intrathecal administration of 131I radiolabelled monoclonal antibody as a treatment for neoplastic meningitis. *Br J Cancer* **62**(4): 637–642.

76. Richardson RB, *et al.* (1990) Dosimetry of intrathecal iodine131 monoclonal antibody in cases of neoplastic meningitis. *Eur J Nucl Med* **17**(1–2): 42–48.

77. Benjamin JC, *et al.* (1989) Cerebral distribution of immunoconjugate after treatment for neoplastic meningitis using an intrathecal radiolabeled monoclonal antibody. *Neurosurgery* **25**(2): 253–258.

78. Kemshead JT, Hopkins KI, Chandler CL. (1996) Treatment of diffuse leptomeningeal malignancy by intrathecal injection of 131I radioimmunoconjugates. *Recent Results Cancer Res* **141**: 145–158.

79. Kramer K, *et al.* (2000) Targeted radioimmunotherapy for leptomeningeal cancer using (131)I-3F8. *Med Pediatr Oncol* **35**(6): 716–718.

80. Bigner DD, *et al.* (1995) Phase I studies of treatment of malignant gliomas and neoplastic meningitis with 131I-radiolabeled monoclonal antibodies anti-tenascin 81C6 and anti-chondroitin proteoglycan sulfate Me1-14 F (ab')2–a preliminary report. *J Neurooncol* **24**(1): 109–122.

81. van Dieren EB, *et al.* (1994) A dosimetric model for intrathecal treatment with 131I and 67Ga. *Int J Radiat Oncol Biol Phys* **30**(2): 447–454.

82. Mohlen KH, Beller FK. (1979) Use of radioactive gold in the treatment of pleural effusions caused by metastatic cancer. *J Cancer Res Clin Oncol* **94**(1): 81–85.

83. Croll MN, Brady LW. (1979) Intracavitary uses of colloids. *Semin Nucl Med* **9**(2): 108–113.
84. Leff A, Hopewell PC, Costello J. (1978) Pleural effusion from malignancy. *Ann Intern Med* **88**(4): 532–537.
85. Fleay RF. (1971) Dosimetry in the use of colloidal isotopes. *Australas Radiol* **15**(4): 388–390.
86. Sklaroff DM. (1965) Radioactive colloid treatment of malignant effusions. *Pa Med J* **68**: 41–43.
87. Botsford TW. (1964) Experiences with radioactive colloidal gold in the treatment of pleural effusion caused by metastatic cancer of the breast. *N Engl J Med* **270**: 552–555.
88. Dybicki J, Balchum OJ, Meneely GR. (1959) Treatment of pleural and peritoneal effusion with intracavitary colloidal radiogold (Au 198). *Arch Intern Med* **104**: 802–815.
89. Lehman J. (1954) Radioactive gold in treatment of malignant effusion. *Miss Valley Med J* **76**(6): 238.
90. Colby MY Jr. (1954) Intracavitary radioactive colloidal gold in the treatment of malignant pleural effusion. *Med Clin North Am* **New York No.**: 1133–1138.
91. Scheer KE. (1964) Radioactive colloids in the treatment of neoplastic effusions in the serous cavities. *Minerva Nucl* **55**: 123–126.
92. Shah JR, Warawdekar MS. (1964) Radio active colloidal gold in the treatment of malignant pleural effusion. *J Assoc Physicians India* **12**: 63–67.
93. Reeve TS, Myhill J. (1962) The role of radioactive isotopes and alkylating agents in the treatment of malignant effusions. *Med J Aust* **49**(2): 245–249.
94. King ER, *et al.* (1952) The use of radioactive colloidal gold (Au198) in pleural effusions and ascites associated with malignancy. *Am J Roentgenol Radium Ther Nucl Med* **68**(3): 413–420.
95. Kalofonos HP, *et al.* (1994) Targeting of tumours with murine and reshaped human monoclonal antibodies against placental alkaline phosphatase: Immunolocalisation, pharmacokinetics and immune response. *Eur J Cancer* **30A**(12): 1842–1850.
96. Kosmas C, Kalofonos HP, Epenetos AA. (1990) Radiolabelled monoclonal antibodies in tumour diagnosis and therapy. *Dev Biol Stand* **71**: 93–102.
97. Malamitsi J, *et al.* (1988) Intracavitary use of two radiolabeled tumor-associated monoclonal antibodies. *J Nucl Med* **29**(12): 1910–1915.
98. Pectasides D, *et al.* (1986) Antibody-guided irradiation of malignant pleural and pericardial effusions. *Br J Cancer* **53**(6): 727–732.
99. Blau N, *et al.* (1977) Massive hemopericardium in a patient with postmyocardial infarction syndrome. *Chest* **71**(4): 549–552.
100. Martini N, *et al.* (1977) Intrapericardial installation of radioactive chromic phosphate in malignant effusion. *AJR Am J Roentgenol* **128**(4): 639–641.
101. Covington EE, Hilaris BS. (1973) P^{32} scans for intracavitary distribution studies. *Am J Roentgenol Radium Ther Nucl Med* **118**(4): 895–899.
102. Wilkinson RH, Jr. (1996) Pleuroperitoneal migration of intraperitoneal phosphorus-32-chromic phosphate therapy for stage I ovarian carcinoma. *J Nucl Med* **37**(4): 636–639.

103. Mahe MA, *et al.* (1999) A phase II study of intraperitoneal radioimmunotherapy with iodine-131-labeled monoclonal antibody OC-125 in patients with residual ovarian carcinoma. *Clin Cancer Res* **5**(10 Suppl): 3249s-3253s.
104. Verheijen RH, *et al.* (2006) Phase III trial of intraperitoneal therapy with yttrium-90-labeled HMFG1 murine monoclonal antibody in patients with epithelial ovarian cancer after a surgically defined complete remission. *J Clin Oncol* **24**(4): 571–578.
105. Alvarez RD, *et al.* (2002) A Phase I study of combined modality (90)Yttrium-CC49 intraperitoneal radioimmunotherapy for ovarian cancer. *Clin Cancer Res* **8**(9): 2806–2811.
106. Alvarez RD, *et al.* (1997) Intraperitoneal radioimmunotherapy of ovarian cancer with 177Lu-CC49: A phase I/II study. *Gynecol Oncol* **65**(1): 94–101.
107. Meredith RF, *et al.* (2001) Intraperitoneal radioimmunochemotherapy of ovarian cancer: A phase I study. *Cancer Biother Radiopharm* **16**(4): 305–315.
108. Meredith RF, *et al.* (2007) Brief overview of preclinical and clinical studies in the development of intraperitoneal radioimmunotherapy for ovarian cancer. *Clin Cancer Res* **13**(18 Pt 2): 5643s–5645s.
109. Meredith RF, *et al.* (1996) Intraperitoneal radioimmunotherapy of ovarian cancer with lutetium-177-CC49. *J Nucl Med* **37**(9): 1491–1496.
110. Rosenblum MG, *et al.* (1999) Phase I study of ^{90}Y-labeled B72.3 intraperitoneal administration in patients with ovarian cancer: Effect of dose and EDTA coadminis-tration on pharmacokinetics and toxicity. *Clin Cancer Res* **5**(5): 953–961.
111. Zhang M, *et al.* (1997) Intravenous avidin chase improved localization of radiolabeled streptavidin in intraperitoneal xenograft pretargeted with biotinylated antibody. *Nucl Med Biol* **24**(1): 61–64.
112. Wahl RL, Liebert M. (1989) Improved radiolabeled monoclonal antibody uptake by lavage of intraperitoneal carcinomatosis in mice. *J Nucl Med* **30**(1): 60–65.
113. Wahl RL, *et al.* (1988) The intraperitoneal delivery of radiolabeled monoclonal anti-bodies: Studies on the regional delivery advantage. *Cancer Immunol Immunother* **26**(3): 187–201.
114. Wahl RL. (1990) Intraperitoneal delivery of monoclonal antibodies. *Cancer Treat Res* **51**: 123–149.
115. Oei AL, *et al.* (2007) Decreased intraperitoneal disease recurrence in epithelial ovar-ian cancer patients receiving intraperitoneal consolidation treatment with yttrium-90-labeled murine HMFG1 without improvement in overall survival. *Int J Cancer* **120**(12): 2710–2714.
116. Lanka VK. (2006) Balloon brachytherapy for brain tumor-radiation safety experiences at the University of Medicine and Dentistry of New Jersey. *Health Phys* **91**(5 Suppl): S83–S86.
117. Chan TA, *et al.* (2005) Treatment of recurrent glioblastoma multiforme with GliaSite brachytherapy. *Int J Radiat Oncol Biol Phys* **62**(4): 1133–1139.
118. Tatter SB, *et al.* (2003) An inflatable balloon catheter and liquid 125I radiation source (GliaSite Radiation Therapy System) for treatment of recurrent malignant glioma: Multicenter safety and feasibility trial. *J Neurosurg* **99**(2): 297–303.
119. Lin LL, *et al.* (2008) Long-term outcome in children treated for craniopharyngioma with and without radiotherapy. *J Neurosurg Pediatr* **1**(2): 126–130.

120. Sadeghi M, Karimi E, Hosseini SH. (2009) Dosimetric comparison of ^{90}Y, ^{32}P, and 186Re radiocolloids in craniopharyngioma treatments. *Med Phys* **36**(11): 5022–5026.

121. Sadeghi, M, Karimi E, Sardari D. (2009) Monte Carlo and analytical calculations of dose distributions in craniopharyngioma cysts treated with radiocolloids containing 32P or 186Re. *Appl Radiat Isot* **67**(9): 1697–1701.

122. Bond WH, Richards D, Turner E. (1965) Experiences with radioactive gold in the treatment of craniopharyngioma. *J Neurol Neurosurg Psychiatry* **28**: 30–38.

123. Zhao R, *et al.* (2010) Treatment of cystic craniopharyngioma with phosphorus-32 intracavitary irradiation. *Childs Nerv Syst* **26**(5): 669–674.

124. Sadeghi M, *et al.* (2007) Dosimetry of (32)P radiocolloid for treatment of cystic craniopharyngioma. *Appl Radiat Isot* **65**(5): 519–523.

125. Hasegawa T, *et al.* (2004) Management of cystic craniopharyngiomas with phosphorus-32 intracavitary irradiation. *Neurosurgery* **54**(4): 813–820; [discussion] 820–822.

126. Shapiro B, Fig LM, Gross MD. (1999) Intracavitary therapy of craniopharyngiomas. *Q J Nucl Med* **43**(4): 367–374.

127. Liu Z, *et al.* (1996) Stereotactic intratumour irradiation with nuclide for craniopharyngiomas. *Chin Med J (Engl)* **109**(3): 219–222.

128. Pollock BE, *et al.* (1995) Phosphorus-32 intracavitary irradiation of cystic craniopharyngiomas: current technique and long-term results. *Int J Radiat Oncol Biol Phys* **33**(2): 437–446.

129. Kumar PP, *et al.* (1986) Retreatment of recurrent cystic craniopharyngioma with chromic phosphorus P^{32}. *J Natl Med Assoc* **78**(6): 542–3, 547–549.

130. Kobayashi, T, Kageyama N, Ohara K. (1981) Internal irradiation for cystic craniopharyngioma. *J Neurosurg* **55**(6): 896–903.

131. Leksell L, Backlund EO, Johansson L. (1967) Treatment of craniopharyngiomas. *Acta Chir Scand* **133**(5): 345–350.

132. Overton, MC 3rd, Sheffel DD. (1963) Recurrent cystic formation in craniopharyngioma treated with radioactive chromic phosphate case report. *J Neurosurg* **20**: 707–710.

133. Julow J, *et al.* (2007) Stereotactic intracavitary irradiation of cystic craniopharyngiomas with yttrium-90 isotope. *Prog Neurol Surg* **20**: 289–296.

134. Van den Berge JH, *et al.* (1992) Intracavitary brachytherapy of cystic craniopharyngiomas. *J Neurosurg* **77**(4): 545–550.

135. Paganelli G, *et al.* (2006) Radioimmunotherapy of brain tumor. *Neurol Res* **28**(5): 518–22.

136. Paganelli G, *et al.* (2001) Pre-targeted locoregional radioimmunotherapy with ^{90}Y-biotin in glioma patients: Phase I study and preliminary therapeutic results. *Cancer Biother Radiopharm* **16**(3): 227–235.

137. Riva P, *et al.* (1999) Loco-regional radioimmunotherapy of high-grade malignant gliomas using specific monoclonal antibodies labeled with ^{90}Y: A phase I study. *Clin Cancer Res* **5**(10 Suppl): 3275s-3280s.

138. Riva P, *et al.* (1994) Intralesional radioimmunotherapy of malignant gliomas. An effective treatment in recurrent tumors. *Cancer* **73**(3 Suppl): 1076–1082.

139. Riva P, *et al.* (1994) Glioblastoma therapy by direct intralesional administration of I-131 radioiodine labeled antitenascin antibodies. *Cell Biophys* **24–25**: 37–43.

140. Riva P, *et al.* (1992) Treatment of intracranial human glioblastoma by direct intratumoral administration of 131I-labelled anti-tenascin monoclonal antibody BC-2. *Int J Cancer* **51**(1): 7–13.

141. Riva P, *et al.* (1995) Local treatment of malignant gliomas by direct infusion of specific monoclonal antibodies labeled with 131I: Comparison of the results obtained in recurrent and newly diagnosed tumors. *Cancer Res* **55**(23 Suppl): 5952s-5956s.

142. Reardon DA, *et al.* (2008) A pilot study: 131I-antitenascin monoclonal antibody 81c6 to deliver a 44-Gy resection cavity boost. *Neuro Oncol* **10**(2): 182–189.

143. Riva P *et al.* (2000) Role of nuclear medicine in the treatment of malignant gliomas: The locoregional radioimmunotherapy approach. *Eur J Nucl Med* **27**(5): 601–609.

144. Hopkins K, *et al.* (1998) Direct injection of ^{90}Y MoAbs into glioma tumor resection cavities leads to limited diffusion of the radioimmunoconjugates into normal brain parenchyma: A model to estimate absorbed radiation dose. *Int J Radiat Oncol Biol Phys* **40**(4): 835–844.

145. Boiardi A, *et al.* (2005) Intratumoral delivery of mitoxantrone in association with 90-Y radioimmunotherapy (RIT) in recurrent glioblastoma. *J Neurooncol* **72**(2): 125–131.

Index